Speech Sound Disorders in Children

In Honor of Lawrence D. Shriberg

Speech Sound Disorders in Children

In Honor of Lawrence D. Shriberg

Edited by
Rhea Paul
Peter Flipsen, Jr.

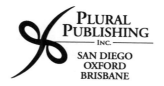

PLURAL
PUBLISHING
INC.

SAN DIEGO
OXFORD
BRISBANE

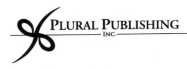

5521 Ruffin Road
San Diego, CA 92123

e-mail: info@pluralpublishing.com
Web site: http://www.pluralpublishing.com

49 Bath Street
Abingdon, Oxfordshire OX14 1EA
United Kingdom

Library of Congress Cataloging-in-Publication Data

Speech sound disorders in children : in honor of Lawrence D. Shriberg / [edited by] Rhea
Paul and Peter Flipsen Jr.
  p. ; cm.
  Includes bibliographical references and index.
  ISBN-13: 978-1-59756-249-2 (alk. paper)
  ISBN-10: 1-59756-249-1 (alk. paper)
  1. Speech disorders in children. I. Shriberg, Lawrence D. II. Paul, Rhea. III. Flipsen, Peter.
  [DNLM: 1. Shriberg, Lawrence D. 2. Speech Disorders—Festschrift. 3. Adolescent. 4. Child.
  5. Speech-Language Pathology—methods—Festschrift. WL 340.2 S7428 2009]
  RJ496.S7S648 2009
  618.92'855—dc22
                                                            2009010342

Contents

Prologue. The Contributions of Lawrence D. Shriberg: A Life's Work   vii
    Rhea Paul and Peter Flipsen, Jr.

Contributors   x

1. **Childhood Speech Sound Disorders: From Postbehaviorism to the Postgenomic Era**   1
   Lawrence D. Shriberg

2. **Explaining Developmental Communication Disorders**   35
   J. Bruce Tomblin and Morten H. Christiansen

3. **Genetic Influences on Speech Sound Disorders**   51
   Barbara A. Lewis

4. **Subgroups, Comorbidity, and Treatment Implications**   71
   Ann A. Tyler

5. **Children's Speech Sound Disorders: An Acoustic Perspective**   93
   Raymond D. Kent, Luciana Pagan-Neves, Katherine C. Hustad, and Haydee Fiszbein Wertzner

6. **Computer Processing for Analysis of Speech Disorders**   115
   John-Paul Hosom

7. **Motor Speech Disorders in Children with Autism**   141
   Shelley L. Velleman, Mary V. Andrianopoulos, Marcil J. Boucher, Jennifer J. Perkins, Keren E. Averback, Alyssa R. Currier, Michael J. Marsello, Courtney E. Lippe, and Richard Van Emmerik

8. **Vocal Production in Toddlers with Autism Spectrum Disorders**   181
   Elizabeth Schoen, Rhea Paul, and Katarzyna Chawarska

9. **Understanding Speech-Sound Change in Young Children Following Severe Traumatic Brain Injury**   205
   Thomas F. Campbell, Christine A. Dollaghan, and Janine E. Janosky

10. **Factors Associated with the Intelligibility of Conversational Speech Produced by Children with Cochlear Implants**   225
    Peter Flipsen, Jr.

Index   247

Prologue
The Contributions of Lawrence D. Shriberg: A Life's Work

Larry Shriberg was our teacher when we were graduate students at the University of Wisconsin-Madison, although we were there nearly 20 years apart. At a time in the history of the field of communication disorders when many were abandoning their traditional role as "speech therapists" and moving toward more trendy topics in language development and disorders, Larry was a bastion of continued commitment to the long-standing core of our profession, concerning the acquisition of the ability to produce the speech of one's community, and the ways in which that process goes awry. When everyone else was teaching clinicians to use child-centered, facilitative play techniques, Larry continued to teach behavioral methods. Larry's stance should not, however, be seen as that of a contrarian. His commitment to evidence-based approaches meant that he believed the data should be examined as carefully as possible before moving from methods that have empirical support to those that just sound sexier. Larry was one of very few investigators who actually studied the effects of various forms of treatment, as well as the effects of clinician's style of presentation. He was also interested from very early in his career in the ways in which psychosocial variables, such as birth order, influenced the acquisition of speech sounds.

What Larry has brought to the study of speech, apart from a deep fascination with every factor that composed and influenced it, has been a profound commitment to data and detail. His research has demonstrated the highest level of attention to multiple sources of information and the value of digging deep within each source for the fullest understanding it could reveal. Larry has long advocated, for example, allophonic level coding of speech production from children, in the belief that only by looking at subtle variations in production could we learn about their source. He has also long believed that it was worth the time and effort it took clinicians to learn these skills because they were critically important in understanding their clients. But he has always searched for ways to make these efforts "doable" in the real world. In the early 1970s, before the wide availability of hand-held calculators, Larry created tables that he distributed to clinicians for converting numbers to percentages. That way, clinicians could easily look up percentages of correct production based on data taken from clinical samples without having to do any long division. Later, he created the PEPPER computer program, and linked it up to the popular SALT program, to help clinicians do phonological analyses more efficiently and to integrate them with language data. In all these efforts, Larry has demonstrated his unwavering commitment to the clinical application of research and his belief that there is no disconnect between the laboratory and clinic.

One of Larry's most enduring contributions to the study of speech has been the development of a principled, data-based approach to classification. His scheme for categorizing disorders of speech sound development, published first over 20 years ago, remains without serious competition. In recent years, Larry has been in the forefront of research on the genetic basis of speech disorders. The path to this endeavor was paved by his interest in classification, and his approach to this study has been no less impressive than his efforts in the earlier stages of his career. He believes that the key to genetic research is the delineation of the most precise phenotype that will allow the linkage of discrete behaviors to specific genes and that the only way to accomplish this is to describe phenomena that may look unitary on the surface, such as developmental speech disorders, at the level of detail that will allow not only subclassificatory schemes, but the isolation of markers that could lead to genetic linkage. In this endeavor, Larry has been unique in both his productivity and originality.

Aside from the quality and quantity of Larry's contribution to our profession, which are both remarkable and with few peers, what motivated us to create this tribute was his effect on not only our careers, which is inestimable, but on our lives. Larry is the staunchest of mentors and the truest of friends. For both of us, Larry has been a career-long guide and presence. Although he may not always be unreservedly positive about everything we do, we always grew—however painfully—as a result of our interactions with him. We each remember meetings when, after reviewing a contribution to a paper we were writing together, Larry looked at us and said, "This just isn't good enough." After we got over the feeling of devastation and embarrassment, we realized he was right, went back to work, and tried

harder. In every case, we turned out better products as a result. It wasn't always easy or comfortable with Larry, but we knew that his insistence on excellence was based on sincere respect and the conviction that we were capable of meeting the high standards he set. We are both convinced that one of the things that made us realize that capability was Larry's refusal to accept anything less from us.

There are few scholars in our field whose web of collaborations extends as widely as Larry's, but nonetheless, being a member of that circle was always a point of pride. We knew that Larry thought we had the right stuff because of his willingness, despite the raft of colleagues with whom he worked, to continue to want to work with us. This was, perhaps, his highest tribute to us, and to everyone with whom he has interacted.

We chose to have Larry lead off this volume with a synopsis of his own work because it reflects what he has always seemed to do, that is, lead the way. Most of us who have worked with him would readily admit that it usually takes considerable effort to keep up with him. Indeed, we both often marvel at Larry's ability to master both the details and the big picture simultaneously. In Chapter 2, Bruce Tomblin has taken Larry as a guide in outlining a move away from simple reductionist accounts of disorders to more mechanistic explanations. Barbara Lewis, a long-time collaborator with Larry, then skillfully highlights the research into the genetic bases for speech sound disorders in Chapter 3. In Chapter 4, Ann Tyler examines the many facets of the comorbidity question and concludes with some practical suggestions about how one might deal with children who have problems that coexist with speech delay. Although Larry's work has long been viewed by some as highly theoretical, anyone who has worked with him knows that his ultimate goal has always been to provide practicing clinicians with useful tools to help real children. Chapter 5 was written by Larry's long-time colleague, Ray Kent along with some of Ray's students and delves into acoustics, an approach to analysis that Larry has whole-heartedly embraced. Having long recognized the limitations of perceptual transcription, Larry began to develop acoustic measures in his lab in the mid-1990s and one look at his most recent list of diagnostic markers makes it obvious that they are serving him well. His most recent work with John-Paul Hosum (Chapter 6) is motivated by his desire to automate his data collection and analysis methods and further improve both the validity and reliability of his measures.

The last four chapters reflect work on some specific populations that has been directly inspired by Larry's work. The first of these (Chapters 7 and 8) both look at autism, a population of great current interest, but do so with an eye to speech production which has received relatively minimal attention thus far. In Chapter 7, Velleman and colleagues look at motor speech disorders in autism. This work bears directly on Larry's recent work as chair of an expert panel put together by ASHA to improve our understanding of the nature of Childhood Apraxia of Speech (CAS); the panel concluded that some instances of CAS may be associated with neurodevelopmental disorders such as autism. In Chapter 8, Schoen et al. use acoustic methods to examine early output in the autism population. The penultimate Chapter 9 represents a homage to Larry's ability to always find the right measure for the job. Campbell and colleagues note that their work on growth curves that is helping them to understand traumatic brain injury in children would not be at all possible without Larry's measures and his willingness to share his data. We chose to conclude with a chapter on intelligibility (Chapter 10) because of the central role of intelligibility in Larry's conception of speech disorder.

Contributors

Mary V. Andrianopoulos, B.S., M.S., Ph.D., CCC-SLP
Associate Professor
Acting Graduate Program Director
Communication Disorders
University of Massachusetts at Amherst
Amherst, Massachusetts
Chapter 7

Keren E. Averback, M.S., CCC-SLP
Sharon, Maine
Chapter 7

Marcil J. Boucher, B.S.
Graduate Student
University of Massachusetts at Amherst
Amherst, Massachusetts
Chapter 7

Thomas F. Campbell, Ph.D.
Professor, School of Behavioral and Brain
  Sciences
Executive Director, Callier Center for
  Communication Disorders
University of Texas at Dallas
Dallas, Texas
Chapter 9

Katyrzyna Chawarska, Ph.D.
Assistant Professor
Yale University School of Medicine
Child Study Center
Yale University
New Haven, Connecticut
Chapter 8

Morten H. Christiansen, Ph.D.
External Professor, Santa Fe Institute
Co-Director, Cornell Cognitive Science
  Program

Associate Professor, Department of
  Psychology
Cornell University
Ithaca, New York
Chapter 2

Alyssa R. Currier, M.A., CCC-SLP
Speech-Language Pathologist
Center for Communication
Sanford, Maine
Chapter 7

Christine A. Dollaghan, Ph.D.
Professor, School of Behavioral and Brain
  Sciences
Callier Center for Communication
  Disorders
University of Texas at Dallas
Dallas, Texas
Chapter 9

Peter Flipsen, Jr., Ph.D., CCC-SLP
Associate Professor of Speech-Language
  Pathology
Department of Communication Sciences
  and Disorders and Education of the Deaf
Idaho State University
Pocatello, Idaho
Chapter 10

John-Paul Hosom, Ph.D.
Assistant Professor
Department of Computer Science and
  Electrical Engineering
Center for Spoken Language Understanding
OGI School of Science and Engineering
Oregon Health and Science University
Beaverton, Oregon
Chapter 6

Katherine C. Hustad, Ph.D., CCC-SLP
Assistant Professor
Department of Communicative Disorders
Waisman Center
University of Wisconsin-Madison
Madison, Wisconsin
Chapter 5

Janine E. Janosky, Ph.D.
Vice Provost for Research and Professor
  of Mathematics
Office of Research and Sponsored Programs
Central Michigan University
Mount Pleasant, Michigan
Chapter 9

Raymond D. Kent, Ph.D.
Professor Emeritus
University of Wisconsin-Madison
Madison, Wisconsin
Chapter 5

Barbara A. Lewis, Ph.D., CCC-SLP
Associate Professor
Department of Communication Sciences
Case Western Reserve University
Cleveland, Ohio
Chapter 3

Courtney E. Lippe, M.A., CFYSLP
Graduate Student
University of Massachusetts at Amherst
Amherst, Massachusetts
Chapter 7

Michael J. Marsello, M.A., CCC-SLP
Research Assistant
University of Massachusetts
Speech Pathologist, Genesis Rehab.
Somerville, Massachusetts
Chapter 7

Luciana Pagan-Neves, M.A.
Graduate Student
Universidade de São Paulo
São Paulo, Brazil
Chapter 5

Rhea Paul, Ph.D., CCC-SLP
Professor
Child Study Center
Yale University School of Medicine
New Haven, Connecticut
Chapter 8

Jennifer J. Perkins, B.S.
Graduate Student
California State University, Northridge
Northridge, California
Chapter 7

Elizabeth Schoen, M.S., CCC-SLP
Research Associate
Yale Child Study Center
Yale University School of Medicine
New Haven, Connecticut
Chapter 8

Lawrence D. Shriberg, Ph.D.
Emeritus Professor of Speech
  Pathology
Department of Communicative
  Disorders
Principal Investigator, The Phonology
  Project
Waisman Center
University of Wisconsin-Madison
Madison, Wisconsin
Chapter 1

J. Bruce Tomblin, Ph.D.
D.C. Spriestersbach Distinguished
  Professor of Liberal Arts and
  Sciences
Department of Communication Sciences
  and Disorders
University of Iowa
Iowa City, Iowa
Chapter 2

Ann A. Tyler, Ph.D.
Western Michigan University
Kalamazoo, Michigan
Chapter 4

Richard Van Emmerik, Ph.D.
University of Massachusetts at Amherst
Department of Kinesiology
Amherst, Massachusetts
Chapter 7

Shelley L. Velleman, BA, M.A., Ph.D.
Associate Professor
Communication Disorders
University of Massachusetts at Amherst
Amherst, Massachusetts
Chapter 7

Haydee Fiszbein Wertzner, Ph.D.
Faculdade de Filosofia
Letras a Ciências Humanas
Universidade de São Paulo
São Paulo, Brazil
Chapter 5

CHAPTER 1

Childhood Speech Sound Disorders: From Postbehaviorism to the Postgenomic Era

LAWRENCE D. SHRIBERG

Introduction

Thanks

I'll never forget the sunny spring day in Madison when Rhea and Peter spilled the beans about this book. What an incredible, wonderful surprise. It took two months before I could get my head around the reality of this gracious gesture and hunker down to begin my writing assignment. Rhea and Peter asked me to sketch the "arc" of my research to date. I've tried to capture that rather wobbly line in the title and content of this chapter, and more personally, in the next few paragraphs. I'm sorry there isn't room to thank people individually by name. I trust that each of you will recognize yourself and your influence in the following brief chronology.

My interest in causality research dates back to the masters program in Communicative Disorders at Boston University, where I found an engaging faculty and a terrific group of fellow students with diverse life experiences. After an aimless series of undergraduate majors at Syracuse University, followed by a string of forgettable jobs, BU was a stimulating and challenging experience. We talked in and out of class about the big stuff (e.g., 'the subsoils of human existence'), which somehow set me on a quest to try to understand the origins of speech disorders of unknown origin. The detective work continued at my first clinical position in Bridgeport, Connecticut—a busy rehabilitation center where clients and their families taught me so much more than I helped them.

At the Lawrence and the Medical Center campuses of the University of Kansas,

I had the good fortune to learn "dust-bowl empiricist" research from a scholarly faculty and a knowledgeable, fun-loving, and very verbal gang of doctoral students. The "postbehaviorism" in the chapter title alludes to this heady period in our discipline when carefully planned and reported treatment research offered the possibility to effect significant behavioral and social change. There is much about the earnest goals of the current focus on evidence-based practice that is reminiscent of the Zeitgeist of this period.

At the Department of Communicative Disorders, University of Wisconsin-Madison and the Communication Processes Unit at the Waisman Center, I have been privileged to have long-term interactions with an extraordinary cohort of academic and clinical colleagues and forward-thinking administrators. I want to acknowledge the contributions of dozens of wonderful alumnae from our research group at the Phonology Project, many doctoral and postdoctoral researchers who have shared their skills and enthusiasm with us, and investigators in Madison and elsewhere with whom I have had the honor of working in past and continuing collaborative projects. One long-term collaborator and good friend I will thank by name is Joan Kwiatkowski, who continues to contribute her immense talent to speech research and to set a standard for clinical efficacy in our university and Phonology Project speech clinics. It's such a joy to share with these colleagues the excitement on the other side of the arc—the boundless opportunities for discovery in the current "postgenomic era."

To Rhea, Peter, and each of the other good friends who have written such lucid papers for this volume—and to Sadanand Singh, a long-time friend and tireless advocate for our discipline—my humble and heartfelt thanks.

Overview

What follows is the latest version of "the Talk." I seem to have been updating variations of this presentation for a very long time. It is an overview of a vision to develop and validate an etiologic classification system for childhood speech sound disorders of currently unknown origin. I first introduce a set of working terms and concepts that constitute the nosological framework for the system. Then, I discuss epidemiologic and other research findings viewed as support for the hypothesis of etiologic subtypes of childhood speech sound disorders.

I hope this review enriches or at least complements each of the thoughtful essays by my colleagues. I thank them in advance for playing nicely with me at points in their discussions where they may need to address the many gaps in theoretical and empirical support for the proposals offered in the following work in progress.

Explanation in Speech Sound Disorders

The American Speech-Language-Hearing Association's recent adoption of the term *speech sound disorders* (SSD) is a welcome solution to the constraints associated with the *articulation disorders versus phonological disorders* dichotomy of the past three decades. The term *SSD* provides a theory-neutral cover term for researchers and clinicians who may, as I do, view SSD as a complex neurodevelopmental disorder. The term *childhood* (or in medical contexts, *pediatric*) *speech sound disorders*, which parallels the term *childhood language disorders*, unifies the study of speech sound disorders of both known (e.g., Down syndrome, cleft palate) and presently unknown origin.

Figure 1–1 is a sketch of four epochs in the history of causality research in childhood speech sound disorders. The first epoch is the 40-year period from the earliest research studies in this country in the 1920s until the many classic studies of the 1950s, in which epidemiologic and descriptive linguistic methods were used to identify and classify children with speech sound errors. Especially toward the end of this period, *distal* causes of speech errors were addressed and research focused primarily on explanatory theories and constructs from articulatory phonetics, speech motor control, and developmental psychology.

In the following perhaps 30-year period, both linguistic descriptions and causal studies of SSD changed markedly. Methods in our discipline included a succession of alternative descriptive, psycholinguistic, and sociolinguistic paradigms from allied disciplines, with markedly decreased interest in the search for distal causes of SSD. Focus clearly shifted to the identification and delineation of core deficits in *proximal* processes that constrain speech acquisition and performance.

A third epoch, lasting perhaps 10 years (note the shrinking shelf-life of epochs), was dubbed the *decade of the brain*. Advances

in neuroimaging and other assessment technologies enabled renewed interest in both distal and proximal causal perspectives underlying SSD, especially, in the present context, as it became possible to describe neural correlates of speech sound processing more directly.

Our discipline is currently enjoying the opportunities presented in a fourth epoch—the postgenomic era. Following the successful conclusion of the Human Genome Project in 2001, continuous technical advances make it possible to study the distal origins of many putative sources of SSD. Overviews of the current period often allude to the "Omics," with levels of explanation proceeding downstream from the genome: Genomics > Transcriptomics > Proteomics > Glycomics > Metabalomics > Epigenomics > Phenomics and others. Vernes et al. (2006) report the first example of functional genetic analyses of a gene underlying one subtype of SSD (*FOXP2*), demonstrating the potential of neurodevelopmental research using systems biology.

We take the perspective that an etiologic classification system for SSD is needed if this highly prevalent disorder (to be discussed) is to participate in the scientific and clinical advances being achieved in other

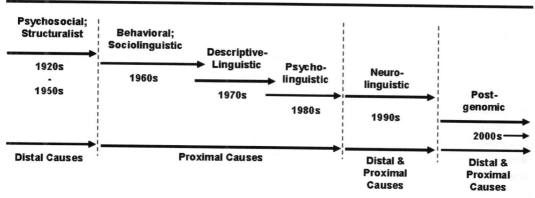

Figure 1–1. Four epochs of causality research in speech sound disorders.

childhood diseases and disorders. The following section describes a research framework proposed for this challenge.

The Speech Disorders Classification System (SDCS)

Speech Disorders Classification System–Typology (SDCS-T)

Figure 1–2 is the Speech Disorders Classification System (SDCS), a framework for research in SSD that has evolved from rudimentary descriptions (Shriberg, 1980, 1982a, 1982b; Shriberg & Kwiatkowski, 1982), a call for speech-genetics research (Shriberg, 1993), and several preliminary presentations (Shriberg, 1994, 1997; Shriberg, Austin, Lewis, McSweeny, & Wilson, 1997b). The left arm of the SDCS, titled SDCS-T, provides a typologic nosology that divides SSD of unknown origin into two subtypes. The more clinically significant subtype is termed *speech delay* (SD) with *delay* highlighting the finding that most children with this subtype of SSD normalize with treatment. The SDCS defines SD as a pattern of speech sound deletions and/or substitutions characteristic of Ingram's (1989) Phonological Stage III that persists past 4 years of age (cf. Shriberg & Kwiatkowski, 1982; Shriberg, Kwiatkowski, & Gruber, 1994). Notice that we use the term SD as one of two subtypes of SSD, whereas SSD and SD typically are used synonymously in the literature. As reviewed shortly, there are few data on the risk and protective factors that predict normalization versus persistence of SD at 6 years of age (Peterson, Pennington, Shriberg, & Boada, in press). Crucially, although speech sound production errors may normalize with treatment, SD places a child at increased

risk for literacy delays (Hesketh, 2004; Leitão & Fletcher, 2004; Raitano, Pennington, Tunick, Boada, & Shriberg, 2004; Shriberg & Kwiatkowski, 1988), lowered self-concept (Barrett & Hoops, 1974), and restricted vocational choices (Felsenfeld, Broen, & McGue, 1994).

The second subtype of SSD of currently unknown origin shown in Figure 1–2 is termed *speech errors* (SE). Children with SE have histories of speech sound distortion errors (for English-speaking children typically on sibilants and rhotics) that are not associated with the risk domains documented for SD and that do not interfere with intelligibility. The prevalence of SE below age 9 is estimated at approximately 5% (Shriberg & Austin, 1998). Reviews of the limited epidemiologic data indicate that after 9 years of age, 1 to 2% of adolescents and adults have one or more of a small set of residual distortion errors from prior SD or SE, errors that may persist for a lifetime (Lewis & Shriberg, 1994).

Speech Disorders Classification System–Etiology (SDCS-E)

The right arm of Figure 1–2 is termed the Speech Disorders Classification System–Etiology (SDCS-E). The SDCS-E provides the conceptual framework and working terms for seven etiologic subtypes of SSD. Table 1–1 includes additional speculation on genetic versus environmental contributions underlying each of seven subtypes. The central claim is that SD and SE do not arise from the same monolithic causal domain and that each includes etiologic subtypes. The hypothesis for SD is that it includes five individual and overlapping etiologies, each with one or more distal and proximal origins with risk and protective factors in both genetic and environmental domains.

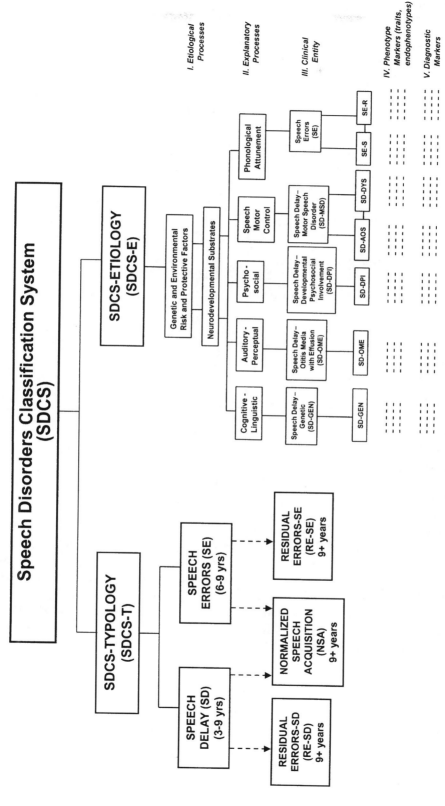

Figure 1–2. A framework for causality research in childhood speech sound disorders.

Table 1–1. Seven Subtypes of Speech Sound Disorders in the Speech Disorders Classification System-Etiology (SDCS-E)

	Working Term	*Abbreviation*	*Primary Origin*	*Processes Affected*
1	Speech Delay–Genetic	SD-GEN	Polygenic/ Environmental	Cognitive-Linguistic
2	Speech Delay–Otitis Media with Effusion	SD-OME	Polygenic/ Environmental	Auditory-Perceptual
3	Speech Delay– Developmental Psychological Involvement	SD-DPI	Polygenic/ Environmental	Affective-Temperamental
4	Speech Delay–Apraxia of Speech	SD-AOS	Monogenic? Oligogenic?	Speech Motor Control
5	Speech Delay– Dysarthria	SD-DYS	Monogenic? Oligogenic?	Speech Motor Control
6	Speech Errors– Sibilants	SE-S	Environmental	Phonological Attunement
7	Speech Errors–Rhotics	SE-R	Environmental	Phonological Attunement
	Undifferentiated Speech Delay	USD	Any of 1–5	Any of 1–5
	Undifferentiated Speech Sound Disorders	USSD	Any 1–7	Any 1–7

The hypothesis for SE is that it includes two subtypes, each based on a different group of environmental risk factors (Shriberg, 1994).

A set of working terms (and their abbreviations) is used to reference children whose speech delay may be due to one or more of the five proposed distal-proximal origins shown in Figure 1–2 and Table 1–1. The five etiologic subtypes of SD are those associated with (a) cognitive-linguistic processing constraints that may be, in part, *genet*ically transmitted (*SD-GEN*); (b) auditory-perceptual processing constraints that are the consequence of the fluctuant conductive hearing loss associated with early recur-rent otitis *m*edia with *e*ffusion (*SD-OME*); (c) affective, temperamental processing constraints associated with *d*evelopmental *p*sychosocial *i*nvolvement (*SD-DPI*); (d) speech motor planning/programming constraints consistent with *a*praxia *o*f speech (*SD-AOS*); and (e) speech motor execution constraints consistent with several forms of *dys*arthria (*SD-DYS*). The term *motor speech disorder* (MSD) is used for children suspected to have either or both of the latter two sensorimotor speech disorders. It is important to underscore the epidemiologic observation that a significant proportion of children with SD have involvement in two or more of the five distal and proximal domains.

The two subtypes of *speech errors* (SE) included in the SDCS-E provide classifications for English speakers who have transient or persistent distortions of sibilants (SE-S) and/or rhotics (SE-R). Changing views of handicap and competing service delivery needs have greatly affected research and applied interests in children and adults with SE. Although SE was well studied in the first two epochs delineated in Figure 1–1, persistent speech sound distortions such as dentalized /s/, lateralized /s/, derhotacized /r/, or velarized /l/ are currently viewed as having negligible or minor social consequences. The causal origins of such allophones and their natural histories, however, remain of considerable theoretical interest. We have proposed a variant of attunement theory (phonological attunement) to account for sociodemographic differences observed between children with SD and SE and between children with each of the two proposed subtypes of SE (Shriberg, 1975, 1994).

The dashes in the lower rows of the right arm in Figure 1–2 are placeholders for the research and applied goals of the SDCS-E. Our aims have been to provide diagnostic markers that discriminate each of the five etiologic subtypes of SD, and to develop binary and quantitative phenotypes and endophenotypes for use in molecular genetic studies. As discussed presently, encouraging progress has been made toward filling in the blanks.

Finally, the two cover terms at the bottom of Table 1–1 are needed to differentiate among research samples. Undifferentiated speech sound disorders (USSD) is a useful class term for speakers who may have either SD or SE. Undifferentiated speech delay (USD) is a useful class term for speakers who have or have had SD, but have not been differentiated on the basis of the proposed etiologic subtypes (e.g., SD-GEN, SD-OME, SD-DPI, SD-AOS, SD-DYS).

Epidemiology of Speech Sound Disorders

Prevalence and Persistence of Speech Delay

Figure 1–3 includes prevalence estimates for USD (i.e., speakers who meet criteria for SD, but are undifferentiated relative to subtypes of SD). Methodological details for

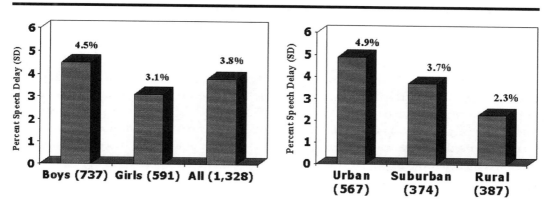

Figure 1–3. Prevalence estimates for Undifferentiated Speech Delay (USD) at six years of age (adapted from Shriberg, Tomblin, & McSweeny, 1999).

the population-based sample from which estimates were obtained are provided in Shriberg, Tomblin, and McSweeny (1999). The prevalence estimate of 3.8% at 6 years of age in the left panel indicates that SD is highly prevalent, with implications for both genetic and environmental explanatory accounts and service delivery needs. Because several of our prospective studies have indicated that approximately 75% of children have normalized their SD by 6 years of age, we estimate that SD occurs in 15 to 16% of children at 3 years of age. A study by Campbell et al. (2003) using the SDCS-T to classify speech disorders cross-validated that projection, reporting a prevalence of SD at age 3 of 15.2%. This latter prevalence estimate is the area approximately equivalent to one-standard deviation below the normal curve, suggesting that speech acquisition is a normally distributed trait with SD reflecting scores below the 16th percentile. From a genetic perspective, as posited in Table 1–1, the mode of genetic transmission for a normally distributed trait is consistent with polygenic, rather than monogenic or oligogenic transmission, in addition to risk associated with environmental sources. The prevalence estimate for males (4.5%) compared to females (3.1%), a ratio of 1.5:1, and the differing prevalence estimates associated with the three geographic strata shown in the right panel in Figure 1–3, further support the need for explanatory models that include both genetic and environmental risk and protective factors. Notice that the prevalence estimate for children from urban strata (4.9%) is more than twice that for children from rural strata (2.3%). Campbell et al. (2003) reported three genetic-environmental risk factors that best predicted SD: male, lower educational level of the mother, and a history of SD in other family members.

The three panels in Figure 1–4 provide preliminary estimates of short- and long-term normalization of SD, with implications for

etiologic subtypes of SD (Lewis & Shriberg, 1994). From 9 to 12 years of age, the period when even severe SD should normalize, about 30% of children shown in the two independent subsamples retained distortions of sibilants and rhotics. That figure dropped to approximately 9% from 12 to 18 years. Rhotic errors persisted after 18 years in 9% of children with prior SD, possibly persisting throughout these individuals' lifetimes.

The normalization/persistence data in Figure 1–4 raise questions of considerable interest for explanatory accounts of SSD. Clinical experience indicates that dentalized and lateralized sibilant errors persist in adults. Yet the preliminary estimates in Figure 1–4, which are based on children who had SD, not SE, indicate persistence primarily of rhotic distortions. If reliable, what explanatory mechanisms might account for this difference in the persistence of subclasses of residual errors? Epidemiologic data using population sampling designs could provide such information, particularly as there are now cohorts of adults with untreated SE due to school districts' contemporary definitions of handicap. Later discussion of research findings in SD-GEN will consider related issues.

Emerging Epidemiologic Data for Subtypes of Speech Sound Disorders

We have been continuously updating epidemiologic and speech findings for the hypothesis of etiologic subtypes of SSD. The entries in Table 1–2 are current estimates for five such variables, based on published and unpublished clinical samples from collaborative studies. The question marks indicate cells for which there presently are no available preliminary estimates, mainly due to the lack of emerging diagnostic markers for some SDCS-E subgroups.

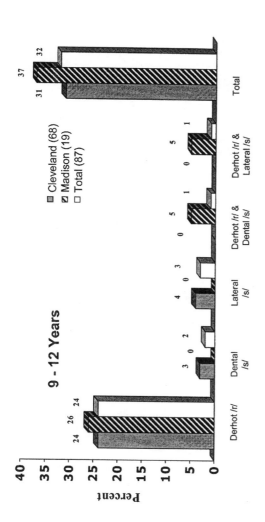

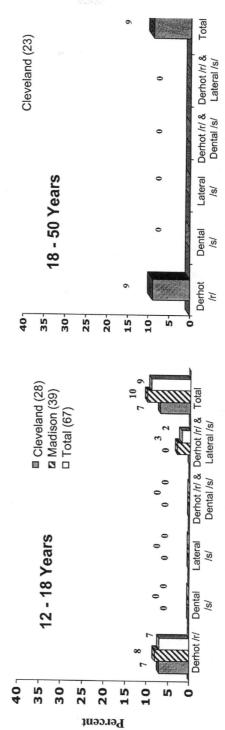

Figure 1–4. Point prevalence estimates for residual speech errors in children with prior SD (RE-SD).

Table 1–2. Epidemiologic Estimates for Seven Proposed Etiological Subtypes of SSD

Variables	Speech Delay (SD)					Speech Errors (SE)	
	SD-GEN	SD-OME	SD-DPI	SD-AOS	SD-DYS	SE-S	SE-R
Clinical Prevalence	56%	30%	12%	<1%	?	?	?
Sex	M > F	M = F	M > F	M > > F	?	M < F	M > F
Delayed Onset of Speech	NO	NO	NO	YES	?	NO	NO
Language Disorder	YES	YES	YES	YES	?	NO	NO
Normalization of Speech	EARLY	?	LATE	LATE	?	Variable	Variable

Clinical Prevalence

The clinical prevalence estimates in Table 1–2 are the percentages of children with speech delay in study samples who met diagnostic criteria for the five proposed etiologic subtypes. These estimates are based on referrals to one university-affiliated speech clinic (Hauner, Shriberg, Kwiatkowski, & Allen, 2005; Shriberg & Kwiatkowski, 1994). Using SDCS inclusionary markers for each proposed subtype (see later discussion), estimates indicate that SD-GEN (56%), SD-OME (30%), and SD-DPI (12%) account for 98% of children referred for assessment/treatment of SD, with the remaining 2% possibly having apraxia of speech and/or dysarthria. Again, these estimates are based on referral rather than population samples, and are not adjusted for overlapping categories. If cross-validated in other clinics, and perhaps in a large epidemiologic study of speech sound disorders, they are presumably informative for research, clinical training, and treatment. Notably, they suggest that the majority of children with SD would best profit from treatment procedures

that address delays in cognitive-linguistic processes (i.e., the proximal causes of SD for SD-GEN; see Figure 1–2 and Table 1–1). They also suggest that a significant percentage of children might require treatment procedures that address alternative or additional speech processing needs.

Sex Ratios

The 1.5:1 boys-to-girls prevalence estimate noted previously for USD (see Figure 1–3) may not obtain for each of the proposed subtypes of SD. It holds for the estimated 68% of children with SD posited to have SD-GEN (56%) or SD-DPI (12%), but not for SD-OME, in which the sex ratio is estimated at 1:1. Boys-to-girls ratios for SD-AOS have been estimated to even more greatly favor boys (Hall, Jordan, & Robin, 1993), but a recent review of 55 cases reported to have genetically-based (i.e., nonidiopathic) SD-AOS occurring in complex neurodevelopmental disorders indicated approximately equal percentages of boys and girls (Shriberg, in press). Finally, as indicated in Table 1–2, preliminary findings of more boys with SE-R (rhotics) errors and more girls with SE-S (sibilant) errors are viewed as support for an attunement theory of SE discussed elsewhere (Shriberg, 1975, 1994).

Onset of Speech

As indicated in Table 1–2, a significant delay in the onset of speech may be one feature that differentiates SD-AOS from the other proposed subtypes. However severe or unintelligible their speech, children in each of the four other proposed subtypes of SD begin speaking at the expected time. The assumption is that for children who are true positives for SD-AOS, the praxis deficit makes speaking inordinately difficult.

Comorbidity of Language Disorder

Entries in the fourth row of Table 1–2 indicate that children in at least four of the five subgroups of SD are at increased risk for language disorder. As with most other domains shown in Table 1–2, there are few data on language impairment in children posited to have a clinical or subclinical type of dysarthria (SD-DYS). Language impairment is a primary feature differentiating children with SD from those with SE. Of considerable interest in recent genetic research is why some children with SD are spared language impairment, and more generally, what are the important genotype-phenotype relationships across verbal disorders (McGrath et al., 2008; McGrath et al., 2007; Miscimarra et al., 2007; Peterson et al., in press).

Normalization/Persistence

Entries in the fifth row of Table 1–2 are estimates of normalization versus persistence of SD, with implications for explanatory

theories and clinical decision making. Presently there are no data on the recovery rates for children differentiated into the five proposed SDCS classifications; retrospective and prospective studies are in process. With the 75% short-term normalization rates for USD referenced previously, and SD-GEN estimated to comprise 56% of clinical referrals, a large percentage of children who normalize may have this subtype of SD. In contrast, the increased severity of involvement in children meeting criteria for SD-DPI (discussed later), and the persistent segmental and especially suprasegmental deficits reported for children with SD-AOS, warrant classifying children in these groups as having late normalization or persistent disorder. Again, data on the natural histories of SE would inform theories of both SE and SD.

Emerging Research Using the SDCS Framework: Overview

To this point, we have proposed that an etiologic classification system for SSD is needed for this highly prevalent disorder to participate in the translational scientific advances emerging for other childhood disorders. What types of evidence in addition to epidemiologic information have been reported supporting the hypothesis of etiologic subtypes of speech sound disorders? The following sections provide brief research overviews and highlight selected methodological and substantive findings. Due to space limitations, the focus is on two of the seven proposed subtypes—SD-GEN and SD-OME—with only brief comment on SD-DPI and SD-AOS. As indicated, there is sparse literature on SD-DYS, and we comment on SE only in the context of the following discussion of SD-GEN.

Emerging Research Using the SDCS Framework: Speech Delay–Genetic (SD-GEN)

Literature Review

Significant recent progress has been made in the molecular genetics of SD. Behavioral genetic research in the previous decade provided strong support for the likelihood of a genetic form of SD based on findings from familial aggregation studies and twin studies (Stromswold, 1998, 2001). Compelling findings from a twin-adoption study (Felsenfeld & Plomin, 1997) provided strong support for genetic, rather than shared or nonshared environmental, sources of risk for SD in families with histories of verbal trait disorders.

The primary molecular genetic research findings to 2008, using a variety of positional cloning and other methods, have been the identification of significant regions of interest for what we term SD-GEN on four chromosomes. Each of these regions also is reported to be a susceptibility locus for language and/or reading disorders. In Lewis et al. (2006), we provide a glossary of common terms in genetics research and a review of findings, focusing on the limited research in speech-genetics compared to the more extensive genetics literature in other verbal trait disorders. A summary table lists findings from 34 linkage studies of language, reading, and spelling impairment that report susceptibility loci on 11 of the 22 autosomes (1–3, 6, 7, 13, 15, 16, 18, 19, 21). In contrast, our review of linkage findings for SD in Lewis et al. includes only four studies reporting significant or suggestive linkage of SD to regions on chromosomes 1 (1p36: Smith, Pennington, Boada, & Shriberg, 2005), 3 (3p12-q13: Stein et al., 2004), 6 (6p22: Smith et al., 2005), and 15 (15q21: Smith et al., 2005; 15q14: Stein et al., 2006). Candidate genes for SD-GEN, based on their association with reading, language, or speech disorders for these proposed studies include loci on chromosomes 3 (*ROBO1*), 6 (*DCDC2, KIAA0319, THEM2*), and 15 (*DYX1C1*). As discussed later, separate literatures continue to address the origins of vocal communication catalyzed by the finding that disruptions in the *FOXP2* gene are associated with reported apraxia of speech. Chapter 3 by Barbara Lewis may also be of interest here.

The Mendelian Inheritance in Man database has created a new entry, *Speech Sound Disorder* (*SSD*: MIM %608445), to archive genetic findings for SSD. Figure 1–5 is a sample of the rich information available in MIM, one of many databases and bioinformatic resources used in genetic research. Interested readers are invited to visit the online version of this database (OMIM: www.ncbi.nlm.nih.gov/omim/) and search on "SSD" for more information on this entry. In this view of a susceptibility region of interest for Speech Sound Disorders on chromosome 3 (11 rows from top), there are two nearby regions of interest and genes associated with other verbal trait disorders: the *DYX5* gene above, and (not shown in this display), the *ROBO1* gene, both of which have been linked to dyslexia.

As indicated previously, a number of recent analyses have explored genotype-phenotype associations within and across verbal domains (McGrath et al., 2007; Miscimarra et al., 2007; Peterson et al., in press). For example, using linkage analyses procedures, Miscimarra et al. (2007) demonstrated that the *DYX8* region (1p34-p36) may include genes with pleiotropic (multiple) effects, including SD, language impairment, and reading disorders. Such findings supporting common genetic influences across verbal domains are consistent with the polygenic-environmental causal model posited for SD-GEN in Table 1–1 and the

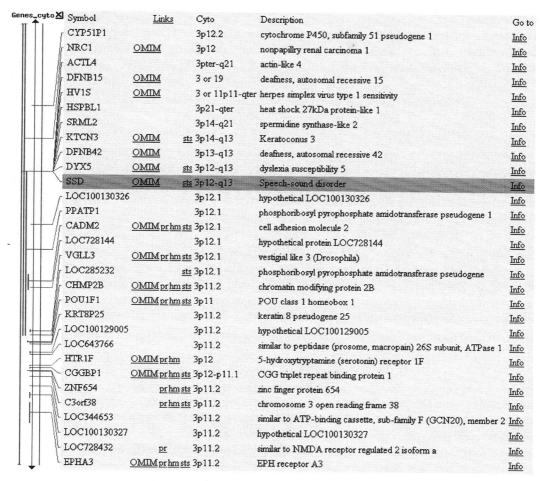

Genes_cyto	Symbol	Links	Cyto	Description	Go to
	CYP51P1		3p12.2	cytochrome P450, subfamily 51 pseudogene 1	Info
	NRC1	OMIM	3p12	nonpapillry renal carcinoma 1	Info
	ACTL4		3pter-q21	actin-like 4	Info
	DFNB15	OMIM	3 or 19	deafness, autosomal recessive 15	Info
	HV1S	OMIM	3 or 11p11-qter	herpes simplex virus type 1 sensitivity	Info
	HSPBL1		3p21-qter	heat shock 27kDa protein-like 1	Info
	SRML2		3p14-q21	spermidine synthase-like 2	Info
	KTCN3	OMIM	sts 3p14-q13	Keratoconus 3	Info
	DFNB42	OMIM	3p13-q13	deafness, autosomal recessive 42	Info
	DYX5	OMIM	sts 3p12-q13	dyslexia susceptibility 5	Info
	SSD	OMIM	sts 3p12-q13	Speech-sound disorder	Info
	LOC100130326		3p12.1	hypothetical LOC100130326	Info
	PPATP1		3p12.1	phosphoribosyl pyrophosphate amidotransferase pseudogene 1	Info
	CADM2	OMIM pr hm sts	3p12.1	cell adhesion molecule 2	Info
	LOC728144		3p12.1	hypothetical protein LOC728144	Info
	VGLL3	OMIM pr hm sts	3p12.1	vestigial like 3 (Drosophila)	Info
	LOC285232	sts	3p12.1	phosphoribosyl pyrophosphate amidotransferase pseudogene	Info
	CHMP2B	OMIM pr hm sts	3p11.2	chromatin modifying protein 2B	Info
	POU1F1	OMIM pr hm sts	3p11	POU class 1 homeobox 1	Info
	KRT8P25		3p11.2	keratin 8 pseudogene 25	Info
	LOC100129005		3p11.2	hypothetical LOC100129005	Info
	LOC643766		3p11.2	similar to peptidase (prosome, macropain) 26S subunit, ATPase 1	Info
	HTR1F	OMIM pr hm	3p12	5-hydroxytryptamine (serotonin) receptor 1F	Info
	CGGBP1	OMIM pr hm sts	3p12-p11.1	CGG triplet repeat binding protein 1	Info
	ZNF654	pr hm sts	3p11.2	zinc finger protein 654	Info
	C3orf38	pr hm sts	3p11.2	chromosome 3 open reading frame 38	Info
	LOC344653		3p11.2	similar to ATP-binding cassette, sub-family F (GCN20), member 2	Info
	LOC100130327		3p11.2	hypothetical LOC100130327	Info
	LOC728432	pr	3p11.2	similar to NMDA receptor regulated 2 isoform a	Info
	EPHA3	OMIM pr hm sts	3p11.2	EPH receptor A3	Info

Figure 1–5. Entry for *Speech Sound Disorders* (%608445) in Mendelian Inheritance in Man (MIM). This figure is included only to illustrate a display from one of the most frequently consulted bioinformatic sources. Definitions for column headings and other terms are available at the online site: www.ncbi.nlm.nih.gov/omim/

contemporary perspective of "generalist genes" (Butcher, Kennedy, & Plomin, 2006).

Phenotypes for SD-GEN

A primary goal of our collaborative genetic research in SD-GEN has been to develop quantitative phenotypes that are sensitive to and specific for this proposed subtype of SD

(Shriberg, 1993). The goal in family-based genetic designs is to assess relevant family members of the proband using measures that provide one or more quantitative indices for each sign of the disorder. Obtaining such information from direct behavioral testing of individuals who are at risk for the disorder, are currently expressing the disorder, or who have normalized prior disorder is preferable to using case records data (Barry, Yasin,

& Bishop, 2007; Lewis et al., 2007; Plante Shenkman, & Clark, 1996). Phenotypes must be sensitive to all levels of severity of expression of the disorder, as adjusted for possible age, gender, and other sociodemographic variables, but they may or may not be specific for it (i.e., they may be narrower or more broad relative to the domain of interest).

Several phenotypes have been used for family members of different ages in collaborative speech-genetics studies. For probands and young siblings assessed during the developmental period (years 3–6) in which misarticulation profiles are especially sensitive and specific for SD, two sets of phenotypes have been productive in the molecular genetic studies with colleagues just reviewed: the binary SDCS-T phenotype (Normal Speech Acquisition [NSA] versus Speech Delay [SD]; Shriberg et al., 1997b) and two continuous phenotypes (*ZPCC* and *ZPCCR*; z-scores for Percentage of Consonants Correct [PCC] and Percentage of Consonants Correct-Revised [PCCR]; Shriberg, Austin, Lewis, McSweeny, & Wilson, 1997a). For ages 6 to 9 years, when speech production errors may be nearly normalized with treatment, two continuous phenotypes developed to be maximally sensitive to persistent SD errors have also been productive: *Speech1* and *Speech2*. The latter two phenotypes (log of the odds and probability of having prior SD, respectively) were obtained from a 7-variable composite derived from a multivariate logistic regression using 17 out of 120 speech metrics that had the highest diagnostic accuracy for a sample of 759 speakers with prior SD (Smith et al., 2005).

Endophenotypes for Verbal Trait Disorders

Significant linkage findings in verbal trait disorders have most often been made to several widely used nonword repetition tasks (Newbury, Bishop, & Monaco, 2005). A significant confound with such tasks in speech-genetics research is that nonword repetition errors cannot be disambiguated from misarticulations. We have reported psychometric and substantive findings for an 18-item syllable repetition task that requires respondents to repeat nonwords comprised of only four Early-8 consonants (/b/, /d/, /m/, /n/) and one nonscored vowel (/ɑ/) in two-, three-, and four-syllable words (e.g., /bɑmɑdɑ/; Shriberg et al., 2008). Responses to this task, titled the Syllable Repetition Task (SRT), and to a comparison measure, the Nonword Repetition Task (NRT; Dollaghan & Campbell, 1998), were obtained from 158 children assessed in a collaborative physiology study, including 95 preschool participants with SD. Findings from three substudies support the construct and concurrent validity of the SRT and its internal reliability. All children had the four consonants in their inventories. Effect sizes estimating its ability to discriminate comorbid expressive language disorder from no language disorder were significant and comparable in magnitudes to those obtained with the NRT.

Additional analyses indicated that the SRT can aid in dissecting the speech processing constraints underlying poor performance on nonword repetition tasks. Briefly, we used differences in item length (2-, 3-, 4-syllable nonwords), error type (within versus across class manner substitutions), and articulatory difficulty (i.e., two-syllable items with homorganic [same place] versus homotypic [same manner] consonants) to assess the level of support for errors reflecting processing constraints at three phases prior to articulatory execution: auditory-perceptual encoding, storage-retrieval, and articulatory planning-programming. Findings provided strong support for auditory-perceptual encoding deficits underlying repetition errors of children with typical and delayed speech, mixed support for memorial processes, and no support for articulatory planning/programming deficits. On memorial processing, although longer SRT words generally were more difficult to imitate correctly, twenty-four percent of the 158 participants (87% of whom had SD) had repetition errors on at least half of the 16 consonant targets in the two-syllable nonwords (e.g., /dɑmɑ/). We interpreted these findings as arguing against a simple memory capacity constraint explanation for poor nonword repetition of these short CVCV words. On auditory-perceptual processing, the substitution errors of children with typical speech-language development more often retained the correct manner feature of the target consonant (e.g., /d/ for /b/, rather than either of the two nasal consonants for /b/) compared to the percentage of within-class substitution errors made by participants with speech-language impairment. We suggest that the SRT may be a useful endophenotypic metric for speech-genetics research, as well as for research with speakers with disorders of any type who have limited phonetic inventories or misarticulations.

Diagnostic Markers for SD-GEN

Recall that as indicated at the bottom of the right arm of the SDCS-E (see Figure 1–2), a primary research need is for diagnostic markers to identify children with one or more of the five proposed subtypes of SD. Diagnostic markers have to be sensitive to SD at all levels of severity of expression. Crucially, unlike phenotype markers, they must be specific for each subtype. We have made some progress identifying diagnostic markers for SD-GEN for use in genetic research.

A Diagnostic Marker for Children with SD-GEN

In Shriberg et al. (2005), we reported diagnostic marker findings for children at risk for SD-GEN. We divided 72 preschool children expressing SD into two groups comparable in age, gender, language status, and speech severity, but differing in family history of speech-language-reading disorder. Group 1 had two or more nuclear family members with histories of or active speech-language-reading disorder, whereas Group 2 had no nuclear family members that met this criterion. Although the two groups were assembled to have similar levels of severity of involvement (Group 1: PCC = 70.0% [10.3]; Group 2: PCC = 71.6% [10.2]), there were statistically significant between-group differences in their absolute and relative percentages of omission errors. Group 1 children, who presumably had higher liabilities for SD-GEN than Group 2 children, had significantly higher percentages of relative omission errors, particularly on the Late-8 (i.e., most difficult) speech sounds. The significant effect size for this latter comparison was 0.86 (C.I. = 0.35–1.37).

In addition to its diagnostic significance, we interpret these findings as support for the core claim (see Figure 1–2 and Table 1–1) that SD-GEN is due to genetically transmitted cognitive-linguistic constraints affecting phonological processing. We propose that speech sound omissions (compared to speech sound substitutions and distortions) reflect significant deficits in encoding and/or storage-retrieval processes. Literature support associating omissions with cognitive constraints includes the widely attested findings of proportionally more speech sound omissions in cognitive disability (e.g., Shriberg & Widder, 1990) and in the higher percentage of omissions in children with comorbid SD and language impairment. Speech sound omissions were also more prevalent in children with lowered performance on the SRT, the nonsense word task described above, which appears to be sensitive to individual differences in cognitive-linguistic aspects of speech processing. The omission marker has been cross-validated in an unpublished study that included 95 participants with SD divided by familial aggregation status.

Acoustic Markers to Recover the Phenotype in Residual Speech Errors

What speech signs or signatures might be used to recover SD versus SE origins in older speakers who have normalized or nearly normalized sibilant or rhotic distortions? Recall in Table 1–1 that SD-GEN is posited to have genetic origins, whereas the distal and proximal origins of SE are posited to be moderated by environmental risk and protective factors.

Figure 1–6 provides summary data from two study series attempting to determine if there were acoustic signatures of former SD versus former SE in speakers with residual distortion errors on rhotics (i.e., RE-R) or sibilants (i.e., RE-S). We tested several groups of adolescents including speakers whose speech histories were documented from our clinic records or school records as having either prior SD or prior SE and control children from the same classrooms. Both narrow phonetic transcription and acoustic methods were used to classify the speech tokens from word lists of speakers with normal or normalized /ɝ/ and those with prior /s/ errors.

As shown in Figure 1–6, /ɝ/ tokens were quantified acoustically by subtracting F2 from F3 and standardizing the result (z-score) using age × sex reference data

(Flipsen, Shriberg, Weismer, Karlsson, & McSweeny, 2001). A zF3–F2 value of 3.0 provided excellent discrimination between tokens transcribed perceptually as correct /ɝ/ productions (<3.0) and derhotacized /ɝ/ productions (>3.0) yielding sensitivity/specificity estimates of 95% and 94%, respectively. Moreover, a zF3–F2 cutpoint of 6.0 provided good discrimination between the perceptually derhotacized /ɝ/ tokens of speakers with RE-SD (<6.0) versus RE-SE (>6.0) speech histories (sensitivity/specificity estimates of 85% and 79%, respectively). Notice that the /ɝ/ tokens from the typical speech control group and the normalized speech group had z-score values below 3.0. Crucially, the /ɝ/ tokens of speakers with RE-SD were mostly below 6.0, whereas the /ɝ/ tokens of speakers with RE-SE were mostly above 6.0. Thus, the persistent /ɝ/ distortions of speakers with prior SE were acoustically most discrepant from typically produced /ɝ/ productions.

As shown in Figure 1–6, trends were in the same direction for /s/ productions of adolescents with former SD versus those with former SE measured acoustically using the first spectral moment (M1; Milenkovic, 1996). All tokens from the adolescent speakers were transcribed as perceptually correct, supporting the previous epidemiologic data indicating fewer residual sibilant than rhotic distortion errors in adolescents. Nevertheless, compared to the perceptually correct /s/ tokens from control speakers, the perceptually correct /s/ tokens from the speakers who had prior SE (see Figure 1–6, lower right panel) had notably higher z Moment 1 values compared to those from the speakers who had prior SD.

These /ɝ/ and /s/ findings suggest the possibility of acoustic signatures that may provide the specificity needed to classify family members correctly for speech-genetics

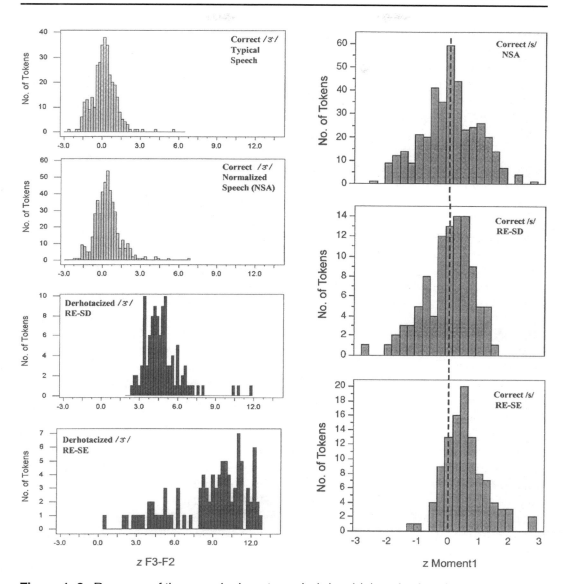

Figure 1–6. Recovery of the speech phenotypes in /ɝ/ and /s/ productions in older speakers. The panels on the left side include the number of tokens at each standardized value (zF3-F2) produced by participants in each of four speaker groups. The panels on the right side include the number of tokens at each standardized value (z Moment 1) produced by participants in each of three speaker groups.

studies. Studies in process are also pursuing implications of the findings in Figure 1–6 in their own right as discussed elsewhere (Karls-son, Shriberg, Flipsen, & McSweeny, 2002; Shriberg, Flipsen, Karlsson, & McSweeny, 2001). There are a number of cognitive and sensorimotor developmental frameworks that would predict that early distortions are more resistant to change than early errors of omission or substitution. Although considered more detrimental for intelligibility than distortion errors, early omissions of or substitutions for Late-8 sounds—as occurs in SD—may actually have a better prognosis for complete normalization than the early speech sound distortions that occur in SE.

Emerging Research Using the SDCS Framework: Speech Delay–Otitis Media with Effusion (SD-OME)

Literature Review

The hypothesis that early recurrent OME places a child at increased risk for SSD is based primarily on the assumption that the fluctuant conductive hearing loss that may accompany OME can affect the development of veridical and stable phonological representations (Shriberg, 1987). As indicated in Table 1–1, such proximal processes are presumed to have their origins in both polygenetic and environmental risk factors. In a review of 27 OME-speech studies, we concluded that support for *correlative* associations among early OME, hearing loss, and speech delay was equivocal, and that support for *causal* associations remained undocumented (Shriberg, Flipsen, et al., 2000). This is essentially the position of several large-scale prospective studies that have concluded that the mild hearing loss that may occur during episodes of early frequent OME is not a risk factor for early or later impairments in speech, language, academics, or social function. Variants of this conclusion have been expressed in a comprehensive literature review (Roberts, Hunter, et al., 2004), a meta-analysis (Roberts, Rosenfeld, & Zeisel, 2004), an updated set of clinical practice guidelines (Rosenfeld et al., 2004), and, most recently, in a long-term follow-up study of cohorts in the Pittsburgh otitis media project (Paradise et al., 2007).

A consistent trend in smaller scale studies of outcomes for children with significant histories of early frequent OME and hearing loss, however, is for study participants to have significantly lowered performance on cognitive and auditory perception tasks. Three research examples illustrate this trend. Nittrouer and Burton (2005) reported that 5-year-old children with histories of OME and low socioeconomic status scored lower than a control group on tasks involving speech perception, verbal working memory, and sentence comprehension. Gravel et al. (2006) reported that OME and early hearing loss was significantly associated with several measures of auditory processing in children assessed at school age, including measures of extended high-frequency hearing and measures assessing brainstem auditory pathways. Majerus et al. (2005) in a study of 8-year-old children with histories of early recurrent OME reported normal performance on short-term memory and new word learning tasks, but small, statistically significant performance decrements on several phonological processing tasks. These latter authors suggested that one negative outcome of OME appears to be ". . . subtle impairments at the level of perceptual-phonologic analysis . . . " (p. 473).

Is Mild Hearing Loss a Risk Factor for Speech Delay?

How can we reconcile the negative risk findings for mild hearing loss reported in the large-scale, prospective studies of OME with the positive risk findings reported from small-scale retrospective or ambispec-tive studies using convenience samples? Review of the hearing loss information in our prior and continuing research collabo-rations prompted us to examine the OME literature for the rationales used to subgroup children by hearing loss histories in both large-group and small-group studies, includ-ing the classic paper by Fria, Cantekin, and Eichler (1985) and the detailed information in Gravel and Wallace (2000). We wondered if the independent variable of *mild* conduc-tive hearing loss based on the pure-tone average (PTA) metric may be the source of important methodological differences among OME outcome studies. Some differences we found in the computation of PTA across OME outcome studies include: (a) the num-ber of frequencies tested (3 or 4), (b) the frequencies used to compute the PTA (.5K, 1K, 2K, or 4K), (c) whether the PTA is used as the index if there is greater than a 20 db HL difference in the better ear between any two frequencies, (d) differences in the cut-off levels used to convert PTA values to the ordinal, adjectival classifications for hearing loss (i.e., *mild* versus *moderate* conductive hearing loss), and (e) other testing differ-ences, including the number of hearing eval-uations available, the age(s) at which one or more PTAs were obtained, methods used to average multiple PTAs or to select the worst PTA as the primary independent variable.

In recent collaborative research, we explored the implications of prior fluctuant hearing loss on speech outcomes in sub-samples of 60 children in each of two pro-spectively assessed otitis media projects: the Chapel Hill (Roberts, Burchinal, Koch, Footo, & Henderson, 1988) and the Pitts-burgh (Paradise et al., 2000) studies. Based on prior collaborative research with the Dallas otitis media study (Shriberg, Friel-Patti, Flipsen, & Brown, 2000) and preliminary

analyses of pure tone averages available in the Chapel Hill and Pittsburgh projects, we defined children as having *typical* hearing or (*negligible* hearing loss) if all of their PTAs during the first three years of life ranged from 0 to 24 dB HL. Participants who had at least one PTA from 35 to 45 db HL dur-ing this period were classified as having *mild-moderate* hearing loss. Participants in each subsample who did not meet either criteria (i.e., 25-34 db HL and above 45 db HL) were excluded from further analyses.

Figure 1–7A provides speech profiles (PCCR calculated on the Goldman-Fristoe Test of Articulation-2 [GFTA-2]; Goldman & Fristoe, 2000) at 3 years of age for the children from the Chapel Hill study. Group 1 (*n* = 9; filled circles) participants had typi-cal hearing levels (0-24 dB HL) as assessed from 6 to 36 months and Group 2 (*n* = 8; open circles) participants had PTAs meet-ing criteria for mild-moderate hearing loss (35-45 dB HL) on at least one audiologic evaluation. Figure 1–7B provides compara-ble GFTA-2 data from the Pittsburgh database (Group 1: *n* = 10; Group 2: *n* = 6). Over half (57%) of the Group 2 participants in the two datasets had hearing loss from 35 to 40 db HL (i.e., within the standard 40 db HL upper limit for mild hearing loss). Two trends in these independent samples are interpreted as support for the hypothesis that mild-moderate hearing loss associated with OME places a child at increased risk for SD.

First, as shown for both datasets, notably in Figure 1–7A, Group 2 participants had markedly lower average percentages of con-sonants correct (i.e., ignoring distortions) compared to participants in Group 1. The statistically significant mean between-group differences for each developmental sound class in the top section of Figure 1–7A (per-centaged separately for Singletons [S], Clus-ters [C], and Total [T]) have a "box" drawn

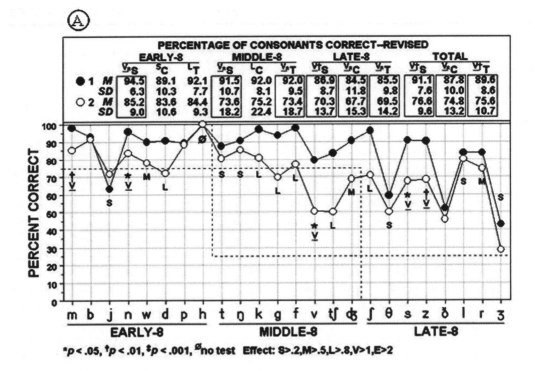

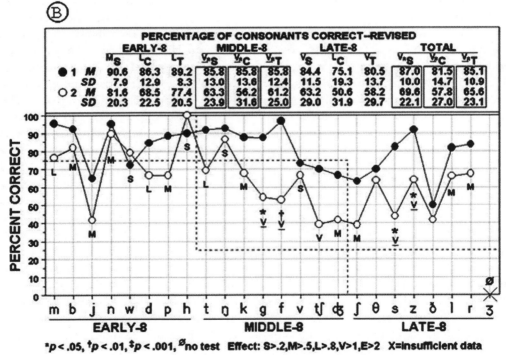

Figure 1–7. Early fluctuant mild-moderate hearing loss as a risk factor for speech delay at three years of age. The data in (**A**) are from the Chapel Hill database (Roberts, Burchinal, Koch, Footo, & Henderson, 1988); the data in (**B**) are from the Pittsburgh database (Paradise et al., 2000).

around them. Conventional inferential statistical symbols and underscored capital letters (*S*: Small; *M*: Moderate; *L*: Large; *V*: Very Large; and *E*: Extremely Large) indicate the magnitudes of significant t-tests and effect sizes, respectively. The significant effect size for the total PCCR was 1.21, especially large for small sample comparisons. Trends for the Pittsburgh data (see Figure 1–7B) were similar, including a significant effect size of 1.29 for total PCCR. Notice that the means for both groups in the two studies are comparable, with most Group 1 children scoring above 85% (typical for 3-year-old children on this speech measure), whereas Group 2 children scored approximately 15–20% lower, in the range reported for children with SD (Shriberg et al., 1997a).

Significant between-group differences in the percentages of correct /s/ and /z/ productions were also evident in both datasets in Figure 1–7. Group 2 participants averaged approximately 20% lower in the atypical 45% to 70% correct range. The magnitudes of the significant effect sizes for the four sibilant comparisons ranged from 1.11 to 1.57. We have reported perceptual (Shriberg & Smith, 1983; Thielke & Shriberg, 1990) and acoustic (Shriberg et al., 2003) data indicating that differences in sibilant production may be one of several possible diagnostic markers of SD-OME. Although considered preliminary due to cell sizes, these are our first data linking mild-moderate hearing loss to later deficits in sibilant production. We interpret findings as reflecting Group 2 participants' reduced attention to the salience of fricative energy in the 4kHz region and above. Again, although the large-scale studies have concluded that mild hearing loss is not a risk factor for SD, over half of the Group 2 children (8/14 = 57%) in these small subsamples had fluctuant hearing loss of 35 to 40 dB HL and all had fluctuant losses below 45 db HL.

Summary and Research Directions

Our current research perspective on the important public health issue in early recurrent OME (i.e., "watchful waiting" versus insertion of tympanostomy tubes) focuses on the need to determine the level and profile of hearing loss that places a child at risk for SD. Auditory perceptual constraints on phonological representations are clearly the relevant primitives in the causal pathways from hearing loss to speech production errors (Clarkson, Eimas, & Marean, 1989), and more generally, in current models of the development (Guenther, 2006) and persistence (Kenney, Barac-Cikoja, Finnegan, Jeffries, & Ludlow, 2006) of speech disorder. If replicated in larger study samples, the findings reviewed may explain why it has been so difficult to document the validity of this proposed subtype of SD. In an invited commentary on the influential Paradise and colleagues 2007 paper, Berman (2007) noted: "Since a hearing loss of 40 dB or higher was uncommon among patients in the study by Paradise and colleagues, it could not address the question of whether this level of hearing loss also leads to impairments" (p. 301). If replicated in prospective studies, the preliminary findings in Figure 1–7 would suggest that an early mild-moderate hearing loss of 35 to 45 dB HL is a risk factor for SD.

Emerging Research Using the SDCS Framework: Speech Delay–Developmental Psychosocial Involvement (SD-DPI)

Literature Review

As indicated previously, due to space constraints we have elected to focus on SD-GEN and SD-OME, with only brief comments on SD-DPI and SD-AOS. The hypothesis of a subtype of SSD in which psychosocial processes are the primary domain in explanatory accounts and central for treatment planning has been difficult to test. As indicated in Table 1–1, such proximal processes are presumed to have their origins in both polygenetic and environmental risk factors. The working term for this proposed etiologic subtype, Speech Delay–Developmental Psychosocial Involvement (SD-DPI), was coined expressly to avoid the concept of psychopathology or emotional disorder. Rather, we have borrowed from the personality and temperament literatures, which include dimensions such as *mood, negative emotionality, approach-withdrawal, distractibility, attention span, task persistence,* and *adaptability*. It has seemed that such constructs have been useful to describe independent variables that are risk factors for successful treatment outcomes in our clinical studies of speech delay (Kwiatkowski & Shriberg, 1993, 1998). Contemporary studies have assessed individual differences in temperament as a risk factor or correlate of delayed language development (e.g., Caulfield, Fischel, DeBaryshe, & Whithurst, 1989; Paul & Kellogg, 1997) and stuttering (Anderson, Pellowski, Conture, & Kelly, 2003; Embrechts, Ebben, Franke, & van de Poel, 2000; Lewis & Goldberg, 1997), but as suggested in Figure 1–1, there have been few studies in recent decades on personality or temperament differences and speech sound disorder.

Diagnostic Markers for SD-DPI

Using parental report and clinical records, we found that 29 of 245 children (12%) seen for speech evaluation and treatment in our university speech clinic during an 18-year period met a set of temperament-based criteria for SD-DPI (Hauner et al., 2005). This percentage of children was larger than we expected; these data are the source of the clinical prevalence entry for SD-DPI in Table 1–2. The SD-DPI groups included children who met criteria for either *approach-related negative affect* or *withdrawal-related negative affect* (Goldsmith, Lemery, & Essex, 2004). We assembled a comparison group of 87 children with speech delay from this database, matched to the SD-DPI group in age, gender, and SDCS classification (i.e., SD or an intermediate classification termed NSA/SD).

Speech analyses using a suite of descriptive measures indicated that children meeting criteria for SD-DPI had significantly more severe speech involvement compared to controls with SD. Their modal profile was an across the board delay of about an additional one year, compared to the control group of children with USD not including SD-DPI. They scored lower than the comparison group in each of the three developmental speech classes (Early-8, Middle-8, Late-8) and had significantly lower total PCC scores ($p <.01$; effect size = .57). Until we computed the clinical prevalence estimate for SD-DPI of 12%, we had assumed that such children would comprise a much smaller percentage of children with SD, and that they would likely have less severe speech delay, at least as compared to children suspected to have SD-GEN and SD-OME.

Although we have not, to date, identified a unique speech or prosody-voice marker for SD-DPI, the unexpected severity feature of SD-DPI is of significant interest for theory and practice. Clearly, more research is needed to cross-validate these initial findings and to design controlled studies of psychosocial processes as possible risk and protective variables in speech delay.

Emerging Research Using the SDCS Framework: Speech Delay–Apraxia of Speech (SD-AOS)

Literature Review

Research and particularly clinical concern for apraxia of speech in children has increased significantly in the past two decades (Shriberg & Campbell, 2003). Whereas *Developmental Verbal Dyspraxia (DVD)* remains the classification term in medical contexts and most other countries, a position statement by the American Speech-Language-Hearing Association (2007) endorsed the term *Childhood Apraxia of Speech (CAS)*. The working term SD-AOS references the same group of children as CAS and these terms will be used synonymously in the following comments.

The primary constraint in CAS research and applied clinical decision making is the lack of a set of inclusionary/exclusionary criteria to classify speakers as positive for this disorder (American Speech-Language-Hearing Association, 2007). From a research perspective, differentiating SD-AOS from dysarthria (SD-DYS) is a major research need discussed elsewhere (Shriberg, in press). Our perspective on this issue is that the problem is due to the focus on CAS as an idiopathic speech disorder, neglecting the potential informativeness of research in CAS as a secondary disorder in complex neurodevelopmental contexts.

Our proposed solution to the circularity (Guyette & Diedrich, 1981) or tautology (McNeil, Robin, & Schmidt, 1997) problem in CAS research and the escalating high rates of false positives in contemporary clinical practice (Shriberg & McSweeny, 2002), is the four-phase research design illustrated in Figure 1–8. In the first ("1") phase, we have begun to describe the core features of apraxia of speech as it occurs in adult AOS, in CAS following pediatric neurologic disorders, and in CAS in complex neurodevelopmental contexts (Potter, Lazarus, Johnson, Steiner, & Shriberg, 2008; Shriberg et al., 2006; Shriberg, Jakielski, & El-Shanti, 2008; Shriberg, Jakielski, & Tilkens, 2009; Shriberg & Potter, 2008). For a related discussion, also see Chapter 7 by Velleman and colleagues in this volume. The assumption is that a disorder of speech praxis should have features that are common to both acquired and developmental subtypes, with developmental issues likely moderating severity of expression of the core features. Critical to this approach is use of a well-developed speech assessment protocol that includes the same perceptual and acoustic measures to assess all forms of CAS across the lifespan. We have developed perceptual- and acoustic-based analytics to test alternative perspectives on the precision and stability of spatiotemporal signs in the speech and prosody-voice profiles of speakers suspected to have apraxia of speech. Findings from the first phase are used in the second phase (see Figure 1–8) to identify and develop the criteria that qualify participants as having idiopathic CAS. Findings from these four forms of CAS are expected to inform third phase studies of the genetic and neural substrates underlying the pathobiology of apraxia of speech (for overviews of *FOXP2* research, see Fisher, 2005, 2006; Fisher, Lai, & Monaco, 2003; for an example of systems biology to early 2008 see Groszer et al., 2008). The fourth phase focuses on applied methods for assessment, treatment, and prevention. Shriberg (in press) includes rationale for the framework and a review of 55 cases of CAS occurring in genetic-based neurodevelopmental contexts.

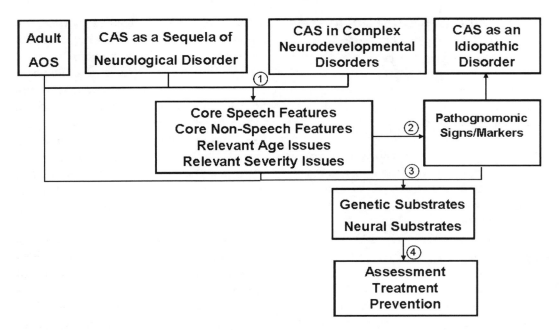

Figure 1–8. A neurodevelopmental framework for research in childhood apraxia of speech. Reprinted with permission from Shriberg, L. D. (in press), A Neurodevelopmental Framework for Research in Childhood Apraxia of Speech. In B. Maassen and P. van Lieshout (Eds.), *Speech Motor Control: New Development in Basic and Applied Research*. Oxford University Press.

Some Translational Needs in SSD

This progress report has described a diagnostic classification system for childhood speech sound disorders and a sample of findings gathered within this framework. To this point, there has been little discussion of clinical issues, specifically, on translating research findings to service delivery contexts. I'll conclude with some personal perspectives on the *why*, *what*, and *how* of these translational needs.

Why Etiologic Classification of SSD?

This chapter's focus on identifying the etiologic causes and clinical signs of subtypes of SSD is essentially similar to the classification perspectives in Duffy's (2005) classic text on motor speech disorders in adults. In his core chapter on differential diagnosis (Chapter 15), Duffy begins with the following quote from Sackett, Haynes, Guyatt, and Tugwell (1991):

> The act of clinical diagnosis is classification for a purpose: an effort to recognize the class or group to which a patient's illness belongs so that, based on our prior experience with that class, the subsequent clinical acts we can afford to carry out, and the patient is willing to follow, will maximize the patient's health. (p. 409)

I obviously agree with Sackett and colleagues and with Duffy on the value of diagnostic classification. As suggested at the outset of this chapter, diagnostic classification is required for children with SSD to fully participate in clinical advances in the postgenomic era, including molecular medicine and other new forms of personalized intervention in pre-emptive, prognostic, and targeted treatment applications. For these clinical goals, a systems biology approach seems to me to be the forward-looking framework for classification, rather than, for example, classification typologies based solely on linguistic descriptions or common speech error patterns. On this point, the long-awaited revision of the Diagnostic and Statistical Manual of the American Psychiatric Association, Version V promised for 2011, reportedly is being reorganized to reflect common genomic and other pathobiological backgrounds as the principle classification axes (Helmuth, 2003).

What Topic Areas in SSD Are Most in Need of Programmatic Studies?

Two figures in this chapter have included placeholder boxes for topic areas in SSD that are in need of programmatic study. The first boxes were included in the right arm of the SDCS (see Figure 1–2): "Genetic and Environmental Risk and Protective Factors" and "Neurodevelopmental Substrates." The second and overlapping boxed topics were echoed as later phase research needs in childhood motor speech disorders (see Figure 1–8): "Genetic Substrates and Neural Substrates" and the translational goals of "Assessment, Treatment, and Prevention." Research in all diseases and disorders pursues these public health topics, of course, but only recently have interdisciplinary projects begun to study the genetic, epigenetic, and neurolinguistic substrates of SSD. I would submit that it is time to recast the long-term dichotomy between SSD of unknown (for-

merly "functional") origin and those of known origin, bringing both together in a consolidated research framework.

Convergence on common genetic, neurodevelopmental, and environmental contributions to typical and atypical speech acquisition should lead to the development of common assessment, treatment, and prevention frameworks. Using an example from research in childhood apraxia of speech, Table 1–3 is a list of complex neurodevelopmental disorders and genetic disruptions in which speakers have been reported to have CAS. As shown in Figure 1–8, we have suggested that such disorders provide a rich source of information on the substrates of CAS, and more generally, of SSD. The descriptions of children's speech in these studies are notably sparse. Most reports continue

Table 1–3. Some Complex Neurodevelopmental Disorders Reporting CAS as a Secondary Sign. Studies are in process for most of the entries in this table.

Autism

Chromosome Translocations

Coffin-Siris syndrome (7q32–34 deletion)

Down syndrome (Trisomy 21)

Rolandic Epilepsy

Fragile X syndrome (*FMR1*)

Joubert syndrome (*CEP290; AHI1*)

Galactosemia

Rett syndrome (*MeCP2*)

Russell-Silver syndrome (*FOXP2*)

Velocardiofacial syndrome (22q11.2 deletion)

Williams-Beuren locus duplication (7q11.23)

to appear in medical journals which, understandably, do not include speech phenotype details even if available (although useful phenotypic details are increasingly appearing in on-line supplements). Again, I think it is no longer tenable to compartmentalize SSD research into those of known and unknown origin in the postgenomic era, when advances in understanding and treatment are likely to emerge from and inform one another.

How Can We Best Improve Service Delivery to Children With SSD?

The "how" questions of translational research necessarily involve new skills and technologies, operationalizing them for use in the field. Among the many instrumental approaches that are candidates for the assessment and treatment of children with SSD, skilled use of acoustic techniques (also see Chapters 7 and 8 in this volume), coupled with competence in narrow phonetic transcription seem to offer the highest possibility for widespread clinical accessibility. As described previously, the assessment protocol we use for diagnostic classification requires a laptop computer and masterslevel skills in phonetic transcription and acoustic analysis.

A key to the success of the work described in this chapter is the identification and verification of risk factors and diagnostic markers for subtypes of SSD. Table 1–4 is a list of 38 risk factors and diagnostic markers that have been assembled through 2008 for the five proposed subtypes of SD. Some are potential entries for the place markers at the bottom right side of Figure 1–2. The entries in Table 1–4 are preliminary; projects in process are completing validation and cross-validation studies of these and other diagnostic markers with comparison acoustic methods. Taken individually, few of the markers have demonstrated sufficient diagnostic accuracy, which would nominally require that they identify at least 90% of the true positives and true negatives for each subtype. We anticipate using a number of statistical techniques to maximize their combined power to accurately classify children's most likely subtype or composite subtype of SD.

Information such as in Table 1–4, which can be obtained using perceptual and acoustic procedures, should be viewed as reflecting only the current report on this continuing conversation on the causal origins of children's speech sound disorders. Once again, I am profoundly grateful to the many people who have shaped and contributed to the thoughts and findings in this report and to the children and their families who continue to participate in studies with us. More generally, I salute the international community of investigators and clinicians who work daily to help children communicate.

Table 1–4. Sample Perceptual, Acoustic, and Case History Risk Factors and Markers for Five Subtypes of Speech Delay Emerging from Studies Using the SDCS Framework*

Risk Factors and Diagnostic Markers	SD-GEN	SD-OME	SD-DPI	SD-AOS	SD-DYS
Familial aggregation of any verbal trait (pedigree interview)	+				
Lower language tests scores	+				
Lower nonword repetition task scores (NRT, SRT)	+				
Higher % relative omissions errors (ROI)	+				
Lower % relative sibilant distortion errors (RDI)	+				
Six or more episodes of OME from 0–2 yrs (medical records)		+			
Mean 3–4 freq. thresholds of at least 35 dB on any evaluation (audiological records)		+			
Higher % backing of fricatives (Siblilant Report)		+			
Smaller Intelligibility-Speech Gap (I-S Gap)		+			
Higher % epenthetic vowels on glides (Diacritic Modification Index)		+			
Higher % glottal stop substitutions (DMI)		+			
Higher % nasal-nasal substitutions (Speech Report 1)		+			
Higher % /h/ insertions/substitutions (Speech Report 1)		+			
Higher % initial consonant deletions (Speech Report 1)		+			
Lower first spectral moment on sibilants (<M1)		+			
History of clinically significant psychosocial issues (case records)			+		
Lower scores on psychological/social skills tests (case records)			+		
Lower aggregate speech competence (PCCR, PVCR)			+		
Late (>2 years) onset of speech (case and clinical records)				+	
Late (>6 years) normalization of SD (clinical records)				+	

continues

Table 1–4. *continued*

Risk Factors and Diagnostic Markers	SD-GEN	SD-OME	SD-DPI	SD-AOS	SD-DYS
Higher % vowel errors				+	
Higher % inconsistent errors on four stability indices				+	
Higher % utterances with inappropriate lexical stress (LSI)				+	
Higher % utterances with inappropriate sentential stress (SSI)				+	
Lower % on Pairwise Variability Index (PVI)				+	
Higher % on Transition Disruption Index (TDR)				+	
Higher % on Syllable Segregation Index (SSI)				+	
Lower ratio on Speech-Pause Index (SPI)				+	
Clinically significant sensorimotor task scores (e.g., tapping rate)					+
Clinically significant oral function task scores (e.g., DDK)					+
Higher % imprecision on Diacritic Modification Index (DMI)					+
Nasal emissions (oral examination; DMI)					+
Smaller planar area for vowels (Vowel Space Index: VSI)					+
Slow articulation and speech rates; by syllable, by phoneme (SRI)					+
Lower Speech Intensity Index (SII)					+
Breathy, strain/strangle; tremulous laryngeal codes (PVSP)					+
Rough voice (jitter, shimmer, harmonics-to-noise ratio) (J, S, HNR)					+
Nasal, denasal, or nasopharyngeal resonance quality (RQA)					+
TOTALS	5	10	3	10	10

*Titles, descriptions, and references for measures and working terms are not included here. Information about most terms can be retrieved using the search function at the Phonology Project Web site: http://www.waisman.wisc.edu/phonology/index.htm .

References

American Speech-Language-Hearing Association. (2007). *Childhood apraxia of speech* [Position statement]. Available from www.asha.org/policy .

Anderson, J. D., Pellowski, M. W., Conture, E. G., & Kelly, E. M. (2003). Temperamental characteristics of young children who stutter. *Journal of Speech, Language, and Hearing Research, 46,* 1221–1233.

Barrett, C. M., & Hoops, H. R. (1974). The relationship between self-concept and the remissions of articulatory errors. *Language, Speech, and Hearing Services in Schools, 2,* 67–70.

Barry, J. G., Yasin, I., & Bishop, D. V. M. (2007). Heritable risk factors associated with language impairments. *Genes, Brain, and Behavior, 6,* 66–76.

Berman, S. (2007). The end of an era in otitis research. *New England Journal of Medicine, 356,* 300–302.

Butcher, L. M., Kennedy, J. K., & Plomin, R. (2006). Generalist genes and cognitive neuroscience. *Current Opinion in Neurobiology, 16,* 145–151.

Campbell, T. F., Dollaghan, C. A., Rockette, H. E., Paradise, J. L., Feldman, H. M., Shriberg, L., et al. (2003). Risk factors for speech delay of unknown origin in 3-year-old children. *Child Development, 74,* 346–357.

Caulfield, M., Fischel, J., DeBaryshe, B., & Whitehurst, G. (1989). Behavioral correlates of developmental expressive language disorders. *Journal of Abnormal Child Psychology, 17,* 187–201.

Clarkson, R. L., Eimas, P. D., & Marean, G. C. (1989). Speech perception in children with histories of recurrent otitis media. *Journal of the Acoustical Society of America, 85,* 926–933.

Dollaghan, C., & Campbell, T. F. (1998). Nonword repetition and child language impairment. *Journal of Speech, Language, and Hearing Research, 41,* 1136–1146.

Duffy, J. R. (2005). *Motor speech disorders: Substrates, differential diagnosis, and management* (2nd ed.). St. Louis, MO: Mosby.

Embrechts, M., Ebben, H., Franke, P., & van de Poel, C. (2000). Temperament: A comparison between children who stutter and children who do not stutter. In H. G. Bosshardt, J. S. Yaruss, & H. F. M. Peters (Eds.), *Proceedings of the Third World Congress on Fluency Disorders: Theory, research, treatment, and self-help* (pp. 557–562). Nijmegen, The Netherlands: University of Nijmegen.

Felsenfeld, S., Broen, P. A., & McGue, M. (1994). A 28-year follow-up of adults with a history of moderate phonological disorder: Educational and occupational results. *Journal of Speech and Hearing Research, 37,* 1341–1353.

Felsenfeld, S., & Plomin, R. (1997). Epidemiological and offspring analyses of developmental speech disorders using data from the Colorado Adoption Project. *Journal of Speech, Language, and Hearing Research, 40,* 778–791.

Fisher, S. E. (2005). Dissection of molecular mechanisms underlying speech and language disorders. *Applied Psycholinguistics, 26,* 111–128.

Fisher, S. E. (2006). Tangled webs: Tracing the connections between genes and cognition. *Cognition, 101,* 270–297.

Fisher, S. E., Lai, C. S. L., & Monaco, A. P. (2003). Deciphering the genetic basis of speech and language disorders. *Annual Review of Neuroscience, 26,* 57–80.

Flipsen, P., Jr., Shriberg, L. D., Weismer, G., Karlsson, H. B., & McSweeny, J. L. (2001). Acoustic phenotypes for speech-genetics studies: Reference data for residual /ɝ/ distortions. *Clinical Linguistics and Phonetics, 15,* 603–630.

Fria, T. J., Cantekin, E. I., & Eichler, J. A. (1985). Hearing acuity of children with otitis media with effusion. *Archives of Otolaryngology, 111,* 10–16.

Goldman, R., & Fristoe, M. (2000). *Goldman-Fristoe Test of Articulation* (2nd ed.). Circle Pines, MN: American Guidance Service.

Goldsmith, H. H., Lemery, K. S., & Essex, M. J. (2004). Temperament as a liability factor for behavioral disorders of childhood. In L. F. DiLalla (Ed.), *Behavior genetics principles: Perspectives in development, personality, and psychopathology*. Washington, DC: American Psychological Association.

Gravel, J. S., Roberts, J. E., Roush, J., Grose, J., Besing, J., Burchinal, M., et al. (2006). Early otitis media with effusion, hearing loss, and auditory processes at school age. *Ear and Hearing, 27*, 353–368.

Gravel, J. S., & Wallace, I. F. (2000). Effect of otitis media with effusion on hearing in the first 3 years of life. *Journal of Speech, Language, and Hearing Research, 43*, 631–644.

Groszer, M., Keays, D. A., Deacon, R. M. J., de Bono, J. P., Prasad-Mulcare, S., Gaub, S., et al. (2008). Impaired synaptic plasticity and motor learning in mice with a point mutation implicated in human speech deficits. *Current Biology, 18*, 354–362.

Guenther, F. H. (2006). Cortical interactions underlying the production of speech sounds. *Journal of Communication Disorders, 39*, 350–365.

Guyette, T. W., & Diedrich, W. M. (1981). A critical review of developmental apraxia of speech. In N. J. Lass (Ed.), *Speech and language: Advances in basic research and practice* (Vol. 5, pp. 1–49). New York: Academic Press.

Hall, P. K., Jordan, L. S., & Robin, D. A. (1993). *Developmental apraxia of speech: Theory and clinical practice*. Austin, TX: Pro-Ed.

Hauner, K. K. Y., Shriberg, L. D., Kwiatkowski, J., & Allen, C. T. (2005). A subtype of speech delay associated with developmental psychosocial involvement. *Journal of Speech, Language, and Hearing Research, 48*, 635–650.

Helmuth, L. (2003). In sickness or in health? *Science, 302*, 808–810.

Hesketh, A. (2004). Early literacy achievement of children with a history of speech problems. *International Journal of Language and Communication Disorders, 39*, 453–468.

Ingram, D. (1989). *Phonological disability in children: Studies in disorders of communication* (2nd ed.). San Diego, CA: Singular.

Karlsson, H. B., Shriberg, L. D., Flipsen, P., Jr., & McSweeny, J. L. (2002). Acoustic phenotypes for speech-genetics studies: Toward an acoustic marker for residual /s/ distortions. *Clinical Linguistics and Phonetics, 16*, 403–424.

Kenney, M. K., Barac-Cikoja, D., Finnegan, K., Jeffries, N., & Ludlow, C. L. (2006). Speech perception and short-term memory deficits in persistent developmental speech disorder. *Brain and Language, 96*, 178–190.

Kwiatkowski, J., & Shriberg, L. D. (1993). Speech normalization in developmental phonological disorders: A retrospective study of capability-focus theory. *Language, Speech, and Hearing Services in Schools, 24*, 10–18.

Kwiatkowski, J., & Shriberg, L. D. (1998). The capability-focus treatment framework for child speech disorders. *American Journal of Speech-Language Pathology: A Journal of Clinical Practice, 7*, 27–38.

Leitão, S., & Fletcher, J. (2004). Literacy outcomes for students with speech impairment: Long-term follow-up. *International Journal of Language and Communication Disorders, 39*, 245–256.

Lewis, B. A., Freebairn, L. A., Hansen, A. J., Miscimarra, L., Iyengar, S. K., & Taylor, H. G. (2007). Speech and language skills of parents of children with speech sound disorders. *American Journal of Speech-Language Pathology, 16*, 108–118.

Lewis, B. A., & Shriberg, L. D. (1994, November). *Life span interrelationships among speech, prosody-voice, and nontraditional phonological measures*. Mini-seminar presented at the Annual Convention of the American Speech-Language-Hearing Association, New Orleans, LA.

Lewis, B. A., Shriberg, L. D., Freebairn, L. A., Hansen, A. J., Stein, C. M., Taylor, H. G., et al. (2006). The genetic bases of speech sound disorders: Evidence from spoken and written language. *Journal of Speech, Language, and Hearing Research, 49*, 1294–1312.

Lewis, K. E., & Goldberg, L. L. (1997). Measurements of temperament in the identification of children who stutter. *European Journal of Disorders of Communication, 32*, 441–448.

Majerus, S., Amand, P., Boniver, V., Demanez, J-P., Demanez, L., & Van der Linden, M. (2005). A quantitative and qualitative assessment of verbal short-term memory and phonological processing in 8-year-olds with a history of repetitive otitis media. *Journal of Communication Disorders, 38,* 473–498.

McGrath, L. M., Hutaff-Lee, C., Scott, A., Boada, R., Shriberg, L. D., & Pennington, B. F. (2008). Children with comorbid speech sound disorder and specific language impairment are at increased risk for attention-deficit/hyperactivity disorder. *Journal of Abnormal Child Psychology, 36,* 151–163.

McGrath, L. M., Pennington, B. F., Willcutt, E. G., Boada, R., Shriberg, L., & Smith, S. D. (2007). Gene *x* environment interactions in speech sound disorder predict language and pre-literacy outcomes. *Development and Psychopathology, 19,* 1047–1072.

McNeil, M. R., Robin, D. A., & Schmidt, R. A. (1997). Apraxia of speech: Definition, differentiation, and treatment. In M. R. McNeil (Ed.), *Clinical management of sensorimotor speech disorders* (pp. 311–344). New York: Thieme.

Milenkovic, P. (1996). *CSpeech* (Version 4) [Computer software]. Madison: University of Wisconsin-Madison, Department of Electrical Engineering.

Miscimarra, L., Stein, C., Millard, C., Kluge, A., Cartier, K., Freebairn, L., et al. (2007). Further evidence of pleiotropy influencing speech and language: Analysis of the DYX8 region. *Human Heredity, 63,* 47–58.

Newbury, D. F., Bishop, D. V., & Monaco, A. P. (2005). Genetic influence on language impairment and phonological short-term memory. *Trends in Cognitive Sciences, 9,* 528–534.

Nittrouer, S., & Burton, L. T. (2005). The role of early language experience in the development of speech perception and phonological processing abilities: Evidence from 5-year-olds with histories of otitis media with effusion and low socioeconomic status. *Journal of Communication Disorders, 38,* 29–63.

Paradise, J. L., Dollaghan, C. A., Campbell, T. F., Feldman, H. M., Bernard, B. S., Colborn, D. K., et al. (2000). Language, speech sound production, and cognition in three-year-old children in relation to otitis media in their first three years of life. *Pediatrics, 105,* 1119–1130.

Paradise, J. L., Feldman, H. M., Campbell, T. F., Dollaghan, C. A., Rockette, H. E., Pitcairn, D. L., et al. (2007). Tympanostomy tubes and developmental outcomes at 9 to 11 years of age. *New England Journal of Medicine, 356,* 248–261.

Paul, R., & Kellogg, L. (1997). Temperament in late talkers. *Journal of Child Psychology and Psychiatry, 38,* 803–810.

Peterson, R. L., Pennington, B. F., Shriberg, L. D., & Boada, R. (in press). *What influences literacy outcome in children with speech sound disorders.* Journal of Speech, Language, and Hearing Disorders.

Plante, E., Shenkman, K., & Clark, M. M. (1996). Classification of adults for family studies of developmental language disorders. *Journal of Speech and Hearing Research, 39,* 661–667.

Potter, N. L., Lazarus, J. C., Johnson, J. M., Steiner, R. D., & Shriberg, L. D. (2008). *Language and motor characteristics of children with galactosemia and speech sound disorders.* Manuscript submitted for publication.

Raitano, N. A., Pennington, B. F., Tunick, R. A., Boada, R., & Shriberg, L. D. (2004). Pre-literacy skills of subgroups of children with speech sound disorders. *Journal of Child Psychology and Psychiatry, 45,* 821–835.

Roberts, J. E., Burchinal, M. R., Koch, M. A., Footo, M. M., & Henderson, F. W. (1988). Otitis media in early childhood and its relationship to later phonological development. *Journal of Speech and Hearing Disorders, 53,* 424–432.

Roberts, J., Hunter, L., Gravel, J., Rosenfeld, R., Berman, S., Haggard, M., et al. (2004). Otitis media, hearing loss, and language learning: Controversies and current research. *Developmental and Behavioral Pediatrics, 25,* 110–122.

Roberts, J. E., Rosenfeld, R. M., & Zeisel, S. A. (2004). Otitis media and speech and language: A meta-analysis of prospective studies. *Pediatrics, 113,* 237–247.

Rosenfeld, R. M., Culpepper, L., Doyle, K. J., Grundfast, K. M., Hoberman, A., Kenna, M. A., et al. (2004). Clinical practice guideline: Otitis media with effusion. *Otolaryngology-Head and Neck Surgery: Official Journal of American Academy of Otolaryngology-Head and Neck Surgery, 130*(Suppl. 5), S95–S118.

Sackett, D. L., Haynes, R. B., Guyatt, G. H., & Tugwell, P. (1991). *Clinical epidemiology: A basic science for clinical medicine* (2nd ed.). Boston: Little Brown.

Shriberg, L. D. (1975, November). *Preliminaries to a social learning theory view of deviant child phonology.* Paper presented at the annual meeting of the American Speech and Hearing Association, Washington, DC.

Shriberg, L. D. (1980). Developmental phonological disorders. In T. J. Hixon, L. D. Shriberg, & J. S. Saxman (Eds.), *Introduction to communicative disorders* (pp. 262–309). Englewood Cliffs, NJ: Prentice-Hall.

Shriberg, L. D. (1982a). Diagnostic assessment of developmental phonologic disorders. In M. Crary (Ed.), *Phonological intervention: Concepts and procedures.* San Diego, CA: College-Hill.

Shriberg, L. D. (1982b). Toward classification of developmental phonological disorders. In N. J. Lass (Ed.), *Speech and language: Advances in basic research and practice* (Vol. 8, pp. 2–18). New York: Academic Press.

Shriberg, L. D. (1987). In search of the otitis media-speech connection. *Journal of the National Student Speech Language Hearing Association, 15,* 56–67.

Shriberg, L. D. (1993). Four new speech and prosody-voice measures for genetics research and other studies in developmental phonological disorders. *Journal of Speech and Hearing Research, 36,* 105–140.

Shriberg, L. D. (1994). Five subtypes of developmental phonological disorders. *Clinics in Communication Disorders, 4*(1), 38–53.

Shriberg, L. D. (1997). Developmental phonological disorder(s): One or many? In B. W. Hodson & M. L. Edwards (Eds.), *Perspectives in applied phonology* (pp. 105–127). Gaithersburg, MD: Aspen.

Shriberg, L. D. (in press). A neurodevelopmental framework for research in childhood apraxia of speech. In B. Maassen & P. van Lieshout, (Eds.), *Speech motor control: New developments in basic and applied research.* Oxford University Press.

Shriberg, L. D., & Austin, D. (1998). Comorbidity of speech-language disorder: Implications for a phenotype marker for speech delay. In R. Paul (Ed.), *The speech-language connection* (pp. 73–117). Baltimore: Paul H. Brookes.

Shriberg, L. D., Austin, D., Lewis, B. A., McSweeny, J. L., & Wilson, D. L. (1997a). The Percentage of Consonants Correct (PCC) metric: Extensions and reliability data. *Journal of Speech, Language, and Hearing Research, 40,* 708–722.

Shriberg, L. D., Austin, D., Lewis, B. A., McSweeny, J. L., & Wilson, D. L. (1997b). The Speech Disorders Classification System (SDCS): Extensions and lifespan reference data. *Journal of Speech, Language, and Hearing Research, 40,* 723–740.

Shriberg, L. D., Ballard, K. J., Tomblin, J. B., Duffy, J. R., Odell, K. H., & Williams, C. A. (2006). Speech, prosody, and voice characteristics of a mother and daughter with a 7;13 translocation affecting FOXP2. *Journal of Speech, Language, and Hearing Research, 49,* 500–525.

Shriberg, L. D., & Campbell, T. F. (Eds.). (2003). *Proceedings of the 2002 childhood apraxia of speech research symposium.* Carlsbad, CA: The Hendrix Foundation.

Shriberg, L. D., Flipsen, P., Jr., Karlsson, H. B., & McSweeny, J. L. (2001). Acoustic phenotypes for speech-genetics studies: An acoustic marker for residual /ɝ/ distortions. *Clinical Linguistics and Phonetics, 15,* 631–650.

Shriberg, L. D., Flipsen, P., Jr., Thielke, H., Kwiatkowski, J., Kertoy, M., Katcher, M., et al. (2000). Risk for speech disorder associated with early recurrent otitis media with effusion: Two retrospective studies. *Journal of Speech, Language, and Hearing Research, 43,* 79–99.

Shriberg, L. D., Friel-Patti, S., Flipsen, P., Jr., & Brown, R. L. (2000). Otitis media, fluctuant hearing loss, and speech-language outcomes: A preliminary structural equation model. *Journal of Speech, Language, and Hearing Research, 43,* 100–120.

Shriberg, L. D., Jakielski, K. J., & El-Shanti, H. (2008). Breakpoint localization using array-CGH in three siblings with an unbalanced 4q;16q translocation and childhood apraxia of speech. *American Journal of Medical Genetics, Part A, 146A,* 2227–2233.

Shriberg, L. D., Jakielski, K. J., & Tilkens, C. M. (2009). *Acoustic and perceptual profiles of*

Childhood Apraxia of Speech in three siblings with an unbalanced 4q;16q translocation. Manuscript in preparation.

Shriberg, L. D., Kent, R. D., Karlsson, H. B., McSweeny, J. L., Nadler, C. J., & Brown, R. L. (2003). A diagnostic marker for speech delay associated with otitis media with effusion: Backing of obstruents. *Clinical Linguistics and Phonetics, 17*, 529-547.

Shriberg, L. D., & Kwiatkowski, J. (1982). Phonological disorders I: A diagnostic classification system. *Journal of Speech and Hearing Disorders, 47*, 226-241.

Shriberg, L. D., & Kwiatkowski, J. (1988). A follow-up study of children with phonologic disorders of unknown origin. *Journal of Speech and Hearing Disorders, 53*, 144-155.

Shriberg, L. D., & Kwiatkowski, J. (1994). Developmental phonological disorders I: A clinical profile. *Journal of Speech and Hearing Research, 37*, 1100-1126.

Shriberg, L. D., Kwiatkowski, J., & Gruber, F. A. (1994). Developmental phonological disorders II: Short-term speech-sound normalization. *Journal of Speech and Hearing Research, 37*, 1127-1150.

Shriberg, L. D., Lewis, B. L., Tomblin, J. B., McSweeny, J. L., Karlsson, H. B., & Scheer, A. R. (2005). Toward diagnostic and phenotype markers for genetically transmitted speech delay. *Journal of Speech, Language, and Hearing Research, 48*, 834-852.

Shriberg, L. D., Lohmeier, H. L., Campbell, T. F., Dollaghan, C. A., Green, J. R., & Moore, C. A. (in press). *A nonword repetition task for speakers with misarticulations: The Syllable Repetition Task*. Journal of Speech, Language, & Hearing Research.

Shriberg, L. D., & McSweeny, J. L. (2002). *Classification and misclassification of childhood apraxia of speech* (Tech. Rep. No. 11). Phonology Project, Waisman Center, University of Wisconsin-Madison.

Shriberg, L. D., & Potter, N. L. (June, 2008). *Speech characteristics of children with galactosemia and persistent speech disorder.* Paper presented at the 12th meeting of the International Clinical Phonetics and Linguistics Association, Istanbul, Turkey.

Shriberg, L. D., & Smith, A. J. (1983). Phonological correlates of middle-ear involvement in speech-delayed children: A methodological note. *Journal of Speech and Hearing Research, 26*, 293-297.

Shriberg, L. D., Tomblin, J. B., & McSweeny, J. L. (1999). Prevalence of speech delay in 6-year-old children and comorbidity with language impairment. *Journal of Speech, Language, and Hearing Research, 42*, 1461-1481.

Shriberg, L. D., & Widder, C. J. (1990). Speech and prosody characteristics of adults with mental retardation. *Journal of Speech and Hearing Research, 33*, 627-653.

Smith, S. D., Pennington, B. F., Boada, R., & Shriberg, L. D. (2005). Linkage of speech sound disorder to reading disability loci. *Journal of Child Psychology and Psychiatry, 46*, 1057-1066.

Stein, C. M., Millard, C., Kluge, A., Miscimarra, L. E., Cartier, K. C., Freebairn, L. A., et al. (2006). Speech sound disorder influenced by a locus in 15q14 region. *Behavior Genetics, 36*, 858-868.

Stein, C. M., Schick, J. H., Taylor, H. G., Shriberg, L. D., Millard, C., Kundtz-Kluge, A., et al. (2004). Pleiotropic effects of a chromosome 3 locus on speech-sound disorder and reading. *American Journal of Human Genetics, 74*, 283-297.

Stromswold, K. (1998). Genetics of spoken language disorders. *Human Biology, 70*, 297-324.

Stromswold, K. (2001). The heritability of language: A review and meta-analysis of twin, adoption, and linkage studies. *Language, 77*, 647-723.

Thielke, H. M., & Shriberg, L. D. (1990). Effects of recurrent otitis media on language, speech, and educational achievement in Menominee Indian children. *Journal of Native American Education, 29*, 25-35.

Vernes, S. C., Nicod, J., Elahi, F. M., Coventry, J. A., Kenny, N., Coupe, A. M., et al. (2006). Functional genetic analysis of mutations implicated in a human speech and language disorder. *Human Molecular Genetics, 15*, 3154-3167.

CHAPTER 2

Explaining Developmental Communication Disorders

J. BRUCE TOMBLIN AND MORTEN H. CHRISTIANSEN

A hallmark of Larry Shriberg's work has been a commitment to the notion that the subtypes or dimensions of developmental speech sound disorders are organized on the basis of their etiology, and that the surface features of these disorders will reflect this multiple causal organization. Certain key points of this perspective are particularly prominent.

First, etiology is key to the study of developmental communication disorders. This statement may sound trite now. But in the 1970s and to some degree even today, some argued that etiology is not relevant, particularly for clinical intervention in behavioral disorders such as developmental speech sound disorders. Shriberg's early research was concerned with psychodynamic factors in speech sound disorders and expanded to include auditory (otitus media), motor (developmental apraxia of speech), and familial/genetic genetic factors. Each of these represented a subtype of developmental speech sound disorder.

A second feature of his work is his emphasis on development and developmental history in understanding the different forms of speech sound disorders. Presumably, different causal factors shape different developmental trajectories and thus, developmental course must be considered.

Finally, Shriberg is known for his concern for careful measurement and description of behavior. Just as etiology is revealed in development, it should be revealed in the fine structure of the behavior of the speaker.

Running through these ideas is the notion that we must develop comprehensive accounts of development and behavior that are grounded in causal explanations. Thus, advancement in our study of human communication and disorders should not merely focus on simple surface accounts of communication behaviors. In this chapter we accept many of Shriberg's key principles as we consider how we might construct a framework for research on developmental communication disorders that is rooted in explanatory sources for individual differences. In so doing we hope to demonstrate that there are alternatives for proceeding with this, and these alternatives have strong roots in several branches of philosophy. Some of the philosophical choices that we will take diverge from those found in Shriberg's work. Consistent with Shriberg, we intend to show that our research rests upon assumptions about communication behavior, development, and individual differences. Additionally, Shriberg's influence can be seen in our adherence to multiple causal systems and developmental history. We will cast these themes into an account that we hope will further scholarship in this field, much as Shriberg has enriched it.

The Challenge of Explanation in Developmental Communication Disorders

Much of science is concerned with generating explanations for observations in the world. And yet for centuries, philosophers have debated the nature of scientific explanation. Within this paper we draw upon some of this literature to present a rather comprehensive framework for conducting scientific research on developmental communication disorders. Our use of the term "developmental communication disorder" is intended to encompass all forms of communication disorders that arise during development, including developmental speech sound disorders which have been the focus of Shriberg's research. Although the factors explaining speech sound disorders may differ from those involving language or fluency, the framework for these explanations is the same. Explaining all forms of developmental disorders is challenging because the affected individual will not previously have had an ambiguous unaffected state. Furthermore, most developmental disorders represent variants in developmental trajectories, and thus they blend in with normal developmental patterns. These are challenges common to characterizing and explaining developmental speech sound disorders, developmental language disorders, and stuttering.

Explanations in science can take various forms, but most focus on either asking how something works or **why** it works as it does (Chater & Oaksford, 1999). In contemporary scientific research, the most common question posed is the "how" question. For example, we can ask how humans produce vocalizations. Our coherent explanation: we use mechanisms of respiration, airflow and pressure, vocal fold dynamics, and acoustic resonance. Note this account does not explain why humans vocalize or why the human larynx is positioned in the vocal tract the way it is. Asking "why" questions of this sort takes us into the realm of teleology (Mayr, 2004) Why questions produce explanations about the role of a system, process or object in serving some end state or goal. Mayr (2004) and Mundale and Bechtel (1996) argue that although one can attempt to generate mechanistic answers to how questions without considering why questions, understanding how mechanisms work ultimately also addresses the systems' functional roles. Therefore why questions become entailed in the how questions. For instance, explaining how the larynx functions in the account above will ultimately incorporate the why as well—the place of the larynx in the vocal tract and the importance of this position in human vocal performance, resulting in a teleologic answer involving evolution (e.g., Lieberman, 2007). Within this paper we aim to address both forms of these explanations as we attempt to answer why and how it is that some children are said to have a developmental communication disorder. The key is that we need to be clear when we are addressing why questions versus how questions.

A Starting Point for Explanation of Developmental Communication Disorders

As we present our model for explanatory research on communication disorders, it may be helpful to establish a prototype of current scientific practice. As with all models, this one aims to capture essential features and highlight the underlying premises. It is unlikely that this model exemplifies the thinking of any particular researcher. Thus, we might view this as an initial model of research practice from which we can build our particular model.

This model begins with the notion that variations in communication development, and resulting communication function, comprise classes of different types of abnormal communication and that each abnormal form of variation contrasts with a normal form of communication. Each class of abnormal communication development is formed by a flaw in the operation of a mechanism necessary for attaining the normal state. The abnormal operations of each these flawed mechanisms will result in distinctive properties (markers) in the communication behaviors (phenotypes) of the affected individuals. Although not often explicitly stated, it seems that the normal state is viewed as largely invariant—or if there is variation in the normal state, it is just the result of noise in the causal system. Scarr (1992) described this view as a platonic conception of normality wherein "individual differences . . . are considered to be unimportant variations on the ideal type" (p. 1). Within this platonic

framework, an organism's healthy state incorporates no variation from the ideal other than functionally unimportant noise. Following from this, illness represents a situation in which the variations are important. Furthermore, presumably the disruptions in the causal systems are no longer noise but rather dysfunctional (broken) systems. Ill health then arises out of these dysfunctional flaws in the causal systems, and ill health can be understood by discovery of these broken systems. Health and ill health, then, represent very different kinds of individual differences.

This perspective, just summarized, is largely consistent with a viewpoint which the philosophy of medicine referred to as neutralism or descriptivism (Boorse, 1977, 1987). This position claims that the constructs of health and ill health refer to natural properties of organisms and not statements reflecting social/cultural values. Within this view it is expected that there are flaws in the causal system that result in disease. In this account, the explanation of ill health requires only one type of explanation that rests primarily on how it is that the processes that give rise to the healthy state are flawed.

Toward an Alternative Explanatory Account

For a number of years, one of us (Tomblin, 2006) has argued against the neutralist model described above and instead advocated a weak normativist position. This model (Figure 2–1) recognizes two somewhat independent systems (biobehavioral and cultural) that each play a role in the explanation of communication disorders. This requirement of two different kinds of explanation is an important distinction between our alternative account and the standard account just described. At the interface of

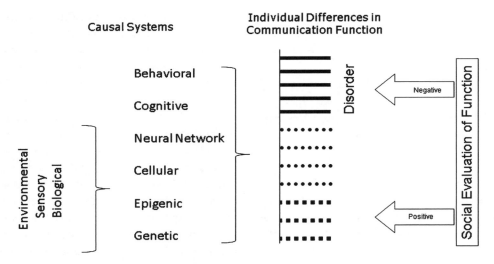

Figure 2–1. Component sources for explanation of communication disorder where individual differences are explained by multiple interactive systems and individual differences are differentially valued via social value systems.

these two explanatory systems are individual differences in communication development and function. A full explanation of a developmental communication disorder requires the use of both the biobehavioral and cultural aspects of this model. The explanatory role of these two domains in relation to individual differences is, we contend, different.

Explaining Disorder via Social Values

On the right-hand side of Figure 2-1, we show that social values are applied to individual differences in communication in such a way that some levels or some forms of communication function have greater negative consequences to the individual than others. The role of social/cultural values in a comprehensive explanation of developmental communication therefore, provides

an explanation for why we claim that a given child presents with a communication disorder. Within our normativist model, we would answer this "why" question by stating "because the child's communication skills place this child at risk for culturally based disvalue." Put simply, the child's differences are likely to result in undesirable outcomes for the child. A normative account accepts the position that concepts of health and illness are inherently value judgments arising from cultural beliefs and the goals societies have for their members. Thus, we can consider health as a state in which one functions within the social expectations of our society; ill health represents an inability to meet these expectations. A developmental communication disorder is a status assigned to the individual by either the individual herself or by others in society based on cultural values. We immediately can see that any explanation of communication disorder must incorporate cultural values and provide statements regarding the relationships between communication performance and the capacity of an individual to participate in socially valued roles.

It can be argued that communication is a universal characteristic of humans, much like bipedalism and opposable thumbs, and thus cultural values are not necessary to claim that limitations in these traits represent ill health. However, if we envision a world without gravity, legs as we know them are of no use. It could be possible that a society in such a world would no longer view the absence of legs as a condition of poor health. Likewise, we might have a world where speech and hearing are not necessary for communication, and therefore their absence is no longer viewed as unhealthy. This last example is not hypothetical, but rather is very well exemplified in the Deaf community where speech and hearing are in some circles disvalued, and lack of hearing and speech do not constitute ill health.

How and why cultural values carve up individual behavioral differences into more or less desirable states is an interesting problem that draws on principles and theories of sociology, particularly social deviance (Erikson, 1962). Thus, construing health and ill health as the normative product of human culture is not dismissive of science. Instead, it points to the necessity of constructing scientific theories that incorporate both why values are applied to behaviors and also why societies would do this. It is most likely that societies will disvalue behaviors that are deleterious to the well-being of the society. If so, as communication becomes important to a society, individual differences in communication skill will become the target of value-based judgments. This implies that the way in which a social group carves up individual differences in communication—along with the functions served by such communication—will differ not only between

societies at a point in time but also within a particular society across time. Today technologic changes have greatly affected our daily lives regarding the amount and import of communication. The bases for social evaluation of behaviors are not arbitrary, and explanations should elucidate the dynamics that produce and support social systems.

Thus, a full explanation of human communication requires understanding how communication functions are directly and indirectly associated with cultural values. The most obvious of these is the importance of communication for interpersonal social interaction. Theorists such as Searle (1989) and Grice (1975), who have broadly addressed facets of pragmatics, have provided an outline of these functions with regard to interpersonal communication settings. Communication also serves to support many other functions in our lives. Indeed, communication is an important means by which we establish and maintain our cultural membership. Thus, it is not just a vehicle for social interaction, it is also a principal means for establishing cultural and subcultural identity. Since communication also serves as the basic tool for instruction and learning, it is a tool of acculturation. We have considerable evidence that children's language and communication abilities are very strongly associated with school outcomes (Bishop & Edmundson, 1987; Hall & Tomblin, 1978; Nation & Aram, 1980; Snowling et al., 2001; Stothard et al., 1998; Young et al., 2002). In fact for children with milder forms of communication disorder, the impact of communication on learning may provide the strongest case for considering these as forms of ill health. Interestingly the distinction made by Shriberg (Chapter 1) between *Speech Delay* and *Speech Errors* highlights this point by noting that the latter is much less likely to be associated with comorbid language and/ or learning problems.

This perspective leads to an important shift in how we study communication disorder. As we noted previously, the prominent strategy has been to assume that by careful study of communication systems, we can identify classes of disorder. That is, the diathesis between "normal" and "abnormal" will be contained in the behavioral system itself; furthermore, this abnormality will extend to the causal systems that affect these behaviors. We contend that the locus of the disorder in a communication disorder will not be found in the characteristics or behavior of the individual, but rather in the cultural context. Thus, the scientific theories used to explain how and why some aspects of communication comprise disorder need not be the same as those used to explain communication function and its individual differences. Thus, we now shift our focus to the second explanatory component in our account, specifically, the factors that give rise to individual differences.

Individual Differences and Communication Disorder

Figure 2–1 shows that individual differences play a central role in our model. Furthermore, we argue that individual differences do not come in two types—one representing abnormal variation based on a defect and the other simply due to noise. Instead, we would argue that all individual differences have the same explanatory basis and the same value within the natural system.

Within an evolutionary perspective, individual differences are the means by which species form, adapt, and survive. Monocultures are well known to be highly vulnerable to the survival of the strain. Furthermore, as future environments cannot be foreseen, all forms of this variation have

equal potential value regarding survival. Thus, there is no place in nature to carve out forms of individual differences that are inherently normal versus disordered. By extension, we should not expect to discover the nature of a communication disorder by simply examining patterns or characteristics or flaws in systems that produce individual differences. In our account, these individual differences become disvalued, and thus disorder exists only in the context of a culture.

We also noted earlier that individual differences within the normal range are often ignored or considered noise. This viewpoint has been particularly prominent with respect to speech and language: it is assumed that full speech and language competence is attained by nearly all adults across languages and that the only individual differences in adulthood are found in those representing speech and language impairments. A common tenet within modern linguistic theory is that spoken language is a universal human trait. Thus, most adult speakers and listeners are treated uniformly with regard to language unless the language system is impaired. This assumption of uniformity of adult language status has then been used to claim that individual differences found during development in typically developing children are temporary and will be resolved by the time the child reaches adulthood. That is, these individual differences represent noise in developmental trajectories. If the differences are not resolved by adulthood when uniformity is expected then they must represent a disordered system. But is this assumption valid? In fact, a vast amount of data in psycholinguistic research has shown that adults do vary on lexical abilities and grammatical processing skills, even among the fairly homogenous population of college-aged adults (see, for instance, Gernsbacher & Faust, 1991; Pearlmutter & Macdonald, 1995).

We have followed a large group of children from kindergarten through age 16—an age most would view as the terminus of child language development. During this time the children's language abilities were measured at five time points: kindergarten, second, fourth, eighth, and tenth grade. After converting the raw scores into Rasch ability scores (Meslevy & Bock, 1990), we examined the growth trajectories of the children who represented a wide range of ability when initially sampled. Figure 2-2 shows that the pattern of language growth over time is remarkably similar regardless of the children's ability level. Individual differences are found at each age level, and there is no evidence that all children within the normal range converge on a common point —leaving individual differences at maturity to those who were initially language impaired. Furthermore, the language ability among children is stable, demonstrating that the variance in language abilities among individuals is not simply measurement error, but rather is systematic and persistent across both development and communication tasks. This stability of relative performance in a coherent behavioral domain is often used as evidence of a behavioral trait. Scarr (1992) for example differentiated between behavioral traits that are enduring and stable across many situations and years versus contextual and situational behaviors that are specific to time and context. Scarr refers to the former stable traits as phenotypes.

We can see now that many individual differences in the development of communication behavior are systematic and therefore should be open to the kind of explanation that draws upon biology, neuroscience and

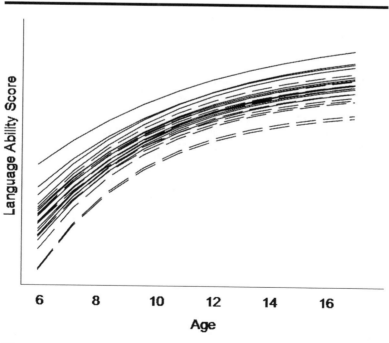

Figure 2–2. A series of language growth trajectories for a random sample of individual during the school years.

cognitive science. The explanatory accounts will not be reserved for explaining developmental communication disorder, but rather will simply explain individual differences in communication development in general. By highlighting the importance of understanding individual differences as potential sources of communication disorders, researchers concerned with such disorders can incorporate theoretical accounts of individual differences into the fields of natural science rather than describing them as ill health. It is to this end that we now consider how such a general theory spanning biology, neuroscience and cognitive science might provide an explanatory framework for individual differences in communication development.

Explanations of Individual Differences That Incorporate Multiple Systems

In the last decade, we have experienced a remarkable change in our ability to ask—and to some degree answer—questions concerning the nature of several systems important to the development and use of language. Cognitive science offers crucial tools involving computational modeling and theories ranging from those that are linguistically and symbolically based to those that are more distributed and statistically based. These tools and theories have resulted in a vibrant discussion of the possible nature of language development, processing, and representation. In addition, a field of cognitive neuroscience has emerged. It is now possible to measure brain function in language usage tasks: event related potentials (ERPs), functional magnetic resonance imaging (fMRI), and recently near-infrared spectroscopy (NIRS). These techniques allow us to examine spatial and temporal properties of brain activity associated with language usage tasks. This ability to study brain function—coupled with continued advances in structural brain imaging such as diffusion tensor imaging—has allowed us to move from merely speculating about brain systems and language to forming data-driven theory. Advances in molecular genetics and biology have also resulted in research concerned with the discovery of genetic bases for cognition, particularly cognitive development and disorders (see also Chapter 3). One cannot ask about genetics and behavior without also asking about cultural and biological environmental influences, which may bring us back to theories of communication development such as usage-based theories (Tomasello, 2003) and exemplar-based approaches (Barsalou, 1990) that are now emphasizing experiential input.

We can see that contemporary scholars in communication sciences and disorders have a rich array of research methods, data, and theory from which to build an account of the origins of individual differences in communication development. In fact, rather than having a shortage of potential explanatory theories we now have an ever expanding array of mechanisms and processes that we can incorporate into a theoretical account of individual differences. The challenge then is how to deal with the complexity that results from this richness of what could be viewed as multiple scientific fields of study. One starting point has been to consider each of these theories as focusing on different explanatory levels or systems for the ultimate product of communication performance. We may conceive of these different methodological and theoretical domains as forming a system comprising levels of explanation as shown in Figure 2–2. In this figure, we hypothesize that there may be at least 7 levels that can be used to study and explain individual differences in communication development.

To begin, we have identified one level that operates in parallel with all the others. This level concerns the sensory, physical, and biological environment of the child. The sensory environment provides the child with stimuli concerning objects and events in the world, including social artifacts such as speech and language. The physical and biological environments comprise a wide range of inputs ranging from gravity to nutritional substances to toxins and even "foreign" beneficial and deleterious flora and fauna that live within us. The genetic level is concerned with heritable biological information contained within DNA sequences as well as transcription and translation of this information into RNA and protein. The epigenetic level is concerned with heritable changes in DNA transcription. The cellular level is concerned in our case with biological functions (metabolism, axon growth, modification synaptic spines, etc.) operating within the neuron. The network level concerns the connectivity of neurons to form the brain, and within these networks the behavior of these neural networks beginning with the synapse. The cognitive level represents mental states and processes that involve such things as learning, memory, recall, intent, representations, etc. The behavioral level concerns all those coherent behavior patterns that yield communication, as well as the change in these patterns that come with development.

Reductionist Explanations of Individual Differences

Once we have identified these levels, we need to determine how each level relates to the others as we attempt to explain individual differences. Some philosophers of science use theory reduction to account for multiple levels of scientific theories and methods. Theory reduction assumes that the scientific statements and data at each level in the hierarchy can independently explain the behavior of the system, but that lower levels provide more explanatory detail than the higher levels, and that theories at higher levels can be translated into comparable theories at more basic levels using bridging laws (Bechtel, 1994); (Mayr, 2004). Thus, all characterizations at a higher level can be also accomplished at a more basic level. This means that each level can explain a phenomenon, but that more basic levels will provide more detail.

The use of theory reduction is called reductionism. For example, we can use any of various levels to describe individual differences in speech production. We can describe speech production broadly using the vocabulary of transcriptional phonetics, finer acoustic descriptions, descriptions of articulatory gestures or even at a more basic level the kinematic features of gestures. Each level is viewed as being concerned with speech sound production, and it should be possible to relate any one level to another. The differences have to do with the grain size of the description, and the choice of level may be determined by the needs of the research question.

An important feature of theory reduction is the implication that a theory at one level can be developed independently of another level. In the prior example regarding speech, it has been common to differentiate phonological theories, transcriptional phonetics, acoustic phonetics, and physiological phonetics. Scholars have been very comfortable working in one of these areas, but with the belief that bridging laws will connect their work to that of others.

Thus, we see a common approach to situations in which there are multiple scientific theories regarding a complex function: identify a level that seems to provide theoretical and methodological strength, and then develop theory through bridging laws to account for a higher level. We see this practice quite clearly in much of the research on developmental communication disorders—linguistic or cognitive data and theory are used to explain speech and language behaviors and development of children with developmental communication disorders. Such a research strategy allows investigators to work within their respective research domain free of the constraints of the other levels. Thus, we can have studies of neural structure, connectivity, and network function associated with individual differences in communication development. Likewise, we can have research on the genetics of these individual differences. However, this approach assumes that a common functional system spans these levels. Since the functional system in this case is the process of speech and language development, we would conclude that there are brain systems for speech and language development and that there might be speech and language genes whose functions can be bridged to brain systems. In fact, this very picture of language development is represented in nativist accounts of language development (Hauser et al., 2002; Pinker, 1994). Reductionism, however, has been broadly and extensively criticized as inadequate either as a description or prescription for scientific inquiry of most complex systems in nature, and biological systems in particular (Hull, 1974).

Mechanistic Explanations of Individual Differences

Many of those who have argued against reductionism in biological and cognitive systems have advocated an alternative approach referred to as mechanistic explanation (Salmon, 1984). A mechanistic explanation, like theory reduction, accepts that complex systems or mechanisms have parts that can even be described in terms of levels (Bechtel, 1994). Bechtel has characterized a mechanism as

> . . . a structure performing a function in virtue of its component parts, component operations, and their organization. The orchestrated functioning of the mechanism is responsible for one or more phenomena. (Bechtel & Abrahamsen, 2005, p. 423)

Thus, mechanisms perform functions and have parts. Each part or submechanism can be considered as having a function as well; however, the functions of submechanisms will not be the same as those of the whole mechanism (Craver, 2001). This was not true with our account of reductionism. Within the context of communication, the function of a gene that in some way influences language development is not the same as the function of cognitive systems. Thus, there will not be bridging rules that allow translation from one level to another, and we would be advised not to talk about genes being language genes or neurons being language neurons (Fisher, 2006).

Much of mechanistic explanation is used to address the "how" questions concerning a system. However, the function of any submechanism must be considered within the context of the broader system (Craver, 2001). The function of vocal folds can be to protect the lungs or to produce the acoustic source for speech, depending on whether we are explaining swallowing and respiration or speech production. The fact that the subsystems can have different roles depending on explanatory accounts leads us to realize that fundamental to explaining how a complex system generates a particular function requires also considering why certain functions come to be. Thus, even in mechanistic accounts of "how" we can be led to consider "why" in order to produce a complete explanation of, for instance, laryngeal function in human vocalization.

The layered structure of complex systems that are often the object of mechanistic accounts allow for the interactions of the functions of different underlying mechanisms. The importance of interactions of components yielding the behavioral functions of the mechanism can be seen in Glennan's definition of a mechanism.

> A mechanism for a behavior is a complex system that produces that behavior by the interaction of a number of parts, where the interactions between parts can be characterized by direct, invariant, change-relating generalizations. (Glennan, 2002, p. 344)

These are not simply additive, such that the mechanism is an aggregation of the parts. Rather, the interactions are nonlinear and often involve cooperative or competitive interactions (Craver, 2001). Thus, mechanisms in this sense produce emergent behaviors.

Using the mechanistic perspective to explain individual differences in communication, we will discover that our way of doing research will change. We cannot assume that there will be simple and predictable ways to move from one level of explanation to another and that each level is concerned with the same thing. Individual differences may not arise from some part being essentially flawed and thus disordered. Rather, the manner in which some subsystem contributes to the variation in communication function is likely to be a feature of a complex interaction, and the "flaw" emerges out of interactions in the system. Sickle cell anemia is associated with a point mutation in the recessive β-globin gene. Although

homozygotes with this mutation are prone to abnormal deformation of the red blood cells (sickling) in situations with low oxygen, this mutation is actually beneficial to heterozygotes exposed to malaria. Thus, the functional characteristics of this mutation depend on (1) the interaction of one allele of the β-globin gene with the homologous allele and (2) whether the person is exposed to malaria. Thus, in our framework, the individual differences in red blood cell function that caused the socially disvalued state of pain and illness are emergent properties arising from system level interactions.

It would be easy at this point to conclude that complex systems defy explanation or that these explanations cannot incorporate any analytic methods or accounts, but rather they can be only global holistic descriptions of complex functions with few details. Admittedly, our explanations will be complex. It is also likely that these explanations may often be incomplete. But it is still possible to functionally decompose a complex system and develop an explanation for the emergence of complex behavior that is grounded on well understood mechanisms. Following is one example of such an explanation.

Long-Term Potentiation, BDNF and Listening Comprehension— A Case Example

A common communication function is that of listening to a passage and later recalling this information. We often describe this as a form of comprehension. In order to accomplish this task, many processes and subprocesses must occur. One of these has to do with the retention of the information that was heard. There is considerable evidence that the hippocampal learning system plays a role in this. This learning system is widely believed to contribute to declarative learning—learning facts or recalling specific events (Squire, 1992). Learning within the hippocampus has been studied extensively within the context of a particular type of neural plasticity called long-term potentiation (LTP) (Bliss & Collingridge, 1993). LTP represents a change in the efficiency of transmission between two neurons at a synaptic site as a product of simultaneous high-frequency firing of the synapse. Thus, it is an example of Hebbian learning. This change in synaptic efficiency can have short term or longer term persistence. In order for this learning to persist over hours and days structural changes must occur in the postsynaptic spine in which the spine actually enlarges. A part of this structural change in response to synaptic activity is dependent upon the actions of proteins. One of these proteins is BDNF which is coded by the *BDNF* gene. Recently, Soule and colleagues (2006) have summarized a model of BDNF action in LTP. In brief, activation of the post synaptic site results in BDNF being secreted where it then docks on both pre and postsynaptic receptors involved in the activity. Within the postsynaptic neuron, this docking triggers an activity-dependent cascade within the neuron that results in increases in another protein called ARC. ARC concentrations in the active synaptic site contribute to the production of actin proteins at the postsynaptic site, resulting in the enlargement of the postsynaptic spine, in turn resulting in consolidation of learning. Thus, secretion of BDNF plays a mechanistic role in memory consolidation. This case about BDNF so far has focused on mechanisms at the neuron (cell) and gene level. The case, however, does move to higher levels in the mechanistic hierarchy. It is well known that in the listening comprehension task described earlier, some

people perform better than others. Recent research has shown that these individual differences in comprehension are associated with allelic variation in the *BDNF* gene (Egan et al., 2003)—a genetic level characteristic. Individuals with one form of the *BDNF* gene secrete less BDNF than those with another form—a cellular characteristic. Those individuals with the BDNF variant associated with less secretion also show lower levels of comprehension than those with the form that is secreted at higher levels. Thus, secreting less BDNF has functional consequences in this cascade from the neuron, to the neural network, through cognitive processes to communication behavior. The effects are not directly upon the language behavior or on a system identified as a language system. Thus, we can't bridge the gene function to language; rather language behaviors and the individual differences therein emerge from the complex mechanistic cascade across these levels. This story about BDNF demonstrates that explanation can be accomplished within a complex system.

Implications for Future Research on Developmental Communication Disorders

This mechanistic approach to explanation of individual differences shows that the manner in which research is conducted in the field of communication disorders will need to change. We can no longer be comfortable reducing the problem to one level of the system and assuming that, in time, we can translate our findings to either higher or lower levels of the causal chain. Rather, we will need to become familiar with theories that span multiple levels of a complex system in a truly interdisciplinary fashion (e.g., Christiansen & Kirby, 2003; Mareschal et al., 2006, see p. 8). Furthermore, we cannot develop research strategies that assume we can work sequentially through these levels as though peeling an onion. Rather, ideally, we should study these systems at multiple levels in parallel. Given that research is often hampered by limited resources, this objective of full parallelism in our research is perhaps not likely. Researchers will have to choose aspects of the problem and prioritize their inquiry based on the availability of resources. This process is likely similar to an artist drawing a picture where a rough sketch of the whole system is developed and then certain local details filled in. In this regard, a researcher may pick a particular level at which the multilevel system is entered. The choice of the entry point should be grounded on good theoretical evidence that the mechanisms at that level are likely to contribute to individual differences in communication development. But another factor is the technologic advances enabling the researcher to obtain data regarding a particular mechanistic level. This latter issue certainly explains why recent advances in neural imaging and molecular genetics have become so prominent. A major constraint on our research in speech and language development is that it can be observed only in humans, thus many molecular and cellular biological techniques cannot be used. However, if we assume that language does not arise from mechanisms that are unique to humans and human language behavior, we can open up our options to the use of animal models as was exemplified by the *BDNF* research.

We also hope to have shown that explanatory accounts of developmental disorders may need to be multifaceted. The explanation of individual differences that utilize the natural sciences of genetics, cognitive neuroscience, and language science will be insufficient for a full account of developmental communication disorder. We need to recognize that an entire additional domain of explanation coming from the social sciences will be needed to understand the social mechanism involving conditions of health and illness. Most importantly, we hope we have shown that all of our research is couched in an extensive network of assumptions and logical arguments that rest on sound philosophical foundations. We can wish that it were simpler and we can try to ignore the metatheoretical context of our research, but we do so at the cost of the important insights that come from seeing the forest in which our small tree of research exists.

We began by noting that the scope of Larry Shriberg's research program was truly ambitious. His research focused on multiple sources for explanations of developmental speech disorders. In this regard, his work has anticipated the likely directions future scholars—as he is indeed a scholar—will need to travel. These new scholars will have at their service the advantages of new and more informative technologies, but they will also face the challenges of incorporating this information into explanatory narratives that respect and exploit the fundamental complexity of speech and language development and disorders.

References

Barsalou, L. W. (1990). On the indistinguishability of exemplar memory and abstraction in category representation. In T. K. Srull & R. S. Wyer (Eds.), *Advances in social cognition: Content and process specificity in the effects of prior experiences* (pp. 61–88). Hillsdale, NJ: Erlbaum.

Bechtel, W. (1994). Levels of description and explanation in cognitive science. *Minds and Machines, 4*, 1–25.

Bechtel, W., & Abrahamsen, A. (2005). Explanation: A mechanist alternative. *Studies in History and Philosophy of Biological and Biomedical Sciences, 36,* 421–441.

Bishop, D. V. M., & Edmundson, A. (1987). Language-impaired 4-year-olds—distinguishing transient from persistent impairment. *Journal of Speech and Hearing Disorders, 52,* 156–173.

Bliss, T. V., & Collingridge, G. L. (1993). A synaptic model of memory: Long-term potentiation in the hippocampus. *Nature, 361,* 31–39.

Boorse, C. (1977). Health as a theoretical concept. *Philosophical Science, 44,* 542–573.

Boorse, C. (1987). Concepts of health. In *Health care ethics: An introduction* (pp. 359–393). Philadelphia: Temple University Press.

Chater, N., & Oaksford, M. (1999). Ten years of the rational analysis of cognition. *Trends in Cognitive Sciences, 3,* 57–65.

Christiansen, M. H., & Kirby, S. (2003). Language evolution: Consensus and controversy. *Trends in Cognitive Science, 7,* 300–307.

Craver, C. F. (2001). Role functions, mechanisms, and hierarchy. *Philosophy of Science, 68,* 53–74.

Egan, M. F., Kojima, M., Callicott, J. H., Goldberg, T. E., Kolachana, B. S., Bertolino, A., et al. (2003). The BDNF val66met polymorphism affects activity-dependent secretion of BDNF and human memory and hippocampal function. *Cell, 112,* 257–269.

Erikson, K. (1962). Notes on the sociology of deviance. *Social Problems, 9,* 307–314.

Fisher, S. E. (2006). Tangled webs: Tracing the connections between genes and cognition. *Cognition, 101,* 270–297.

Gernsbacher, M. A., & Faust, M. E. (1991). The mechanism of suppression: A component of general comprehension skill. *Journal of Experimental Psychology, 17,* 245–262.

Glennan, S. (2002). Rethinking mechanistic explanation. *Philosophy of Science, 69,* S342–S353.

Grice, H. P. (1975). Logic and conversation. In P. Cole & J. Morgan (Eds.), *Syntax and semantics: Volume 3, Speech acts* (pp. 43–58). New York: Academic Press.

Hall, P. K., & Tomblin, J. B. (1978). A follow-up study of children with articulation and language disorders. *Journal of Speech and Hearing Disorders, 43,* 227–241.

Hauser, M. D., Chomsky, N., & Fitch, W. T. (2002). The faculty of language: What is it, who has it, and how did it evolve? *Science, 298,* 1569–1579.

Hull, D. (1974). *The philosophy of biological science.* Englewood Cliffs, NJ: Prentice-Hall.

Lieberman, P. (2007). The evolution of human speech: Its anatomical and neurological bases. *Current Anthropology, 48,* 39–66.

Mareschal, D., Johnson, M., Sirois, S., Spratling, M., Thomas, M., & Westermann, G. (2006). *Neuroconstructivism: How the brain constructs cognition.* Oxford: Oxford University Press.

Mayr, E. (2004). *What makes biology unique? Considerations on the autonomy of a scientific discipline.* Cambridge, UK: Cambridge University Press.

Meslevy, R. J., & Bock, R. D. (1990). *BILOG 3: Item analysis and testing scoring with binary logistic models.* Mooresville, IN: Scientific Software.

Mundale, J., & Bechtel, W. (1996). Integrating neuroscience, psychology, and evolutionary biology through a teleological conception of function. *Minds and Machines, 6,* 481–505.

Nation, J. E., & Aram, D. M. (1980). Preschool language disorders and subsequent language and academic difficulties. *Journal of Communication Disorders, 13,* 159–179.

Pearlmutter, N. J., & Macdonald, M. C. (1995). Individual differences and probabilistic constraints in syntactic ambiguity resolution. *Journal of Memory and Language, 34,* 521–542.

Pinker, S. (1994). *The language instinct.* New York: William Morrow and Company.

Salmon, W. C. (1984). *Scientific explanation and the causal structure of the world.* Princeton, NJ: Princeton University Press.

Scarr, S. (1992). Developmental theories for the 1990s—development and individual-differences. *Child Development, 63,* 1–19.

Searle, J. R. (1989). *Speech acts: An essay in the philosophy of language.* Cambridge: Cambridge University Press.

Snowling, M. J., Adams, J. W., Bishop, D. V. M., & Stothard, S. E. (2001). Educational attainments of school leavers with a preschool history of speech-language impairments. *International Journal of Language and Communication Disorders, 36,* 173–183.

Soule, J., Messaoudi, E., & Bramham, C. R. (2006). Brain-derived neurotrophic factor and control of synaptic consolidation in the adult brain. *Biochemical Society Transactions, 34,* 600–604.

Squire, L. R. (1992). Memory and the hippocampus: A synthesis from findings with rats, monkeys, and humans. *Psychology Reviews, 99,* 195–231.

Stothard, S. E., Snowling, M. J., Bishop, D. V. M., Chipchase, B. B., & Kaplan, C. A. (1998). Language-impaired preschoolers: A follow-up into adolescence. *Journal of Speech Language and Hearing Research, 41,* 407–418.

Tomasello, M. (2003). *Constructing a language: A usage-based theory of language acquisition.* Cambridge, MA: Harvard University Press.

Tomblin, J. B. (2006). A normativist account of language-based learning disability. *Learning Disabilities: Research and Practice, 21,* 8–18.

Young, A. R., Beitchman, J. H., Johnson, C., Douglas, L., Atkinson, L., Escobar, M., et al. (2002). Young adult academic outcomes in a longitudinal sample of early identified language impaired and control children. *Journal of Child Psychology and Psychiatry, 43,* 635–645.

CHAPTER 3

Genetic Influences on Speech Sound Disorders

BARBARA A. LEWIS

Introduction

In the past decade, studies on the genetics of speech and language disorders and the comorbid conditions of dyslexia, ADHD, and other learning disabilities have appeared in the behavioral literature and the molecular genetic literature, as well as the popular press. It is no longer surprising or controversial that speech and language disorders to some degree are genetically mediated. With rapid advances in technology, we have quickly moved from studies that merely documented familial aggregation for disorders, to studies searching for candidate chromosome regions where genes that may influence speech and language disorders reside, and on to the identification of candidate genes themselves. Several studies have begun to focus on the expression of these genes in the brain and have sought to trace their conservation in primates and other species. As the story of the genetics of speech and language disorders unfolds,

researchers have just begun to grasp the biological complexity of relating a gene to a behavior as complex as speech and language (see Chapter 2 for a broader discussion of this complexity). Drawing a direct connection between genes and speech and language is difficult as genes do not code for specific language skills such as syntax, phonology, semantics, or pragmatics, nor do they code for specific brain areas that subserve speech and language. Rather, they code for proteins that direct molecular processes in cells and ultimately affect brain development (Ramus, 2006). Despite the complexities of the neurogenetics of speech and language disorders and the seemingly endless combinations of genes that may give rise to a disorder, the genetics of speech and language disorders are relevant to the practice of speech and language pathology. This chapter will serve to summarize what is known about the genetics of speech and language disorders and the possibilities that uncovering genes might hold for understanding these disorders.

Why Study Genetics?

Genetic studies of speech and language disorders have both clinical applications as well as theoretical implications. One of the primary clinical applications of genetic studies is the early identification of children at risk for disorders so that intervention can begin at a young age. Communication disorders are highly prevalent in the United States with approximately 42 million people or 1 in 6 reporting some type of communication disorder. These disorders have high personal and societal costs with estimates in the U.S. ranging from $30 to $154 billion in special education, medical costs, and lost productivity annually. Data compiled by the Individuals with Disabilities Education Act (IDEA) Part B for the 2000 to 2001 school year (Agency for Healthcare Research and Quality, 2006) indicated that 1,093,808 children received services for speech or language disorders in the schools (U.S. Department of Education, 2002). More than half of these children encounter later academic difficulties in language, reading, and spelling (Aram & Hall, 1989; Bishop & Adams, 1990; Flax et al., 2003; Lewis, Freebairn, & Taylor, 2000; Shriberg & Austin, 1998) and often require other types of remedial services, with 50% to 70% exhibiting general academic difficulty through grade 12 (Gierut, 1998). Early intervention may reduce the long-term costs of speech and language disorders and reduce the number of children who experience communication difficulties and academic failure in school.

A second clinical application of the study of genetics is to validate current clinical practices and suggest new therapies. Current diagnostic categories that are largely based on behavioral observations may be validated by genetic information and new diagnostic categories may be established. Genetic subtypes of disorders may present with distinctive phenotypes and dictate a particular course of therapy (Shriberg, Flipsen, Karlsson, & McSweeny, 2001; Shriberg et al., 2005). Therapy techniques may be tailored to fit individual differences associated with genetic subtypes and the resultant underlying deficits. See also Tyler (Chapter 4) for further discussion of treatment implications and subtypes. Furthermore, understanding the genetics of a disorder may also serve to illuminate environmental contributions to the disorder that then may be modified. Finally, understanding the genetics of a disorder may suggest the cognitive overlap of co-morbid disorders such as reading, spelling, ADHD, and learning disabilities. Several studies have already suggested genetic overlap of speech sound disorders, language impairment, and reading disorders (Smith, 2007; Smith, Pennington, Boada, & Shriberg, 2005; Stein et al., 2004; Stein et al., 2006). It is likely that more genes that have general rather than specific effects (generalist genes) on speech, language, and reading skills will be identified (Plomin & Kovas, 2005). Ultimately, it is the hope that understanding the etiology of speech and language disorders will result in improved prognosis and treatment.

Genetic studies of speech and language disorders also will contribute to our theoretical understanding of speech and language disorders (Lewis et al., 2006). The molecular genetic pathology may shed light on neurobehavioral processes that underlie both typical and atypical speech and language. Identification of key genetic pathways, that is, proteins coded by genes, and the resulting metabolic structure, signaling, transcriptional regulation, or other cellular pathways, may serve to bolster our knowledge of the biological basis of speech and language. Genetics may help to pinpoint the emergence of the capacity for language in evolutionary studies (Culotta, 2005). Homologue forms of genes are found in other species that may have similar functions. For example, mouse pups with a knockout for the *FOXP2* gene (a gene associated with speech disorders) showed disruptions in ultrasonic vocalization that interfered with the communication between pup and mother (Shu et al., 2005). Genes associated with speech may have been under evolutionary selective pressure that led to the development of modern man. Bridging the gap between genetics, brain imaging, and neuropsychology will provide a comprehensive understanding of these disorders.

Challenges to Genetic Studies of SSD

There are many challenges to the genetic study of speech and language disorders. First, there is a lack of life span measures that may be used to assess family members of different ages, although as Shriberg notes in Chapter 1, some attempts are being made to develop protocols that can be used with both children and adults. Often, researchers rely on historical reports of disorders for older siblings and parents. These reports may be inaccurate or incomplete. Speech and language disorders follow a developmental trajectory. Thus, the phenotypes change with age and the genetic influences on these phenotypes may differ in early childhood, school age, adolescence, and adulthood. Statistical models are needed that can adjust for changes in the phenotype over time. Environmental correlates of speech and language disorders are not well understood; thus, parceling out genetic influences from environmental influences may be difficult. Parents with a history of a speech or language disorder may provide a deviant linguistic environment and thus both genetic and environmental influences are intertwined. Finally, there is the complexity of speech and language itself that

makes genetic studies a challenge. Numerous biochemical and physiologic processes and anatomical structures as well as numerous cognitive skills are related to speech and language. Each of these biological and cognitive processes may be under different genetic control and may be differentially heritable.

Speech Sound Disorders as a Complex Trait

Speech sound disorders (SSD), like most language-learning disorders, represent a complex trait; that is, SSD results from the aggregate contribution of an unknown number of genes interacting with each other and with the environment. No single gene is responsible for the majority of cases or deficit of any particular developmental disorder. Rather, multiple heterogeneous effects of risk genes may act alone or together to give rise to multiple profiles of skills culminating in the same diagnosis (i.e., SSD) and general impairment on the surface. The environment may work in concert with an individual's genotype to either contribute to the disorder or to protect from the disorder. These environmental effects may be unique to individuals (nonshared environment) or shared with other individuals in the environment. Furthermore, the nature and severity of the disorder might vary at different developmental stages; genes may be turned on and off during the life span. Different components of this complex phenotype may be linked to distinct genetic loci. Below we review some components (i.e., endophenotypes, measurable intermediate traits assumed to provide a closer link to the biological substrate of a disorder) of the phenotype for SSD and their relation to comorbid disorders such as language impairment (LI) or reading disorder (RD).

Phenotypes and Endophenotypes for SSD

SSD is a complex behavioral disorder characterized by speech-sound production errors associated with deficits in articulation (speech motor), phonological processes, and cognitive-linguistic skills. The behavioral phenotypes associated with SSD are not static; rather they follow a developmental trajectory. SSD is often comorbid with deficits in expressive and/or receptive language, (i.e., LI) at early childhood and later with RD at school-age. Approximately 38% to 62% of children with SSD also have LI and about 68% of children with LI also present with RD (Lewis et al., 2000). Previous research suggests that developmental problems in domains associated with speech and language acquisition place a child at risk for RD (Bird, Bishop, & Freeman, 1995; Bishop & Adams, 1990; Catts, 1993; Flax et al., 2003; Lahey, Edwards, & Munsen, 2001; Larrivee & Catts, 1999; Lewis et al., 2000; Ratiano, Pennington, Tunick, Boada, & Shriberg, 2004; Rvachew, Ohberg, Grawberg, & Heyding, 2003; Snowling, 2001).

The comorbidity of SSD, LI, and RD may be explained by common underlying neuropsychological processes (Bishop, 2001; Pennington, 2006; Stein et al., 2004). SSD, LI and RD are all associated with deficits in phonological awareness and phonological memory. RD is also associated with processing speed. Phonological memory is a correlate of LI. Several studies have suggested that deficits in speech sound production result in deficient phonological representations of sounds which in turn impact reading and spelling development (Bishop & Edmundson, 1987; Leitão & Fletcher, 2004; Pennington, 2006). Figure 3–1 depicts a model of the overlap of processes involved

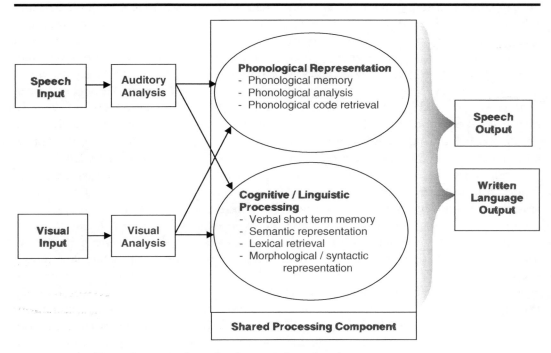

Figure 3–1. Shared processing of written and spoken language.

in spoken and written language. Although speech relies on auditory input and reading relies on visual input, both speech and reading share underlying phonological representations and cognitive linguistic processes.

This model is in agreement with Pennington's (2006) multiple cognitive deficit model of developmental disorders that argues that the comorbidity of SSD and RD arises from a shared cognitive deficit in phonological representations which interacts with other non-shared cognitive deficits to produce the symptoms that distinguish these two disorders. Distinct subtypes of SSD may be explained by a multiple deficit model. This model would predict that children with SSD without comorbid RD have a phonological deficit but compensate for it via other cognitive protective factors. Children with combined SSD and RD do not necessarily have a more severe phonological deficit, but have additional cognitive risk factors that result in RD. These cognitive deficits are, in part, genetic.

Our genetic linkage studies have supported common genetic influences, or pleiotropy, (i.e., multiple phenotypes that are influenced by one gene or locus) for SSD, LI and RD, but have also revealed evidence for disorder specific genetic influences. To identify genetic susceptibility loci for SSD, model-free sib-pair approaches to linkage were conducted on regions of chromosome 1, 3, 6, and 15. These chromosome regions have also been associated with RD. Genotyping was performed on the data from 463 sibling pairs. In our initial analysis (Stein et al., 2004) we observed that speech-sound production and phonological encoding was influenced by a locus on chromosome 3. Quantitative trait measures such as the Goldman-Fristoe Test of Articulation (GFTA; Goldman & Fristoe, 1986), Percent Consonants Correct (Shriberg, Austin, Lewis, McSweeny, & Wilson, 1997), Multisyllabic Word Repetition (Catts, 1986), Nonsense Word

Repetition (Kamhi & Catts, 1986), and the Rapid Naming of Colors (Denckla & Rudel, 1976) also linked to chromosome 3. A locus on chromosome 15 (DYX1) demonstrated linkage for speech production and oral motor skills (Stein et al., 2006). Finally, we examined a region on chromosome 1 (DYX8) that was previously linked to single word decoding and spelling (Miscimarra et al., 2007). There was some evidence on this chromosome for an association with articulation, receptive vocabulary, listening comprehension, and sentence imitation.

These findings are in agreement with a linkage study conducted by Smith et al. (2005) on 111 probands with SSD and 76 siblings. They examined linkage of SSD to loci on chromosomes 1, 6, and 15. Although linkage to chromosome 1 (1p36) did not reach significance for any of the traits, the articulation test, GFTA, approached significance. Articulation, however, did link significantly to a region on chromosome 6 (6p22). Both the articulation and nonword repetition linked significantly to a region on chromosome 15 (15p21). Although the possibility of separate genes for SSD and RD in these regions cannot be ruled out, it is more likely that RD and SSD share genes in these regions that may influence neurologic functions. Thus, component skills or endophenotypes, both unique and shared with SSD and RD, have been linked to the same chromosome regions.

Endophenotypes for SSD, RD, and LI

Skills unique to SSD include deficits in speech motor skills and speech sound planning, as well as some aspects of auditory perception and auditory discrimination. Skills potentially affecting both SSD and spoken and written language include cognitive and linguistic processes and phonological processing: the ability to form, maintain, and manipulate phonological representations. Behaviorally defined clinical phenotypes of SSD, RD, and LI are postulated to result from core cognitive deficits or endophenotypes with a specific genetic etiology (Gottesman & Gould, 2003; Inoue & Lupski, 2003). Endophenotypes are less genetically complex than a clinical disorder and are influenced by fewer environmental factors. Presumably, endophenotypes are facets of a clinical phenotype, and therefore are simpler than the clinical phenotype and more directly related to the underlying genetic basis for the disorder than the clinical phenotype. The endophenotype is hypothesized to involve fewer genes than the clinical phenotype, simplifying the genetic analysis. Yet, an endophenotype may be affected by one or more of the genes that make an individual susceptible to a disorder (Almasy & Blangero, 2001; Doyle et al., 2005; Gottesman & Gould, 2003; Skuse, 2001). Subtypes of SSD may result from various combinations of deficits impacting these endophenotypes.

Motor skills. Oral-motor skills are an example of a trait that may be influenced by both genes that make unique contributions to SSD and by genes that contribute to overall neurodevelopmental maturity. Several studies have demonstrated that children with speech and language disorders present with poorer motor skills than normally developing children (Bishop, 1990, 2002; Bishop & Edmunson, 1987; Visser, 2003). High rates of comorbidity of SSD, LI, RD, and motor incoordination suggest that slow motor performance may be an indicator of a general underlying neurodevelopmental immaturity rather than a true motor disorder (Bishop, 2002). As shown in

Table 3-1, there is some evidence that oral motor skills are heritable.

Phonological memory. Phonological memory refers to coding information phonologically for temporary storage in working or short-term memory (Gathercole & Baddeley, 1990; Torgesen, 1996). Deficits in phonological memory impair an individual's ability to learn both spoken and written new words (Bishop, Adams, & Norbury, 2006). Phonological short-term memory may be under genetic influence as suggested by family aggregation and twin studies (Torgesen, 1996) (see Table 3-1).

Phoneme awareness. Phoneme awareness is the ability to manipulate phonemes in spoken words and awareness of the sound structure of language. Deficits in phoneme awareness have been identified as one of the strongest earliest predictors of RD (Nathan, Stackhouse, Goulandris, & Snowling, 2004; Pennington & Lefly, 2001; Tunick & Pennington, 2002). Other studies have demonstrated that children with SSD both with and without additional language impairment perform more poorly than controls on phoneme awareness measures (Raitano et al., 2004). Thus, phoneme awareness is a useful endophenotype for RD as well as SSD. Phoneme awareness has been associated with several chromosome regions (see Table 3-1).

Speed of processing. Speed of processing refers to the rate at which information (either auditory or visual) is processed. Several investigators have proposed that children with LI and/or RD have a

Table 3–1. Genetic Evidence for the Core Domains and Endophenotypes of SSD

Core Domain	Component Skills	Heritability	Linkage to	References
Speech sound production	Articulation	.37–.97	1p36, 1p33-32, 3p12-q12 6p22-21, 7q31, 15q14-21	Miscimarra et al., 2007 Stein et al., 2004 Smith et al., 2005 Lai et al., 2001 Stein et al., 2006
Phonological encoding	Nonword repetition	.61	3p12-q12 6p22-21	Stein et al., 2004 Smith et al., 2005
Language	Total language	.38–.76	1p36	Miscimarra et al, 2007
	Semantics	.52	6p22-21 13q21	Grigorenko et al., 2000 Bartlett et al., 2002
	Syntax	.30–.82	16q23.1-24.1 19q13	SLI Consortium, 2004 SLI Consortium, 2004
Reading	Reading composite	.30–.72	1p34-36 3p12-13	Rabin et al., 1993 Nopola-Hemmi et al., 2001
	Decoding	.80	6p21.3 6p22.3-21.3 13q21	Cardon et al., 1994 Grigorenko et al., 1997 Bartlett et al., 2002
	Rapid naming	.44–.64	15q21 6p22.3-21.3	Grigorenko et al., 1997 Grigorenko et al., 1997
	Spelling	.21–.62	1p34-p36 6p21.3	Tzenova et al., 2004 Grigorenko et al., 2000

Endophenotypes

Core Domain	Component Skills	Heritability	Linkage to	References
Oral motor skill		.37	7q31 15q14-21	Lai et al., 2001 Stein et al., 2006
Phonological memory		.36–.71	1p34-36 3p12-13 3p12-q13 6p22-21 16q23-24	Miscimarra et al., 2007 Nopola-Hemmi et al., 2001 Stein et al., 2004 Grigorenko et al., 1997 SLI Consortium, 2004
Phonological awareness		.55–.83	1p 3p12-13 6p22-21 18p11.2	Grigorenko et al., 2000 Nopola-Hemmi et al., 2001 Grigorenko et al., 1997 Fisher et al., 2002
Speed of processing		.70	6q11-q12	Finkel et al., 2005

generalized slowing of information processing when compared to control children (Kail, 1994; Lahey et al., 2001; Miller, Kail, Leonard, & Tomblin, 2001; Tallal, Miller, Jenkins, & Merzenixh, 1997). In our previous work (Stein et al., 2004) on SSD, rapid naming of colors, a speed of processing task, demonstrated linkage to a region of chromosome 3 also associated with RD. Other studies have also demonstrated rapid naming to be heritable (see Table 3–1).

Genetic Influences on the Developmental Trajectory of SSD

These endophenotypes as well as the clinical manifestations (core symptom domains) of SSD differ with age. At early childhood, SSD may be comorbid with LI. At school age, the SSD may be persistent or recovered, with or without comorbid LI and RD. At adolescence/adulthood residual speech sound errors may be observed accompanied by LI and/or RD. Spelling difficulties (included under RD) may be present in isolation or with other comorbid conditions. A key question is whether genes play a role in the changes in traits (i.e., core symptom domains and endophenotypes) over time. To date, longitudinal genetic studies of speech and language disorders have not been conducted. Most linkage studies have been performed using data from a single time point, which cannot demonstrate genetic influences on developmental trajectories, change over time, or cohort effects (de Andrade, Gueguen, Visvikis, Sass, & Amos, 2002). Longitudinal genetic studies are needed to investigate genetic and environmental factors that influence long-term average (data averaged over several repeated measurements) and changes over time for these complex phenomena.

Furthermore, observations over time can provide more accurate information on progression of the disorder from one stage to another (such as early childhood SSD and later school-age RD). The onset of a disorder and the progression of the disorder may be triggered and/or regulated by different genes. Genes that contribute to the progression of diseases (for example, moderate SSD to mild SSD to recovery) are defined as slope genes. Slope genes influence the rate of change in the value of a trait within a subject.

Analysis of longitudinal pedigree data is complicated by the simultaneous existence of the serial correlation over time and the familial correlation within the same pedigree. In linkage methods that use data from one single time point, the correlation structure can be modeled easily because only familial correlation exists. The correlation structure in a longitudinal linkage study is much more complex than in a linkage study that examine a single time point because of the additional temporal correlation among the trait values within the same subject. Analysis methods must jointly model the serial timewise and familial correlations to estimate genetic and longitudinal effects simultaneously. Statistical methods to perform longitudinal genetic analyses are needed so that genetic effects on the developmental trajectory of SSD may be understood. Although genes that influence the developmental rate and course of SSD have not yet been identified, several candidate genes for speech, language, and reading disorders have been described.

Candidate Genes for Cognitive-Linguistic Traits

Few genetic studies have examined SSD as an outcome variable, though several genes show association with component traits that are common to SSD and RD. This is not surprising, because as described by Fisher and Francks (2006) these genes do not directly code for the ability to speak, read or acquire language, but rather for processes such as cell-to-cell communication and proliferation of cells that when disrupted lead to SSD. In the past year, four genes associated with RD have shown to effect neuronal (axonal) migration. The proteins encoded by these genes may be functionally linked. The mechanisms that relate neuronal migration to specific processes that are disrupted in RD are still unknown. However, comparable abnormalities in young rodent brains cause auditory and cognitive deficits (Galaburda, Lo Turco, Ramus, Fitch, & Rosen, 2006). These genes may result in brain changes that cause phonological processing and auditory processing abnormalities that impact RD as well as SSD. Below we review these genes with the most promising links to SSD and its component traits.

FOXP2

Studies of a large 3-generation family with a SSD, designated as the KE family, identified the gene locus for affected family members' orofacial apraxia and associated speech-language disorders to a region at 7q31 and identified the causative gene as a brain-expressed transcription factor, that is, a gene that produces proteins that regulate the translation of other genes into proteins. The gene was named *FOXP2*. Individuals who carried the mutant *FOXP2* allele presented a variety of deficits, including apraxia of speech and SSD, as well as impairments in IQ, LI, and RD (Lai, Fisher, Hurst, Vargha-Khadem, & Monaco, 2001). Findings from neuroimaging studies of the KE family suggest that the *FOXP2* gene has pleiotropic effects on multiple aspects of brain devel-

opment, accounting for the co-occurrence of SSD, LI, and RD in the family.

Several studies of individuals with SLI failed to find the *FOXP2* mutation (Newbury et al., 2002; O'Brien, Zhang, Nishimura, Tomblin, & Murray, 2003), whereas other studies identified changes or deletions in the *FOXP2* region (MacDermot et al., 2005; Zeesman et al., 2006). Although the *FOXP2* mutation has been found in only a few families and does not account for the majority of SSD, these findings confirm the existence of genes that influence SSD.

Roundabout 1 (ROBO1)

A locus on chromosome 3, DYX5 for RD susceptibility, originally identified by a Finnish group (Hannula-Jouppi et al., 2005), demonstrated pleiotropy with SSD and RD in our dataset (Stein et al., 2004). A translocation patient with RD contributed genetic material used to clone a gene from the DYX5 locus called ROBO1 (Hannula-Jouppi et al., 2005). Disruption in this gene, which guides axons to receptors, interferes with neuronal axon growth across the midline between brain hemispheres (Andrews et al., 2006).

KIAA0319 and Doublecortin 2 (DCDC2)

One of the earliest reports for dyslexia pointed to a region on chromosome 6 (Cardon et al., 1994). Since then two genes, *KIAA0319* and *DCDC2*, have been implicated in RD at this locus (Cope et al., 2005; Deffenbacher et al., 2004; Francks et al., 2004; Meng et al., 2004; Paracchini et al., 2006; Schumacher et al., 2006; Smith et al., 2005). These genes are separated by a relatively small distance on the chromosome, and there is a debate in the literature as to which gene is responsible for RD (Grigorenko et al., 2003). Experiments with mice show that both genes disrupt neuronal migration (Meng et al., 2005; Paracchini et al., 2006). *KIAA0319* has a very specific spatial-temporal expression, a disruption which leads to an impairment in neural migration necessary for the formation of the cerebral neocortex. Although the function of *DCDC2* is not known, it contains two regions seen in DCX genes, which are necessary for neuronal migration, although the action of *DCDC2* appears to be less direct. Moreover, *DCDC2* localizes to the region of the brain thought to be critical for fluent reading.

DYX1C1 (formerly known as EKN1, a locus on 15q)

DYX1C1 (DYX1 Candidate 1) was associated with dyslexia in a Finnish population (Nopola-Hemmi et al., 2000). The *DYX1C1* locus, on 15q, has been identified as a candidate gene for developmental dyslexia and has been associated with short-term verbal memory deficits (Marino et al., 2005). Most recently, the *DYX1C1* region has been linked to articulation and phonological memory (Smith et al., 2005). We also report linkage to 15q14 for oral motor skills, articulation and phonological memory (Stein et al., 2006). *DXY1C1* is expressed in many tissues including those of the cortical neurons and white matter glial cells (Taipale et al., 2003). Its protein target and functional role in the brain is unknown. However, as with *DCDC2* and *KIAA0319*, a disruption in this gene affects neural migration (Wang et al., 2006).

Genetic Influence on Neuronal Migration

The genes identified thus far are thought to influence neuronal migration. To date, specific cognitive processes are not known to

be influenced by these candidate genes. Nor is the expression of these genes restricted to areas of the brain related to phonology, speech or language (Meng et al., 2005). Neuronal migration is one of the most fundamental processes in brain development. The intricate cytoarchitecture of the brain results from the coordination of millions of neurons. Genetic mechanisms control the migration of different types of neurons; similar mechanisms are suggested regardless of their morphology, pattern of migration, and location in the brain (Marin, Valdeolmillos & Moya, 2006). Neuronal migration is a multistep process. It is initiated by a chemotactic response that leads to cell polarization and extension of the leading process, followed by somal translocation. Rearrangements in adhesive elements of the plasma membrane lead to overall movement of the neuron. The influence of genes on neural migration may affect cognitive processes or endophenotypes that underlie several developmental disorders including SSD, LI, and RD. It is important to note, however, that although neural structures may be genetically determined, neural activity maintains and shapes these structures (Ramus, 2006). Thus, although we are genetically prewired we are not genetically hard-wired and environment (including interventions) may shape the development of our neural structures and thus, our speech and language skills (Ramus, 2006). Functional imaging studies may provide a window to neural processing differences in individuals with genetic subtypes of SSD.

Functional Imaging Studies

Once candidate genes or genomic changes related to SSD have been found, the next challenge is to test them functionally, especially when the function is largely human specific. Functional magnetic imaging studies (fMRI) may identify neurologic processes that are more proximal to the genes and the related biological processes than the phenotype of SSD itself. Genes may not affect all the endophenotypes related to SSD equally; Neurobiological measures (e.g., measures of neuroanatomy, neurochemistry, or functional organization) may yield mediating levels of analysis between gene and behavioral phenotype (Pugh, 2006). MRI and fMRI studies (e.g., measures of neuroanatomy or functional organization) can inform us of the neurobiology that exists between the gene and behavioral phenotype. Sex specific effects of genes may be observed. Functional imaging studies have been shown to be of great importance in exploring mechanisms of developmental disorders such as specific language impairment, dyslexia, attention deficit disorders, and autism. Individual differences in activation patterns across subsets of brain regions may be linked to individual differences in core deficits in behavioral performance, suggesting different approaches to remediation. Imaging studies of dyslexia have demonstrated changes in neural processing of reading tasks after intervention suggesting normalizing and compensatory changes (Aylward et al., 2003; Eden et al., 2004; Shaywitz et al., 2004; Temple, Deutsch, & Poldrack, 2003). Few intervention studies have been conducted for speech and language disorders. One such study by Boberg et al. (1983) showed differences in cortical activation patterns before and after an intensive behavioral intervention for stuttering.

Functional imaging studies provide evidence that increased levels of activation, spread of activation, or recruitment of homologous areas in the right hemisphere are linked to task complexity in participants without speech, language, or reading disorders. Individuals with disorders, however, may demonstrate hypoactivation and/or less clear lateralizations than normals. A large number of studies indicate that reading disordered readers tend to underactivate both left hemisphere temporoparietal and left hemisphere ventral occipitotemporal regions (Paulesu et al., 2001). Results suggest a less functional network for individuals with these disorders (Marin et al., 2006). Overactivation of brain areas could reflect the recruitment of a compensatory circuit to counter dysfunction within the normal circuit, the use of an alternative behavioral strategy, or simply extra cognitive effort or attention. An fMRI study of children with SLI suggested a less functional network for individuals with SLI than normal controls (Weismer, Plante, Jones, & Tomblin, 2005). However, this study did not distinguish individuals with SSD from those without SSD.

To date, few fMRI studies have examined individuals with SSD. One study of young children with speech delay (ages 2–7 years) showed right hemisphere activation when the child listened to his mother's voice, whereas age-matched controls showed the expected activation in the left hemisphere (Bernal & Altman, 2003). Patients with speech delay may have difficulty transferring information from the left to right hemisphere, which could suggest a dysfunction in the corpus callosum (Fabbro, Libera, & Tavano, 2002).

Another fMRI study was conducted on members of the KE family (the family demonstrating a heritable apraxia of speech described above) employing a covert (silent) verb generation task and an overt (spoken) verb generation task (Liegeois et al., 2003). Unaffected family members showed a typical left-dominant activation of Broca's area in the generation tasks and a more bilateral distribution in the repetition tasks. Affected members showed a more posterior and more extensive bilateral activation in all tasks.

These reports are consistent with structural abnormalities reported that include low levels of gray matter density in the inferior frontal gyrus, the head of the caudate nucleus, the precentral gyrus, the temporal pole, and the cerebellum, whereas abnormally high levels of gray matter density were found in the posterior superior temporal gyrus (Wernicke's area), the angular gyrus, and the putamen (Liegeois et al., 2003). Affected members of the KE family display highly atypical brain activation when repeating words. The *FOXP2* gene may have a role in the development of a putative frontostriatal network involved in learning and/or planning and execution of speech motor sequence.

Thus, there is some evidence that genes influence neural processes that underlie speech and language skills. These effects may have a lifelong impact on the individual and influence occupational, social, and academic outcomes.

Genetic Influences on Outcomes of Individuals with SSD

To date, few studies have examined adult outcomes of early childhood SSD and no study has examined outcomes in the context of known genetic influences. In a recent workshop on the epidemiology of communication disorders, NIDCD identified a life span perspective of communication disorders as a priority for research including educational achievement, occupational performance, social participation, and quality of life (Workshop on Epidemiology of Communication Disorders, March 29–30, 2005). In early adulthood the individual experiences transitions to new activities and social roles. Data are needed on the association of early

communication disorders to problems and difficulties with this transition. Below is a review of adolescent and adult outcomes of early childhood SSD.

Occupational/Behavioral Difficulties

One of the few studies of adult outcomes of SSD by Felsenfeld, Broen, and McGue (1992) followed 24 adults with a history of SSD and 24 adults without a history of SSD who, as children, participated in the Templin Longitudinal Study designed to collect normative data on articulation skills. Results showed that adults with a history of SSD performed more poorly than adults without a history of SSD on measures of articulation, and receptive and expressive language. Furthermore, adults with a history of SSD reported that they required more remedial services throughout their academic careers and completed fewer years of formal education than adults without earlier SSD. The groups did not differ in nonverbal reasoning skills, employment status (i.e., full, part-time, or unemployed), or job satisfaction (Felsenfeld, Broen, & McGue, 1992; Felsenfeld, McGue, & Broen, 1995). However, the groups differed on their occupational classification based on the Hollingshead Four Factor Index of Social Class. Specifically, the adults with a history of SSD occupied jobs requiring fewer skills than the adults without histories of SSD. Such long-term educational, social, and economic consequences for the affected individual may result from residual difficulties in reading and spelling that persist into adulthood. However, written language skills were not assessed in the Felsenfeld study. In our study we confirmed that parents with a history of SSD had poorer outcomes than parents without a history

(Lewis et al., 2007). Another recent adult follow-up of 17 men in their mid 30's with a history of a severe language disorder in childhood revealed persistent deficits in theory of mind, verbal short-term memory, and phonological processing, together with social difficulties and an increased risk of psychiatric disorders (Clegg, Hollis, Mawhood, & Rutter, 2005). However, this study did not classify the participants according to the presence or absence of a history of SSD.

Studies of younger individuals with LI have suggested behavioral and social difficulties at school-age and early adolescence (Botting & Conti-Ramsden, 2000; Cantwell & Baker, 1987; Conti-Ramsden & Botting, 2004; Fujiki, Brinton, & Todd, 1996; Redmond & Rice, 1998). Problems with social relationships and other behavioral difficulties may persist after the language difficulties have supposedly resolved (Redmond & Rice, 1998).

Academic Difficulties

Studies that have followed children with early childhood SSD to school-age have found later academic difficulties in 50 to 75% of their samples (Aram & Hall, 1989; Bishop & Adams, 1990; King, Jones, & Laskey, 1982; Lewis et al., 2000; Shriberg & Austin, 1998). This comorbidity of reading and written language difficulties with SSD, supports the notion of generalist genes with broad cognitive influences. Our follow-up study of young children with these disorders revealed that 18% of participants with an isolated SSD had reading problems in mid-elementary school, compared with 75% of those with combined SSD and language impairment (LI) (Lewis et al., 2000). Linguistic deficits and reading and spelling problems persist for even longer periods for some children (Lewis et al., 2007).

In one of the few studies of adult outcomes of childhood speech-language impairments (Young et al., 2002) participants with LI performed significantly lower than control subjects on all areas of academic achievement, including literacy and mathematics. Furthermore, higher rates of learning disabilities were observed in the LI group than in the SSD or control groups. Despite the more pervasive deficits of the LI group, participants with histories of SSD scored lower than controls in real-word decoding indicating that individuals with SSD alone have some long-term deficits. In another follow-up study of adolescents (Weiner, 1974) children whose speech errors were characterized by nondevelopmental error processes had weaknesses in phonological awareness, reading, and spelling. We also found that individuals with isolated SSD scored poorer on spelling measures relative to their other academic skills (Lewis, O'Donnell, Freebairn, & Taylor, 1998).

Several studies have suggested that children with persistent SSD may have different outcomes than children whose problems resolve by school-age (Bishop, Price, Dale, & Plomin, 2003). Children whose problems had resolved by 5½ years performed less well on tests of phonological processing and literacy skills. Furthermore, evidence for differences in etiology between persistent and nonpersistent SSD is provided by Bishop et al. (2003) who showed that heritability of LI was higher for children with persistent LI than for those with language delays that normalized during early childhood. However, Bishop et al. (2003) did not examine persistent SSD independent of LI. Few studies considered SSD apart from LI and most studies did not follow participants into adulthood nor did they assess the functional significance of early SSD at adulthood. Studies did not assess multiple symptom dimensions at each time point. Finally, no study to date has examined outcomes based on genetic influences and, thus, the groups examined mostly likely were heterogeneous in their etiology.

Summary and Future Directions

In summary, some SSDs are under genetic influences that are most likely polygenic, that is, under the control of many genes that work in concert and form genetic networks. These genes may affect underlying endophenotypes or cognitive processes that have broad influences on speech, language, and reading skills. Genes identified to date have been shown to influence neural migration and development and are likely to have broad rather than narrow effects on speech and language skills. Finally, genes are turned on and off during the individual's life span and thus impact the developmental trajectory of the individual affecting both the rate and outcome of skills. The effects of a SSD may be lifelong resulting in poorer occupational, social, and academic outcomes than those for individuals without SSD. Early identification and treatment is needed to minimize the impact of these disorders. In the future, an individual's genetic makeup may, in part, direct the course of therapy and inform the prognosis for improvement. Tools such as fMRI may be used to chart the course of therapy. A clear understanding of the genetic influences on neurologic processing and the resulting behavioral phenotypes will allow educators and therapists to identify at risk children early, to make more accurate prognoses, and to tailor treatments to address the individual's underlying cognitive/linguistic deficits. Ultimately, such research may lead to prevention of SSD and related reading impairments.

References

Agency for Healthcare Research and Quality, U.S. Department of Health and Human Services. (2006). *Criteria for determining disability in speech-language disorders. Evidence Report/Technology Assessment.*

Almasy, L., & Blangero, J. (2001). Endophenotypes as quantitative risk factors for psychiatric disease: Rationale and study design. *American Journal of Medical Genetics, 105,* 42–44.

Andrews, W., Liapi, A., Plachez, C., Camurri, L., Zhang, J., Mori, S., et al. (2006). Robo1 regulates the development of major axon tracts and interneuron migration in the forebrain. *Development, 133*(11), 2243–2252.

Aram, D. M., & Hall, N. C. (1989). Longitudinal follow-up of children with preschool communication disorders: Treatment implications. *School Psychology Review, 18,* 487–501.

Aylward, E. H., Richards, T. L., Berninger, V. W., Nagy, W. E., Field, K. M., Grimme, A. L., et al. (2003). Instructional treatment associated with changes in brain activation in children with dyslexia. *Neurology, 61,* 212–219.

Barlett, C. W., Flax, J. F., Logue, M. W., Vieland, V. J., Bassett, A. S., Tallal, P., et al. (2002). A major susceptibility locus for specific language impairment is located on 13q21. *American Journal of Human Genetics, 71,* 45–55.

Bernal, B., & Altman, N. R. (2003). Speech delay in children: A functional MR imaging study. *Radiology, 229*(3), 651–658.

Bird, J., Bishop, D., & Freeman, N. (1995). Phonological awareness and literacy development in children with expressive phonological impairments. *Journal of Speech and Hearing Research, 38,* 446–462.

Bishop, D. V. (1990). Handedness, clumsiness and developmental language disorders. *Neuropsychologia, 28*(7), 681–690.

Bishop, D. V. (2001). Genetic influences on language impairment and literacy problems in children: Same or different? *Journal of Child Psychology and Psychiatry, 42* (2), 189–198.

Bishop, D. V. (2002). Motor immaturity and specific speech and language impairment: Evidence for a common genetic basis. *American Journal of Medical Genetics*, *114*(1), 56–63.

Bishop, D. V. & Adams, C. (1990). A prospective study of the relationship between specific language impairment, phonological disorders and reading retardation. *Journal of Child Psychology and Psychiatry*, *31*, 1027–1050.

Bishop, D. V., Adams, C. V., & Norbury, C. F. (2006). Distinct genetic influences on grammar and phonological short-term memory deficits: Evidence from 6-year-old twins. *Genes, Brain, and Behavior*, *5*(2),158–169.

Bishop, D. V., & Edmundson, A. (1987). Specific language impairment as a maturational lag: Evidence from longitudinal data on language and motor development. *Developmental Medicine and Child Neurology*, *29*(4), 442–459.

Bishop, D. V., Price, T. S., Dale, P. S., & Plomin, R. (2003). Outcomes of early language delay: II. Etiology of transient and persistent language difficulties. *Journal of Speech, Language, and Hearing Research*, *46*, 561–575.

Boberg, E., Yeudall, L. T., Schopflocher, D., & Bo-Lassen, P. (1983). The effect of an intensive behavioral program on the distribution of EEG alpha power in stutterers during the processing of verbal and visuospatial information. *Journal of Fluency Disorders*, *3*, 245–263.

Botting, N., & Conti-Ramsden, G. (2000). Social and behavioral difficulties in children with SLI. *Child Language Teaching and Therapy*, *16*(2), 105–120.

Cantwell, D. P., & Baker, L. (1987). Clinical significance of childhood communication disorders: Perspectives from a longitudinal study. *Journal of Child Neurology*, *2*(4), 257–264.

Cardon, L. R., Smith, S. D., Fulker, D. W., Kimberling, W. J., Pennington, B. F., DeFries, J. C. (1994). Quantitative trait locus for reading disability on chromosome 6. *Science*, *266*, 276–279.

Catts, H. W. (1986). Speech production/phonological deficits in reading-disordered children. *Journal of Learning Disabilities*, *19*, 504–508.

Catts, H. (1993). The relationship between speech-language impairment and reading disabilities. *Journal of Speech and Hearing Research*, *36*, 948–958.

Clegg, J., Hollis, C., Mawhood, L., & Rutter, M. (2005). Developmental language disorders—a follow-up in later adult life: Cognitive, language, and psychosocial outcomes. *Journal of Child Psychology and Psychiatry*, *46*(2), 128–149.

Conti-Ramsden, G., & Botting, N. (2004). Social difficulties and victimization in children with SLI at 11 years of age. *Journal of Speech, Language, and Hearing Research*, *47*, 145–161.

Cope, N., Harold, D., Hill, G., Moskvina, V., Stevenson, J., Holmans, P., et al. (2005). Strong evidence that KIAA0319 on chromosome 6p is a susceptibility gene for developmental dyslexia. *American Journal of Human Genetics*, *76*(4), 581–591.

Culotta, E. (2005). What genetic changes made us uniquely human? *Science*, *309*, 91.

de Andrade, M., Gueguen, R., Visvikis, S., Sass, G., & Amos, C. I. (2002). Extension of variance components approach to incorporate temporal trends and longitudinal pedigree data analysis. *Genetic Epidemiology*, *22*, 221–232.

Deffenbacher, K. E., Kenyon, J. B., Hoover, D. M., Olson, R. K., Pennington, B. F., DeFries, J. C., et al. (2004). Refinement of the 6p21.3 quantitative trait locus influencing dyslexia: Linkage and association analysis. *Human Genetics*, *115*, 128–138.

Denckla, M. B., & Rudel, R. G. (1976). Naming of object-drawings by dyslexic and other learning disabled children. *Brain and Language*, *3*, 1–15.

Doyle, A., Faraone, S. V., Seidman, L. J., Willcutt, E. G., Nigg, J., Waldman, I. D., et al. (2005). Are endophenotypes based on measures of executive functions useful for molecular genetic studies of ADHD. *Journal of Child Psychology and Psychiatry*, *46*, 774–803.

Eden, G. F., Jones, K. M., Cappell, K., Gareau, L., Wood, F., Zeffiro, T., et al., (2004). Neural changes following remediation in adult developmental dyslexia. *Neuron*, *44*, 411–422.

Fabbro, F., Libera, L., & Tavano, A. (2002). A callosal transfer deficit in children with developmental language disorder. *Neuropsychologia*, *40*(9), 1541–1546.

Felsenfeld, S., Broen, P. A., & McGue, M. (1992). A 28-year follow-up of adults with a history of a moderate phonological disorder: Linguistic and personality results. *Journal of Speech and Hearing Research, 35,* 1114-1125.

Felsenfeld, S., McGue, M., & Broen, P. A. (1995). Familial aggregation of phonological disorders: Results from a 28 year follow-up. *Journal of Speech and Hearing Research, 38,* 1091-1107.

Finkel, D., Reynolds, C. A., McArdle, J. J., Pedersen, N. L. (2005). The longitudinal relationship between processing speed and cognitive ability: Genetic and environmental influences. *Behavior Genetics, 35*(5), 535-549.

Fisher, S. E., & DeFries, J. C. (2002). Developmental dyslexia: Genetic dissection of a complex cognitive trait. *Nature Review Neuroscience, 3,* 767-780.

Fisher, S. E., & Francks, C. (2006). Genes, cognition and dyslexia: Learning to read the genome. *Trends in Cognitive Science, 10*(6), 250-257.

Flax, J. F., Realpe-Bonilla, T., Hirsch, L. S., Brzustowicz, L. M., Bartlett, C. W., Tallal, P. (2003). Specific language impairment in families: Evidence for co-occurrence with reading impairments. *Journal of Speech, Language, and Hearing Research 46,* 530-543.

Francks, C., Paracchini, S., Smith, S. D., Richardson, A. J., Scerri, T. S., Cardon, L. R., et al. (2004). A 77-kilobase region of chromosome 6p22.2 is associated with dyslexia in families from the United Kingdom and from the United States. *American Journal of Human Genetics, 75*(6), 1046-1058.

Fujiki, M., Brinton, B., & Todd, C. (1996). Social skills of children with specific language impairment. *Language, Speech, and Hearing in the Schools, 25,* 195-202.

Galaburda, A. M., LoTurco, J., Ramus, F., Fitch, R. H., & Rosen, G. D. (2006). From genes to behavior in developmental dyslexia. *Nature Neuroscience, 9*(10), 1213-1217.

Gathercole, S. E., & Baddeley, A. D. (1990). Phonological memory deficits in language disordered children. Is there a casual connection? *Journal of Memory and Language, 29,* 349-367.

Gierut, J. A. (1998). Treatment efficacy: Functional phonological disorders in children. *Journal of Speech Language and Hearing Research, 41,* S85-S100.

Goldman, R., & Fristoe, M. (1986). *The Goldman-Fristoe Test of Articulation (GFTA).* Circle Pines, MN: American Guidance Services.

Gottesman, I. I., & Gould, T. D. (2003). The endophenotype concept in psychiatry: Etymology and strategic intentions. *American Journal of Psychiatry, 160*(4), 636-645.

Grigorenko, E. L., Wood, F. B., Meyer, M. S., Hart, L. A., Speed, W. C., Shuster, A., et al. (1997). Susceptibility locus for distinct components of developmental dyslexia on chromosomes 6 and 15. *American Journal of Human Genetics, 60,* 27-39.

Grigorenko, E. L., Wood, F. B., Golovyan, L., Meyer, M., Romano, C., & Pauls, D. (2003). Continuing the search for dyslexia genes on 6p. *American Journal of Medical Genetics B: Neuropsychiatric Genetics, 118,* 89-98.

Grigorenko, E. L., Wood, F. B., Meyer, M. S., & Pauls, D. L. (2000). Chromosome 6 p influences different dyslexia cognitive related processes. *American Journal of Human Genetics, 66,* 715-723.

Hannula-Jouppi, K., Kaminen-Ahola, N., Taipale, M., Eklund, R., Nopola-Hemmi, J., Kaariainen, H., et al. (2005). The axon guidance receptor gene ROBO1 is a candidate gene for developmental dyslexia. *PLoS Genetics, 1*(4), e50.

Inoue, K., & Lupski, J. R. (2003). Genetics and genomics of behavioral and psychiatric disorders. *Current Opinions of Genetic Development, 13*(3), 303-309.

Kail, R. (1994). A method for studying the generalized slowing hypothesis in children with specific language impairment. *Journal of Speech and Hearing Research, 37*(2), 418-421.

Kamhi, A. G., & Catts, H. W. (1986). Toward an understanding of developmental language and reading disorders. *Journal of Speech and Hearing Disorders, 51,* 337-347.

King, R. R., Jones, C., & Laskey, E. (1982). In retrospect: A fifteen-year follow-up report of speech-language disordered children. *Language, Speech and Hearing Services in the Schools, 13,* 24-32.

Lahey, M., Edwards, J., & Munson, B. (2001). Is processing speed related to severity of language impairment? *Journal of Speech and Hearing Research, 44,* 1354-1361.

Lai, C. S., Fisher, S. E., Hurst, J. A., Vargha-Khadem, F., & Monaco, A. P. (2001). A forkhead-domain gene is mutated in a severe speech and language disorder. *Nature, 413*(6855), 519–523.

Larrivee, L. S., & Catts, H. W. (1999). Early reading achievement in children with expressive phonological disorders. *American Journal of Speech-Language Pathology, 8*, 118–128.

Leitão, S., & Fletcher, J. (2004). Literacy outcomes for students with speech impairment: long-term follow-up. *International Journal of Language and Communication Disorders, 39*(2), 245–256.

Lewis, B. A., Freebairn, L. A., Hansen, A. J., Miscimarra, L., Iyengar, S. K., & Taylor, H. G. (2007). Speech and language skills of parents of children with speech-sound disorders. *American Journal of Speech-Language Pathology, 16*, 108–118.

Lewis, B. A., Freebairn, L. A., & Taylor, H. G. (2000). Academic outcomes in children with histories of speech sound disorders. *Journal of Communication Disorders, 33*, 11–30.

Lewis, B. A., O'Donnell, B., Freebairn, L. A., & Taylor, H. G. (1998). Spoken language and written expression- interplay of delays. *American Journal of Speech-Language Pathology, 7*, 77–84.

Lewis, B. A., Shriberg, L. D., Freebairn, L. A., Hansen, A. J., Stein, C. M., Taylor, H. G., & Iyengar, S. K. (2006). The genetic bases of speech sound disorders: Evidence from spoken and written language. *Journal of Speech, Language and Hearing Research, 49*, 1294–1312.

Liegeois, F., Baldeweg, T., Connelly, A., Gadian, D. G., Mishkin, M., & Vargha-Khadem, F. (2003). Language fMRI abnormalities associated with FOXP2 gene mutation. *Nature Neuroscience, 6*(11), 1230–1237.

MacDermot, K. D., Bonora, E., Sykes, N., Coupe, A. M., Lai, C. S., Vernes, S. C., et al. (2005). Identification of FOXP2 truncation as a novel cause of developmental speech and language deficits. *American Journal of Human Genetics, 76*, 1074–1080.

Marin, O., Valdeolmillos, M., & Moya, F. (2006). Neurons in motion: Same principles for different shapes? *Trends in Neuroscience, 29*, 655–661.

Marino, C., Giorda, R., Luisa Lorusso, M., Vanzin, L., Salandi, N., Nobile, M., et al. (2005). A family-based association study does not support DYX1C1 on 15q21.3 as a candidate gene in developmental dyslexia. *European Journal of Human Genetics, 13*, 491–499.

Meng, H., Smith, S. D., Hager, K., Held, M., Lui, J., Olson R. K., et al. (2005). DCDC2 is associated with reading disability and modulates neuronal development in the brain. *Proceedings of the National Academy of Science of the United States of America, 102*, 17053–17058.

Miller, C. A., Kail, R., Leonard, L. B., & Tomblin, J. B. (2001). Speed of processing in children with specific language impairment. *Journal of Speech, Language, and Hearing Research, 44*, 416–433.

Miscimarra, L., Stein, C., Millard, C., Kluge, A., Cartier, K., Freebairn, L., et al. (2007). Further evidence of pleiotropy influencing speech and language: Analysis of the DYX8 region. *Human Heredity, 63*, 47–58.

Nathan, L., Stackhouse, J., Goulandris, N., & Snowling, M. J. (2004). The development of early literacy skills among children with speech difficulties: A test of the "critical age hypothesis." *Journal of Speech, Language and Hearing Research, 47*(2), 377–391.

Newbury, D. F., Bonora, E., Lamb, J. A., Fisher, S. E., Lai, C. S., Baird, G., et al. (2002). FOXP2 is not a major susceptibility gene for autism or specific language impairment. *American Journal of Human Genetics, 70*, 1318–1327.

Nopola-Hemmi, J., Myllyluoma, B., Haltia, T., Taipale, M., Ollikainene, V., Ahonen T., et al. (2001). A dominent gene for developmental dyslexia on chromosome 3. *Journal of Medical Genetics, 38*, 658–664.

Nopola-Hemmi, J., Taipale, M., Haltia, T., Lehesjoki, A. E., Voutilainen, A., Kere, J. (2000). Two translocations of chromosome 15q associated with dyslexia. *Journal of Medical Genetics, 37*, 771–775.

O'Brien, E. K., Zhang, X., Nishimura, C., Tomblin, J. B., & Murray, J. C. (2003). Association of specific language impairment (SLI) to the region of 7q31. *American Journal of Human Genetics, 72*, 1536–1543.

Paracchini, S., Thomas, A., Castro, S., Lai, C., Paramasivam, M., Wang, Y., et al. (2006). The chromosome 6p22 haplotype associated with dyslexia reduces the expression of KIAA0319, a novel gene involved in neuronal migration. *Human Molecular Genetics*, *15*(10), 1659–1666.

Paulesu, E., Demonet, J. F., Fazio, F., McCrory, E., Chanoine, V., Brunswick, N., et al. (2001). Dyslexia: Cultural diversity and biological unity. *Science*, *291*, 2165–2167.

Pennington, B. F. (2006). From single to multiple deficit models of developmental disorders. *Cognition*, *101*, 385–413.

Pennington, B. F., & Lefly, D. L. (2001). Early reading development in children at family risk for dyslexia. *Child Development*, *72*, 816–833.

Plomin, R., & Kovas, Y. (2005). Generalist genes and learning disabilities. *Psychological Bulletin*, *131*, 392–617.

Pugh, K. (2006). A neurocognitive overview of reading acquisition and dyslexia across languages. *Developmental Science*, *9*(5), 448–450.

Rabin, M., Wen, X. L., Hepburn, M., Lubs, H. A., Feldman, E., & Duara, R. (1993). Suggestive linkage of developmental dyslexia to chromosome 1p34-p36. *Lancet*, *342*, 178.

Raitano, N. A., Pennington, B. F., Tunick, R. A., Boada, R., & Shriberg, L. D. (2004). Pre-literacy skills of subgroups of children with speech sound disorders. *Journal of Child Psychology and Psychiatry*, *45*(4), 821–835.

Ramus, F. (2006). Genes, brain, and cognition: A roadmap for the cognitive scientist. *Cognition*, *101*, 247–269.

Redmond, S., & Rice, M. (1998). The socioemotional behaviors of children with SLI: Social adaptation or social deviance? *Journal of Speech, Language, and Hearing Research*, *41*, 688–700.

Rvachew, S., Ohberg, A., Grawburg, M., & Heyding, J. (2003). Phonological awareness and phoneme perception in 4-year old children with delayed expressive phonology skills. *American Journal of Speech-Language Pathology*, *12*, 463–471.

Schumacher, J., Anthoni, H., Dahdouh, F., Konig, I. R., Hillman, A. M., Kluck, N., et al. (2006). Strong genetic evidence of DCDC2 as a susceptibility gene for dyslexia. *American Journal of Human Genetics*, *78*(1), 52–62.

Shaywitz, B. A., Shaywitz, S. E., Blachman, B., Pugh, K. R., Fullbright, R. K., Skudlarski, P. et al. (2004). Development of left occipito-temporal systems for skilled reading in children after a phonologically-based intervention. *Biological Psychiatry*, *55*, 926–933.

Shriberg, L. D., & Austin, D. (1998). Comorbidity of speech-language disorder: Implications for a phenotype marker for speech delay. In R. Paul (Ed.), *The speech-language connection* (pp. 73–117). Baltimore: Paul H Brookes.

Shriberg, L. D., Austin, D., Lewis, B. A., McSweeny, J. L., & Wilson, D. L. (1997). The percentage of consonants correct (PCC) metric: Extensions and reliability data. *Journal of Speech, Language, and Hearing Research*, *40*, 708–722.

Shriberg, L. D., Flipsen, P. J., Jr., Karlsson, H. B., & McSweeny, J. L. (2001). Acoustic phenotypes for speech-genetics studies: An acoustic marker for residual /er/ distortions. *Clinical Linguistics and Phonetics*, *15*, 631–650.

Shriberg, L. D., Lewis, B. A., Tomblin, J. B., McSweeny, J. L., Karisson, H. B., & Sheer, A. R. (2005). Toward diagnostic and phenotype markers for genetically transmitted speech delay. *Journal of Speech, Language, and Hearing Research*, *48*, 834–852.

Shu, W., Cho, J. Y., Jiang, Y., Zhang, M., Weisz, D., Elder, G. A., et al. (2005). Altered ultrasonic vocalization in mice with a disruption in the Foxp2 gene. *Proceedings of the National Academy of Sciences of the USA*, *102*(27), 9643–9648.

Skuse, D. H. (2001). Endophenotypes and child psychiatry. *British Journal of Psychiatry: The Journal of Mental Science*, *178*, 395–396.

Smith, S. D. (2007). Genes, language development, and language disorders. *Mental Retardation and Developmental Disabilities Research Reviews*, *13*, 96–105.

Smith, S. D., Pennington, B. F., Boada, R., & Shriberg, L. D. (2005). Linkage of speech sound disorder to reading disability loci. *Journal of Child Psychology and Psychiatry*, *46*, 1057–1066.

Snowling, M. J. (2001). From language to reading and dyslexia. *Dyslexia*, 7, 37–46.

Stein, C. M., Millard, C., Kluge, A., Miscimarra, L. E., Cartier, K. C., Freebairn, L. A., et al. (2006). Speech sound disorder influenced by a locus in 15q14 region. *Behavior Genetics*, 36, 858–868.

Stein, C. M., Schick, J. H., Taylor, H. G., Shriberg, L. D., Millard, C., Kundtz-Kluge, A., et al. (2004). Pleiotropic effects of a chromosome 3 locus on speech sound disorder and reading. *American Journal of Human Genetics*, 74, 283–297.

Taipale, M., Kaminen, N., Nopola-Hemmi, J., Haltia, T., Myllyluoma, B., Lyytinen, H., et al. (2003). A candidate gene for developmental dyslexia encodes a nuclear tetratricopeptide repeat domain protein dynamically regulated in brain. *Proceedings of the National Academy of Science USA*, 100, 11553–11558.

Tallal, P., Miller, S. L., Jenkins, W. M., & Merzenixh, M. M. (1997). The role of processing developmental language-based learning disorders: Research and clinical implications. In B. A. Blachman (Ed.), *Foundations of reading acquisition and dyslexia: Implications for early interventions* (pp. 49–66). Mahwah, NJ: Lawrence Erlbaum Associates.

Temple, E., Deutsch, G. K., & Poldrack, R. A. (2003). Neural deficits in children with dyslexia ameliorated by behavioral remediation: Evidence from functional MRI. *Proceedings of the National Academy of Sciences*, 100, 2860–2865.

The SLI Consortium. (2004). Highly significant linkage to SLI locus in an expanded sample of individuals affected by specific language impairment. *American Journal of Human Genetics*, 74, 1225–1238.

Torgesen, J. K. (1996). A model memory from an information processing perspective: The special case of phonological memory. In G. R. Lyon & N. A. Krasnegor (Eds.), *Attention, memory and executive function* (pp. 157–184). Baltimore: Brookes.

Tunick, R. A., & Pennington, B. F. (2002). The etiological relationship between reading disability and phonological disorder. *Annals of Dyslexia*, 52, 117–124.

Tzenova, J., Kaplan, B. J., Petryshen, T. L., & Fields, L. L. (2004). Confirmation of a dyslexia susceptibility locus on chromosome 1p34-p36 in a set of 100 Canadian families. *American Journal of Medical Genetics, Part B*, 127B, 117–124.

U.S. Department of Education. (2002). *To assure the free appropriate public education of all Americans: Twenty-fourth annual report to Congress on the implementation of the Individuals with Disabilities Education Act.*

Visser, J. (2003). Developmental coordination disorder: A review of research on subtypes and comorbidities. *Human Movement Science*, 22(4–5), 479–493.

Wang, Y., Paramasivam, M., Thomas, A., Bai, J., Kaminen-Ahola, N., Kere, J., et al. (2006). DYX1C1 functions in neuronal migration in developing cortex. *Neuroscience*, 143, 515–522.

Weiner, P. S. (1974). A language-delayed child at adolescence. *Journal of Speech and Hearing Disorders*, 39, 202–212.

Weismer, S. E., Plante, E., Jones, M., & Tomblin, J. B. (2005). A functional magnetic resonance imaging investigation of verbal working memory in adolescents with specific language impairment. *Journal of Speech, Language, and Hearing Research*, 48, 405–425.

Workshop on Epidemiology of Communication Disorders [NIDCD Funding for Research]. (2005). 3-29-0005.

Young, A. R., Beitchman, J. H., Johnson, C., Douglas, L., Atkinson, L., Escobar, M., et al. (2002). Young adult academic outcomes in a longitudinal sample of early identified language impaired and control children. *Journal of Child Psychology and Psychiatry*, 43(5), 635–645.

Zeesman, S., Nowaczyk, M. J., Teshima, I., Roberts, W., Cardy, J. O., Brian, J., et al. (2006). Speech and language impairment and oromotor dyspraxia due to deletion of 7q31 that involves FOXP2. *American Journal of Medical Genetics*, 140, 509–514.

CHAPTER 4

Subgroups, Comorbidity, and Treatment Implications

ANN A. TYLER

Results of genetic studies of speech sound disorder, language impairment, and reading disorders suggest that etiologic subgroups of speech only, language only, reading only, or comorbid deficits among these domains may correspond to unique or shared genetic traits. (See also Chapters 1 and 3) Reported rates of comorbidity between speech sound disorder and language impairment range from 40 to 60% for preschool children. This group is also most likely to later display a comorbid reading disability. Evidence increasingly suggests that early interventions should target multiple skill areas, particularly in subgroups with more diverse impairments. Yet intervention research has just begun to compare interventions for their success in stimulating multiple skills, including phonological awareness, in subgroups. This chapter focuses on evaluating interventions for their effectiveness in producing gains in a wide range of skills including; phoneme awareness, speech production, grammatical performance, and early reading performance.

The timing and intensity of such interventions are discussed with respect to the presenting profile of deficits and strengths. Factors such as severity or temperament that influence variability in response to treatment are presented.

The classification of types or subgroups of speech sound disorder (SSD) has been of interest in the last decade as the heterogeneity in this population is increasingly recognized. Not surprisingly, the search for subtypes that potentially are associated with unique phenotypes (physical or behavioral traits) intensifies as we acknowledge the genetic bases of speech and language disorders and enter the Postgenomic Era. Shriberg's focus on etiology and genetic factors in childhood SSDs is at the forefront of this quest. Shriberg (2004; Chapter 1) has not minimized the clinical necessity of accurate differential diagnosis, but rather suggests that such diagnosis is key to evidence-based practice and drives the search for validated diagnostic markers for disorder subtypes.

With the ultimate goal being prevention of childhood speech sound disorders, and a long-term goal being the provision of treatment that is optimally designed for a specific subtype, Shriberg views the identification of cause (etiology) as a critical step in differential diagnosis. Whether the underlying difficulty of SSD is viewed as one of phonetics or phonemics, articulatory versus organizational (cognitive-linguistic), or motor versus perceptual there has been an implied search for etiology for many decades.

Yet, a classification system based on etiology and the medical model is just one of three commonly proposed classificatory systems applied to speech sound disorders. A second type of system is based on physiologic data or on psycholinguistic processing and the search for levels of breakdown in the processing chain (Stackhouse & Wells, 1997). In this type of system, performance on specific tasks is proposed to explain specific deficits according to the processing requirements of the task. A third classification system is one that is symptomatic in nature, although it may allude to linguistic theory (e.g., phonological processes). Such a system must rely on behavioral measures that may or may not prove valid in operationalizing underlying processes. The latter two systems focus more squarely on symptoms and proximal causes of possible subtypes of speech sound disorder. Major examples of these different types of classification systems are reviewed beginning with Shriberg's framework for seven subtypes of SSD. Within this framework there are two broad categories of undifferentiated SSDs, speech delay and speech errors; speech delay is characterized by speech sound deletions, substitutions, and distortions and risk for literacy deficits, whereas speech errors are characterized by sound distortions only and no risk for literacy deficits. The speech delay category is further subdi-

vided into five possible subtypes with different proposed processes affected, and as yet unidentified phenotype markers: Speech Delay—Genetic; Speech Delay—Otitis Media with Effusion; Speech Delay—Developmental Psychosocial Involvement; Speech Delay—Apraxia of Speech; and Speech Delay—Dysarthria. The etiologic origins are proposed to be an interaction between many genes and the environment for the first three subtypes listed above, and single or a few genes for the two speech motor involvement subtypes. The speech error category is divided into Speech Errors—Sibilants and Speech Errors—Rhotics with suggested environmental origins.

In contrast to an etiologic based classification system, Dodd's (1995) frequently cited classification system relies on speech symptomatology and is based in psycholinguistic theory. The nature of phonological processes or error patterns, along with the child's consistency in producing three repetitions of 25 single and multisyllabic words are considered in assigning children to four different subtypes. One subtype is termed Phonological Delay and is characterized by the presence of a set of phonological error patterns that are typical during normal development and thus, observed in children of a younger chronologic age. A second subtype, termed Consistent Deviant Phonological Disorder, is differentiated by the child's use of unusual phonological processes alongside those seen during typical development, as well as less than 40% variability on the 25-word repetition task. The 40% criterion is established by different productions across two or more of the three repetitions for 10 or more of the 25 words. A third subtype, the Inconsistent Deviant Phonological Disorder group is differentiated from the Consistent group by its 40% or greater variability on the word repetition task and the presence of both unusual and typical, developmental processes. The final subtype is termed Articulation Disorder and is characterized by perceptually incorrect productions of selected phones, such as /s/ or /r/. There is an additional category for Developmental Verbal Dyspraxia (childhood apraxia of speech or CAS), although certain speech characteristics of this group may overlap those of the inconsistent group. Dodd (1995) outlines several specific differentiating symptoms for the apraxia group.

In an examination of a clinical sample of 1,100 referrals to a pediatric speech and language service in the United Kingdom, Broomfield and Dodd (2004) found that of the 320 with "primary" speech disability, 57.5% displayed phonological delay, 20.6% had consistent deviant phonological disorder, 9.4% had inconsistent deviant phonological disorder, and 12.5% had articulation disorder. There is, however, no evidence regarding the diagnostic accuracy, sensitivity, and specificity of Dodd's system in differentiating subtypes.

Shriberg's research has focused on the identification of diagnostic markers that have sufficient predictive values, sensitivity and specificity, and diagnostic accuracy to differentiate subtypes in the SSD framework. To this end, he and his colleagues have proposed unique markers based on perceptual and acoustic analysis of manifest speech for the majority of subtypes (Hauner, Shriberg, Kwiatkowski, & Allen, 2005; Karlsson, Shriberg, Flipsen, & McSweeny, 2002; Shriberg, Campbell, Karlsson, Brown, McSweeny, & Nadler, 2003; Shriberg, Flipsen, Kwiatkowski, & McSweeny, 2003; Shriberg, Green, Campbell, McSweeny, & Scheer, 2003; Shriberg, Kent, Karlsson, McSweeny, Nadler, & Brown, 2003). Although Shriberg's framework is causally based, clearly identifiable and mutually exclusive etiologies are not yet apparent. Thus, there appears to be overlap in the subtypes and the possibility that a particular

case can belong to more than one subtype. For example, a child with a positive family history may also have a profile that is positive for otitis media with effusion. Further, the speech delay—genetic subgroup may be a misnomer as Shriberg, Lewis, Tomblin, McSweeny, Karlsson, and Scheer (2005) clearly acknowledge that there are genetic contributions to each of the proposed subtypes. Similarly, examination of pre- and perinatal, audiologic, and family history risk factors did not differentiate specific factors for Dodd's different subgroups of SSD. The extent of overlap among risk factors in clinical cases, or lack thereof, may make it difficult to clearly identify a subgroup according to etiologic factors (Fox, Dodd, & Howard, 2002).

Genetic studies eventually may validate proposed subtypes or conversely reveal new diagnostic subtypes. Lewis et al. (2006) suggest that many genes contribute to SSD, some of which affect SSD uniquely, and others which share an influence on spoken and written language. Lewis et al. propose a conceptual framework for considering genetic influences on SSD that may affect unique or shared traits. That is, genetic influences may affect skills unique to SSD, such as motor planning, skills that are shared by both SSD and language, such as phonological working memory, as well as skills that are both unique and shared. Multiple subtypes of SSD might follow from such a framework and show a variety of overlaps with deficits in written and spoken language, that is, reading disability and language impairments. Results of genetic studies of SSD, language impairment, and reading disorders suggest that clinical subgroups of speech only, language only, reading only or comorbid deficits among these domains may correspond to unique or shared genetic traits. It may be particularly useful from a treatment perspective to consider such single or comorbid deficit subgroups.

Comorbidity

Although the two aforementioned classification systems delineate subtypes based
on suspected etiology and surface speech
error patterns, they do not directly address
observations of comorbid deficits. Reported
rates of comorbidity between speech sound
disorder and language impairment range
from 40 to 60% for preschool children.

Further inspection of Shriberg and
Dodd's research samples, however, shows
that several of their proposed subtypes have
reported evidence of comorbid expressive
or expressive and receptive language deficits
(Broomfield & Dodd, 2004; Shriberg, 2007;
Shriberg & Austin, 1998).

Comorbid Language Deficits

In an investigation of children (age $M = 4;9$)
exhibiting SSD from families with increased
genetic load, defined as two or more nuclear
family members affected, versus those with
no affected members, Shriberg et al. (2005)
reported that 62.5% of the genetic group
had comorbid language impairment. The
nongenetic group had 47.9% with comorbid language impairment. Even the speech
delay—apraxia subtype is often reported to
display concomitant language impairment.
In a study of 248 twin pairs ($M = 6$ years)
involving parent report on children's speech
and language histories, 44% of the affected
cases had both speech and language difficulties whereas 40% had isolated speech difficulties (DeThorne et al., 2006). With respect
to comorbid language deficits within each
of Dodd's subtypes, 23 to 40% had comprehension deficits, 34 to 67% had expressive
deficits, and 51 to 63% had vocabulary
deficits (Broomfield & Dodd, 2004). The
phonological delay group had the smallest
percentages for each of the comorbid deficit

areas, whereas the inconsistent group had
the largest percentages (40–63%). Further,
case history interviews indicated parent/
sibling history of developmental speech/
language difficulty for 20 to 25% of each
subtype. Regardless of classification system
used to delineate subtypes, the groups
appear to overlap with respect to comorbid
language impairment and genetic origin.

Thus, from some of the largest clinical
samples of children identified for their SSD,
there is clear evidence suggesting an increased probability of comorbid language
impairment, particularly as genetic load and
severity increases. It is imperative that we
carefully assess both speech and language
to adequately describe population samples
along these variables to understand and treat
these children effectively. Unfortunately, participant samples in studies of the nature of
both speech and language disorders often
exclude children who displayed a concomitant communication disorder or fail to report
the abilities in the nonprimary linguistic
domain. When children are initially identified
for their "primary" (i.e., reason for referral)
deficit in either speech or language, it is
now paramount that skills in the nonprimary domain be assessed and described. It
would also be advantageous for researchers
to report numbers of participants excluded
from selection and for what reasons.

Similarly, genetic studies have often been
limited to examining one type of communication difficulty rather than considering
comorbid impairments. Recent evidence,
however, shows linkage of SSD to chromosomal regions previously identified for associations to language impairment and reading
disability (Lewis et al, 2006). Shriberg (2004,
2007; Chapter 1) estimates that the speech
delay–genetic (SD-GEN) subtype represents
the largest proportion of undifferentiated
SSDs and proposes that the neurodevelopmental processes affected in this subtype

are cognitive-linguistic. Such a proposed source of difficulty also would likely manifest in phenotypic variants with concomitant language and/or reading impairment. All these pieces of evidence come together to suggest that it is unlikely that various subtypes are distinct with respect to underlying neurodevelopmental processes affected or etiology. In fact, many of the children in the clinical population of SSD likely share genetic traits, fitting with Shriberg et al.'s proposal of polygenic origins.

Comorbid Speech Deficits

Additional evidence of the comorbidity of speech and language deficits comes from investigations of children selected from populations attending language units or special schools for children with speech and language impairment in the United Kingdom, the Netherlands or Canada. These investigations typically have employed factor and cluster analyses to identify test scores/tasks that cluster together from a large battery of standardized measures. Subgroups are then imputed from the factors that reflect particular clustering of speech and language scores. Most importantly, this work has revealed that, across different measures used, there appears to be a clustering of speech sound production tasks with certain expressive language tasks, a clustering of receptive and expressive syntactic and vocabulary tasks, and a clustering of certain language and information processing or auditory perception tasks. Subgroups that have been proposed based on these analyses separate primarily language deficits (e.g., Lexical-Semantic, Lexical-Syntactic) from mixed morphosyntactic and speech deficits (e.g., Speech Production, Expressive, Phonologic-Syntactic), pragmatic or comprehension/processing deficits (e.g., Semantic-Pragmatic,

Syntactic-Sequential) and speech only difficulties (e.g., Phonological programming). In these clinical samples, when individual cases were assigned to clusters, those reflecting both speech sound production problems and language difficulties encompassed one-third to one-half of the samples.

Conti-Ramsden, Cruthley, and Botting's (1997) cluster analysis of the scores from 229 randomly selected seven-year-old children attending language-based classrooms in England produced six significantly different clusters. Five of these clusters closely matched those previously identified by Rapin and Allen (1983, 1988), whose deficit terminology was used. Those clusters suggestive of comorbid speech and language deficits described by Botting and Conti-Ramsden (2004) included Cluster 3 (Expressive; $n = 29$) and Cluster 5 (Phonologic-syntactic; $n = 84$). The Expressive cluster was characterized by poor performance on grammar comprehension, story retelling, word reading, and articulation tasks with good expressive vocabulary. Cluster 5 was characterized by poor performance across all tasks. The latter cluster appears to reflect overall more severe performance and also was the largest subgroup of the 213-participant sample.

Van Daal, Verhoeven, and van Balkom (2004) performed principal components factor analyses on scores from a battery of 20 tasks administered to 110 four-year-olds, randomly selected from those attending special schools for children with severe speech and language impairments in the Netherlands. Four factors were identified which Van Daal et al. interpreted to support previously identified clusters (Botting & Conti-Ramsden, 2004; Rapin & Allen, 1983). Similar to Botting and Conti-Ramsden's Clusters 3 and 5, Van Daal et al. identified a Speech Production factor characterized by low scores on articulation, word and nonsense word repetition, sentence repetition, and narrative tasks. Van Daal et al. even suggest that speech sound production difficulties affected performance on expressive language tasks in this group with comorbid language deficits.

Domain Relationships

It is tempting to view our clinical samples as ones that are circumscribed by speech and language skills that are highly associated, perhaps unlike those in the normal population. Marquardt and Saxman (1972) found that although articulation and language comprehension had a correlation of .44 in a group of 30 children with articulation disorders, correlation of these measures in typically developing children did not reach significance. Examination of the bivariate correlations in Van Daal et al. (2004) shows that correlations among the various language measures and the articulation measure do not exceed .36. In Tyler et al.'s (2003) sample of 40 preschool children (age $M = 4;3$), selected specifically for speech and language performance more than one SD below the mean, the correlation between percent consonants correct (PCC; Shriberg & Kwiatkowski, 1982) and mean length of utterance (MLU; Brown, 1973) was .133 and the correlation between the Bankson-Bernthal Test of Phonology (Bankson & Bernthal, 1990) Word Inventory standard score and expressive language standard score was .09.

We further examined performance profiles in this group of 40 to determine if either the domain of speech or expressive language was relatively more delayed. Standard scores for speech (BBTOP) and MLU, from spontaneous language samples that exceeded 200 utterances, were converted to z-scores. In order to make comparisons among domains, scores that were ≥.75 standard deviations apart were considered to be indicative of performance that was discrepant between the two domains. Forty

percent of the sample showed discrepant performance suggesting that one domain was relatively less impacted than the other, confirming a similar result found in a smaller sample (Tyler & Watterson, 1991). In more than 60% of the cases, performance in speech was better than expressive language performance. This may portend the finding of long-term normalization by age 9;0 in 90% of population samples of children with SSD, alongside the observation that in many studies of school-age children with SLI, speech performance falls within the normal range. Upon follow-up of the sample when children were in third to fifth grade, however, 17 of the 28 (61%) who could be located were receiving some type of special education services.

Comorbid Reading Deficits

Research on literacy achievement and speech and language disorders suggests that it is precisely the group with comorbid speech and language impairment that is at greatest risk of reading disability, in comparison to the group with only speech disorders (Catts, 1993; Catts, Fey, Zhang, & Tomblin, 2001; Snowling, Bishop, & Stothard, 2000). Follow-up of preschool children with comorbid speech and language disorder found 75% experienced reading difficulties in mid-elementary school (Lewis, O'Donnell, Freebairn, & Taylor, 2002). Similarly, 63% with comorbid disorders scored more than one SD below the mean in reading and/or spelling at the end of first grade (Nathan, Stackhouse, Goulandris, & Snowling, 2004). Within the broader domain of phonological awareness, the awareness of phonemes as individual units is highly predictive of later reading and writing success. Furthermore, research has shown that children with speech and language impairments demonstrate poor phonological awareness skills in comparison to their typically developing peers (Gillon, 2000; Raitano, Pennington, Tunick, Boada, & Shriberg, 2004; Rvachew, Ohberg, Grawburg, & Heyding, 2003). The poor prognosis regarding early literacy achievement is also evident in the literature exploring genetic bases of speech and language disorders. For example, in families at high risk, early problems in spoken language predict later reading difficulties (Raitano et al., 2004). Furthermore, assessment of reading-related skills in 6-year-old twins indicated that those at risk for poorest performance were ones with reported histories of difficulty across both receptive and expressive language and articulation (De Thorne et al., 2006).

To summarize then, the implications of both genetic research in SSD and research exploring subtypes of speech and language impairment are that the children represented in large numbers on speech-language pathologists' (SLPs) caseloads are likely to have comorbid deficits. The finding that as many as one half of the samples from populations attending special language units exhibited comorbid speech deficits corresponds to the estimated 40 to 60% of children with SSD who exhibit a concomitant language deficit. In these studies, it is important to recognize such groups likely represent the severest of what constitute clinical samples. The finding that a large number of seven-year-olds in special language classrooms exhibit comorbid deficits suggests the intractable nature of increased severity posed by multiple deficits. It is precisely this clinical population for which aggressive, efficient treatment programs are needed.

Treatment Implications

The long-term outcome for our clinical population with respect to continued impairment, communication status, and educational and occupational results is guarded (Aram, Ekelman, & Nation, 1984; Aram & Hall, 1989; Felsenfeld, Broen, McGue, 1994; Tallal, Ross, & Curtiss, 1989). The majority of children identified as language impaired (with or without accompanying speech impairments) at age five in a longitudinal study of a community sample of 142, maintained that classification at 18 to 20 years of age (Johnson et al., 1999). Thus, many of the children that speech-language pathologists will encounter on their caseloads and who will pose the greatest challenges for the effectiveness of our interventions have a variety of potential long-term co-occurring deficits. They may be experiencing any of the following: (1) isolated speech difficulties with early literacy difficulties; (2) speech *and* language difficulties with early literacy difficulties; (3) language and early literacy difficulties; or (4) speech and language, but no early literacy difficulties. What are the implications for treatment from these observations?

If our long-term goal is not only to improve these children's functional communication performance, but also their academic achievement, how should we consider these co-occurrences in intervention during the preschool period? First it appears that we would need to achieve the highest degree of efficiency possible as we consider the scientific evidence for efficacy of potential interventions. Second, we must ask if several domains can be treated together without sacrificing efficiency. These are questions for which currently we have little empirical evidence to guide our decision making. Third, we must consider if treatment for one domain will have indirect effects on another; will it facilitate gains across multiple interacting domains? For example, might we expect to achieve generalization from speech intervention to grammar or from grammar intervention to speech intelligibility or from phonological awareness intervention to speech?

Simple perusal of the text titles in Brookes Publishing's Communication and Language Intervention Series demonstrates our field often separates treatment for language disorders and SSDs. Recent publications include *Treatment of Language Disorders in Children* (McCauley & Fey, 2006) and *Phonological Disorders in Children: Clinical Decision-Making in Assessment and Intervention* (Kamhi & Pollock, 2005). Certainly, there are isolated chapters that focus on the inclusive range of linguistic domains (Norris & Hoffman, 2005), but these are small in number. Similarly, the evaluation of behavioral interventions in the communicatively impaired population has typically focused more on the efficacy of intervention within a specific linguistic domain, using a population selected for impairment in only that domain, than on interactions between aspects of the linguistic system, such as phonology and morphosyntax. Interventions that produce gains in a nontargeted domain provide an indirect method of treating multifaceted errors. If clinicians could anticipate cross-domain generalizations as a result of intervention focused on just one skill area, treatment efficiency may be increased.

Theoretical and Empirical Bases

When we consider the broad areas of speech, language, and early literacy, what theoretical basis do we have for expecting to achieve gains in multiple domains from a particular intervention? We know, for example, that specific phonological *error* patterns, such as final consonant deletion or cluster reduction, may prevent accurate production of grammatical morphemes such as the plural *–s*, past tense *–ed*, or third person singular. We can expect, therefore, that if we target elimination of these error patterns there should be improvement in those affected grammatical morphemes. In this example, speech intervention should have an affect on one aspect of language, morphosyntax.

Conversely, would intervention focused on language, have an effect on speech? Drawing on a transactional model of speech and language development, we could hypothesize that a procedure such as conversational recasting has the potential to achieve gains across domains of vocabulary, grammar, and phonology. Once recasting facilitates improvements in speech intelligibility, this provides a richer scaffold for recasts that incorporate more advanced linguistic structures (Camarata & Nelson, 2006). Finally, would phonological awareness intervention not only ameliorate later reading difficulties, but also affect changes in speech intelligibility? We might hypothesize this to be the case because bringing a child's attention to the sound structure of words may help establish more accurate phonological representations which, in turn, may lead to improved speech intelligibility.

Empirical Bases

An evidence-based practice perspective requires that a scheme for classifying the scientific rigor in a body of evidence be used when critically judging clinical procedures and outcomes for adoption to particular cases. The higher ranked the evidence, the greater the strength or quality is thought to be involved. High-level studies, often recommended as evidential, establish control ideally through randomization and an untreated, control group. Meta-analyses of multiple well-designed, control group studies also provide useful critical summarization of scientific evidence regarding the efficacy of particular types of interventions (Law, Garrett, & Nye, 2004). Intervention research involving multifaceted deficits can be examined for its adherence to high-level rigorous methodologies. First, returning to the question about gains across multiple domains, does speech sound intervention affect language? Several case and single subject design studies have shown beneficial effects on morphologic gains from the treatment of speech errors that prevented realization of certain morphemes (Fey & Stalker, 1986; Tyler & Sandoval, 1994). These results, however, have not been replicated in randomized, control-group studies. Secondly, can language intervention affect speech intelligibility? In studies with random or semi-random assignment to experimental and control groups, we find evidence of both beneficial and negligible effects of intervention for lexical targets and grammatical targets on speech production (Fey, Cleave, Ravida, Long, Dejmal, & Easton, 1994; Girolametto, Pearce, & Weitzman, 1997; Matheny & Panagos, 1978; Tyler, Lewis, Haskill, & Tolbert, 2002). Analysis of effect sizes from some of these studies has found that the effects of language intervention on speech appeared larger than those of speech intervention on language (Garrity & Hoffman, 2005).

Tyler et al. (2002) hypothesized that their morphosyntactic intervention, which focused specifically on finite morphemes such as past tense -ed, copula, and third person singular regular (Haskill, Tyler, & Tolbert, 2001), resulted in phonological gains because of its indirect focus on final cluster forms. Sweat (2003) further compared phonological changes involving final clusters and the final consonant inventory for participants in the morphosyntax intervention and those in the phonological intervention from the Tyler et al. study. Findings revealed that the morphosyntax group had significantly greater final cluster accuracies in spontaneous speech for regular past tense and contractible copula morphemes than did the phonology group, after 12 weeks

of intervention. Although there was no significant group difference for the number of sounds added to the final inventory, there was a trend for the morphosyntax group to have more participants add both age-appropriate and later developing sounds to their inventories. Thus, it can be hypothesized that repeated practice of finite morpheme targets results in indirect practice of final clusters and an accompanied increase in their accuracy in spontaneous language. It is not known if a morphosyntax intervention focused on finite morphemes can facilitate change in less marked aspects of phonology (i.e., basic clusters, singletons), or in awareness of final phonemes, as well as in finite morphology.

Scheduling Domains. Another obvious question we can pose about the need for a variety of interventions to focus on multiple deficit areas is how we might schedule treatment for these areas together. That is, could one area be treated for awhile and subsequently the others in blocks; could we alternate treatment focused on different areas weekly? These questions were addressed for the domains of speech and morphosyntax in a controlled study of 47 participants with random assignment for experimental groups. Importantly, participants were selected to exhibit clinical deficits in both speech and language. The experimental groups differed in how speech and language goals were scheduled, either in blocks, alternating weekly, or simultaneously (Tyler et al., 2003). Although no single goal attack strategy produced significantly greater change in speech performance, the schedule of alternating speech and language treatment weekly produced the greatest change in morphosyntax.

Results are less ambiguous with regard to the effects of phonological awareness intervention on speech production change.

Several studies suggest that phonological awareness intervention facilitates improvement in speech production (Dodd & Gillon, 2001; Gillon, 2000; Hesketh, Adams, Nightingale, & Hall, 2000), although this may not always parallel the improvement made in phonological awareness (Harbers, Paden, & Halle, 1999). As noted by Stackhouse, Wells, Pascoe, and Rees (2002), separating articulation and phonological awareness interventions can be problematic because traditional articulation therapy often requires some level of metaphonological analysis.

Phonological awareness intervention, however, has not been considered in a broader test of treatments focused on multiple deficit areas. Although preliminary research suggests that phoneme awareness can be successfully stimulated in preschool children (Gillon, 2002, 2005), with associated success in early reading and spelling experiences, the large subgroup with co-occurring speech and language impairments (i.e., increased severity) has not been examined. Similarly, it is not known if phoneme awareness can be stimulated in children with co-occurring speech and language impairment and if it will lead to successful early reading and spelling, improved phonology, and/or changes in grammar.

In our laboratory we are engaged in an ongoing project with goals to: (1) examine gains in specific areas targeted by different interventions, as well as the extent of indirect gains in non-targeted areas; and (2) determine if phoneme awareness can be stimulated in preschool children who have co-occurring speech and language impairments. The following section highlights some of this ongoing work.

Indirect Speech, Language, or PA Gains.
A total of 31 children participated, 18 in the United States and 13 in New Zealand; data discussed below are from the U.S. children.

Criteria for inclusion in the study were as follows: (a) documentation of speech performance at least one standard deviation below the mean on the Goldman-Fristoe Test of Articulation-2 (GFTA-2; Goldman & Fristoe, 2000); (b) documentation of expressive language score at least one standard deviation below the mean on the Structured Photographic Expressive Language Test-Preschool 2 (SPELT-P2; Dawson, Stout, Eyer, Tattersall, Foukalsrud, & Croley, 2005) and/or 1.5 standard deviations below the mean MLU for the child's age based on Miller and Chapman's (2000) normative data; (c) documentation of receptive vocabulary within one and one-half standard deviations from the mean on the Peabody Picture Vocabulary Test–III (PPVT-III; Dunn & Dunn, 1997); (d) normal functioning on oral motor assessment (Robbins & Klee, 1987); (e) neurologic, behavioral, hearing, and motor skills reported within normal limits; and (f) within the age range of 4;0 to 4;6 at the commencement of the study. For the 18 U.S. children the mean standard score on the PPVT-III was 96, mean score on the SPELT-P2 was 67, and mean score on the GFTA-2 was 64.

Cohorts of five, six, or eight children entered the project at different starting points throughout the 2005 to 2006 year. Children were matched on age and severity of speech/language disorder and randomly assigned to phoneme awareness (PA) or the alternating speech and language intervention (Tyler et al., 2003). Participants received two, 6-week blocks of treatment separated by a 6- to 7-week break from treatment. Intervention occurred in small groups of 2 to 3 children scheduled twice weekly for 50 minutes. The PA intervention targeted early phoneme awareness and letter knowledge with integration of speech sound targets. The alternating intervention targeted morphosyntax, in particular finite morphemes, and speech sounds (clusters, velars, fricatives) in alternate weeks. Data collection sessions occurred at pre-treatment, mid-treatment (after 1st block) and post-treatment (after 2nd block). Measures consisted of: phonological awareness and letter knowledge probes (seven tasks); target sound probes; finite morpheme composites (FMC) and MLU from spontaneous language sample analysis (using SALT); and percent consonants correct (PCC, Shriberg & Kwiatkowski, 1982) from the GFTA-2 words supplemented with 25 additional words from Dodd's (1995) variability task.

Immediate post-treatment assessments involving administration of the Pre-Reading Inventory of Phonological Awareness (PIPA; Dodd, Crosbie, McIntosh, Teitzel, & Ozanne, 2003), the Clinical Evaluation of Language Fundamentals-Preschool 2 (CELF-P2; Wiig, Secord, & Semel, 2004), and GFTA-2 + supplementary words for phonological analysis were also completed for all participants. Analyses and scores were generated so that change in all linguistic skills; phoneme awareness, speech production, grammatical performance, and early reading performance could be examined. Cursory examination of children's probe results, their FMC and PCC results, and PIPA scores suggests that both interventions facilitated improvements in speech production. PCC for the PA intervention group increased from a mean of 46.66 to 59.07 post-treatment; for the alternating group, PCC increased from a mean of 44.86 to 58.98.

The PA intervention appears to have facilitated specific change in phoneme awareness and letter knowledge skills that did not result from the alternating intervention. On the phoneme identity probe, mean percent correct increased from 37% to 61% for the PA group, although for the alternating group, accuracy increased from 43% to 51%. On the letter knowledge probe, mean percent correct for the PA group increased

from 31% to 60%; for the alternating group, accuracy increased from 32% to 37%. The alternating intervention facilitated change in grammatical skills that was not observed from the PA intervention. Mean MLU for the alternating intervention group increased from 2.65 to 3.68 post-treatment and for the PA group increased from 3.19 to 3.61. Similarly, the finite morpheme composite increased from 26% to 39.25% for the alternating group, while it increased from 29.22% to 31% for the PA group. These preliminary results suggest that while change specific to the skill areas targeted was observed from both interventions, these children with severe impairments in both speech and language remain significantly below age expectations.

Planned follow-up assessments as participants receive formal Kindergarten instruction will aid in determining the extent of PA influence on early literacy. Should the early PA intervention prove to have a protective effect on risk for early literacy difficulty, results would support other data suggesting that it be provided in the preschool years for this population (Gillon, 2005). Speech intelligibility appears to improve when incorporated in PA intervention at a rate similar to that achieved in other intervention configurations (Tyler et al., 2003). Language, however, appears to need specific intense focus as the greater change observed in the alternating intervention group did not bring performance within age-range expectations.

Case

To demonstrate the general pattern of improvements noted above, as well as blocks of shifting intervention focus, a case example is provided. John was 4;6 when he was referred to the university speech and hearing clinic due to concerns about his speech intelligibility. He was diagnosed with both a speech and language impairment. His standard score on the PPVT-III was 92, but standard score on the SPELT-P2 was 44 and on the receptive core of the CELF-P2 was 81. His MLU in morphemes from a spontaneous language sample was 2.52. In this sample, John's use of finite morphemes that mark tense and agreement, reflected in a composite percent accuracy, was 12%. His standard score on the GFTA-2 was 64 and his PCC calculated from these stimulus words, supplemented with 25 additional words from Dodd's (1995) variability task was 44%. John also completed phonological awareness and speech probes; these results are displayed in Table 4-1.

As part of the intervention comparison study, John was randomly assigned to receive the alternating speech-language intervention. Language goals targeted copula and auxiliary *to be* forms, past tense *-ed*, and third person singular. Speech sound goals targeted /s/ clusters and final /f, m, z, t/. These goals were alternated weekly during two, 6-week intervention blocks, so that there were three weeks of a focus on speech goals and three with a focus on language goals in each block. Both speech and language intervention procedures involved elicited production and naturalistic focused stimulation activities. Phonological awareness and speech probes were repeated at the end of the first 6-week block and subsequently, at the end of the 12 weeks of intervention. These results are also displayed in Table 4-1. It can be seen that although he did not receive explicit phoneme awareness intervention, some of John's phonological awareness skills appeared to improve, especially phoneme identity. His production of final consonants in untrained probe words also improved, although /s/ clusters did not show substantial change.

A post-treatment assessment was completed two weeks after the final probe and comparison to pre-treatment results is pro-

Table 4–1. Case Example Performance on Phonological Awareness and Speech Probes

Task	Probe 1	Probe 2 (6-wk post)	Probe 3 (12-wk post)
Rhyme Detection	20%	10%	40%
Letter Name	100%	100%	100%
Phoneme Identity	50%	30%	60%
Phoneme Identity with Words	100%	100%	100%
Blending	60%	60%	80%
Segmentation	0%	20%	0%
Letter Knowledge	100%	100%	100%
Speech Probes: pattern accuracy	FCD—35% /s/ CR—18%	FCD—63% /s/ CR—29%	FCD—75% /s/ CR—29%

FCD = final consonant deletion; CR = cluster reduction.

vided in Table 4–2. John's PCC increased considerably to 60%; although his GFTA-2 standard score change little. His MLU increased slightly, but his finite morphemes showed no change. Results from the post-treatment administration of the PIPA for peer group comparison suggested that the majority of John's phonological awareness skills were below the normal range for his age. The discrepancy between this performance and that on the probe measures (see Table 4–1) appears to be due to increased difficulty of task requirements on the PIPA. It may be important that letter-sound knowledge skills, likely a result of his preschool curriculum, are a strength. To summarize broadly, John's speech had improved, his language changed little, and his early literacy skills remained at risk at the end of the intervention study period.

John continued to receive services through the university clinic during the next semester during which the focus was on morphologic targets for approximately half of the weeks, followed by a focus on phoneme awareness, phoneme identity, blend-ing and segmentation. This plan was devised due to continued low performance in language, demonstrated by a standard score of 79 on the Comprehensive Assessment of Spoken Language (Carrow-Woolfolk, 1999) with a specific syntax subtest score of 69 and risk of early literacy difficulties. The PIPA was administered again at the end of the semester so results could be compared to those from its previous administration (see Table 4–2). John's scores in alliteration awareness and sound isolation improved to fall in the lower end of the normal range (Basic rating). His accuracy for the production of selected finite morphemes, copula and past tense, increased to 86% in spontaneous environments. In addition, John's PCC increased by 11% to 71%.

Long-Term Outcomes and Ongoing Decision-Making

The focus of John's intervention and his response highlight several important points regarding decision-making for positive long-term outcomes in children with co-occurring

Table 4–2. Assessment Data for Case Example

	Pretreatment	Post-treatment	Follow-up
Test Age	4;6	5;0	5;6
GFTA-2	64	68	—
PCC	44%	60%	71%
MLU	2.52	2.68	3.84
Finite morphemes	12%	3%	86%
PIPA/alliteration	—	10–14	30–34
PIPA/sd isolation	—	10–14	30–34
PIPA/segmentation	—	20–24	20–24

GFTA-2 = Goldman-Fristoe Test of Articulation-2; PCC = percent consonants correct; MLU = mean length of utterance; PIPA = Pre-Reading Inventory of Phonological Awareness (percentile range).

deficits. These include, but are not limited to: (1) the need to focus on multifaceted skills; (2) the importance of clinically significant change; (3) the importance of close monitoring of response to intervention; (4) the potential importance of intensity or "dosage" in intervention (McCauley & Fey 2006); and (5) the role of temperament or "fit" in influencing response to intervention. First, with respect to long-term outcome, it is clear that even at the age of 5;6, after not quite one year of twice-weekly treatment, John continues to display deficits in speech, language, and early literacy. All of these areas continue to need attention. John has not yet entered Kindergarten by which time's end, short-term normalization of speech skills would be a positive prognostic indicator (Nathan et al., 2004; Rvachew, Chiang, & Evans, 2007). Evidence suggests that those children who enter school with speech and language problems are more likely than other children to have poor outcomes, socially, academically, and occupationally. This suggests the need for continued shifting focus and close monitoring of change.

Second, the obvious need to accelerate John's growth in several areas indicates that we must determine if clinically significant change is occurring. That is, treatment should accelerate the growth curve by producing greater than expected change if John is to approach his peer group. Relative gains should be greater for John than would be observed in the population sample that functions within the normal range. An example of clinically significant change would be a post-intervention score that exceeds the standard error of measurement 95% confidence interval of a pre-intervention score.

The third factor in decision-making follows guidelines from the responsiveness to intervention model currently advocated in educational settings (Batsche, 2006). Data derived from assessments and progress monitoring should be used to inform instructional decisions. With respect to monitoring change in multiple domains, as is necessary in the case of John, a combination of standardized measures, criterion-referenced "probes," and contextually-based procedures should be used. These should be designed to detect gains in not only the treated domain, but possible generalization to an untreated domain as well. For example, after a block of phonological awareness intervention, speech sound production, and intelligibility should be monitored.

Information obtained from close monitoring should be used to support decisions regarding the fourth variable that has a potential impact on long-term outcomes, what McCauley and Fey (2006) call dosage. This refers to the frequency of treatment sessions as well as the frequency of targeting goals within a session. The frequency of treatment sessions as it relates to long-term outcome has received little research attention and is another factor in efficiency. For preschoolers with speech and language impairments, an increased number of individual sessions has been reported to lead to greater functional gains (Jacoby, Lee, Kummer, Levin, & Creaghead, 2002). Intense blocks of treatment, with daily sessions, have also been associated with greater long-term gains and maintenance of those gains in studies of language and reading interventions (Gillam, Loeb, Friel-Patti, Hoffman, Brandel, & Champlin, 2005; Torgeson, Alexander, Wagner, Rashotte, Voeller, & Conway, 2001). Although block scheduling was advocated in the schools long ago, there has been little systematic investigation of gains associated with intensive block intervention as compared to more traditional scheduling. Close progress monitoring might reveal, for example, that relative gains in speech sound production are small after PA intervention, necessitating a change in focus to speech intelligibility. It would appear that careful scheduling of intense treatment blocks holds promise as a mechanism for not only increasing the frequency of treatment sessions, but for focusing on different deficit areas for concentrated time periods.

Finally, the role of temperament and goodness-of-fit in the therapeutic relationship are variables that influence response to intervention and have also received little attention in our intervention research. Shriberg and colleagues were some of the first to address these related variables in their investigation of capability-focus (Kwiatkowski & Shriberg, 1998). Capability was characterized by the child's psycholinguistic profile of strengths and weaknesses; focus was operationalized as a child's disposition for speech change as reflected in attention, motivation, and support needed in a clinician-directed speech task within a behavioral paradigm. The task was a trial-teaching, or stimulability, one using different levels of extrinsic reinforcement aimed at teaching target sounds. A child with high focus could maintain attention and persist in the face of difficulty, whereas a child with low focus became distracted and discouraged. These behavioral descriptors are precisely those used in the temperament literature to describe children who show a cluster of traits that may lead them to be perceived as low achieving learners.

Researchers have observed a moderate relationship between temperament and educational success that is hypothesized to be a function of how children score on a "task orientation" factor (Keogh, 1989). This factor is relevant for tasks that require a high degree of attention and focus, such as those required for educational success and not unlike clinician-directed tasks used in speech-language intervention. Martin (1989a, 1989b) speculates that the temperament characteristics of high activity, high distractibility, and low persistence may act to alter how efficiently a child learns, in explaining their relationship to lower achievement. Similarly, the child with low persistence, high distractibility, and high activity may do less well in a directive speech-language intervention that requires high task orientation. As an example, what explains the differential response to treatment of the two same-aged children whose initial linguistic capabilities are displayed in Figure 4–1? Child A made a 25% gain in PCC and a 66% gain in FMC whereas Child B gained 4% in PCC and 2% in FMC. It is quite likely that the children's different temperaments in concert with that of their clinician, or the goodness-of-fit in the therapeutic relationship, may have influenced these vastly different outcomes. Kwiatkowski and Shriberg (1998) found they could better predict individual differences in intervention outcomes when they added their measure of focus to the construct of capability. In particular,

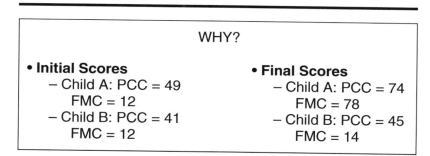

Figure 4–1. Initial linguistic capabilities of two same-aged children.

accuracy of classification for nonmaximal outcomes increased. They also reported that, even with different capabilities accounted for, children whose focus was low showed a greater likelihood of demonstrating poorer outcomes.

Decisions for Long-Term Outcomes: Preliminary Suggestions

Where do we begin when faced with a preschooler who has a comorbid speech and language deficit, and a positive family history, indicating increased risk for literacy and academic difficulties? Preliminary guidelines are presented in Figure 4–2. First, with prevention foremost, our goal should be to facilitate normalized speech by school entry, or age 5;0 to 6;0. Second, careful evaluation of assessment results to construct a profile of strengths and weaknesses is necessary

to determine prioritization of speech, language, or early literacy domains. The area of language would be implicated if the child is relatively young (2;0 to 3;0), if language appears relatively more delayed than speech, or if comprehension is lower than expressive language. As language is treated, generalization to phonotactic forms potentially influenced by grammatical forms should be monitored. For example, a focus on plural forms might influence the correct production of certain final clusters, which may in turn facilitate addition of new sounds to the child's repertoire.

Speech would be a priority for treatment if speech error patterns, in particular omissions of final consonants, prevent realization of language forms. With such a focus, untrained sounds affected by the targeted error pattern, as well as the accuracy of grammatical morphemes should be monitored. For example, if final /s/ and /k/ are target sounds, other final stops and frica-

---

Preliminary Suggestions: Preschooler with Speech and Language Delay

- **Treat just the *language***
  - If language is relatively more delayed
  - If comprehension is low
  - If young
- **Treat just the *speech***
  - If speech error patterns prevent realization of language forms, target the speech – omissions in particular
- **Treat *both* speech and language**
  - Alternate goals weekly: if both language and speech appear similarly, and even moderate-severely impaired
- **Treat just PA**
  - If speech is severe
  - If child is in prekindergarten year

Figure 4–2. Preliminary guidelines when faced with a preschooler with increased risk for literacy and academic difficulties.

tives should be monitored along with the production of possessives. Intervention should focus on both speech *and* language in alternate weeks if both appear moderate-severely impaired as development progresses (3;0 to 4;0). Untrained sounds and morphemes could be monitored, along with PA, for indirect gains. Finally, if the child is in his or her pre-kindergarten year, is experiencing PA delays, and speech remains impaired, a period of phonological awareness intervention is warranted. Generalization to untrained sounds affected by error patterns indirectly targeted through the PA intervention could be expected.

We might envision a course of early intervention in which a toddler first receives twice weekly sessions or an intense block focused on language (with consideration of phonetic inventory), followed by a period of alternating focus on both speech and language goals. In the prekindergarten year the child receives an intense summer block of PA treatment followed by a break and then another intense block of speech and language focus prior to school entry. The bottom line is that multiple skill areas need attention and the clinician must continually monitor progress across these areas to insure that growth is accelerated. As gains are made, the clinician must be prepared to change the focus of intervention, as well as to consider the dosage of intervention and its goodness-of-fit.

References

Aram, D., Ekelman, B., & Nation, J. (1984). Preschoolers with language disorders: Ten years later. *Journal of Speech and Hearing Research, 27,* 232–244.

Aram, D. M., & Hall, N. E. (1989). Longitudinal follow-up of children with preschool commu-nication disorders: Treatment implications. *School Psychology Review, 18,* 487–501.

Bankson, N., & Bernthal, J. E. (1990). *Bankson-Bernthal Test of Phonology.* Austin, TX: Pro-Ed.

Batsche, G. (2006). *Response to intervention: Policy considerations and implementation.* Alexandria, VA: National Association of State Directors of Special Education.

Botting, N., & Conti-Ramsden, G. (2004). Characteristics of children with specific language impairment. In L. Verhoeven & H. van Balkom (Eds.), *Classification of developmental language disorders: Theoretical issues and clinical implications* (pp. 23–38). London: Lawrence Erlbaum Associates.

Broomfield, J., & Dodd, B. (2004). The nature of referred subtypes of primary speech disability. *Child Language Teaching and Therapy, 20,* 135–151.

Brown, R. (1973). *A first language.* Cambridge, MA: Harvard University Press.

Camarata, S., & Nelson, K. (2006). Conversational recast intervention. In R. McCauley & M. Fey (Eds.), *Treatment of language disorders in children* (pp. 237–264) Baltimore: Brookes.

Carrow-Woolfolk, E. (1999). *Comprehensive assessment of spoken language.* Circle Pines, MN: American Guidance Service.

Catts, H. (1993). The relationship between speech-language impairments and reading disabilities. *Journal of Speech and Hearing Research, 36,* 948–958.

Catts, H. W., Fey, M. E., Zhang, X., & Tomblin, J. B. (2001). Estimating the risk of future reading difficulties in kindergarten children: A research-based model and its clinical implications. *Language, Speech, and Hearing Services in Schools, 32,* 38–50.

Conti-Ramsden, G., Crutchley, A., & Botting, N. (1997). The extent to which psychometric tests differentiate subgroups of children with SLI. *Journal of Speech, Language, and Hearing Research, 40,* 765–777.

Dawson, J., Stout, C., Eyer, J., Tattersall, P., Foukalsrud, J., & Croley, K. (2005). *Structured Photographic Expressive Language Test–Preschool 2.* Dekalb, IL: Janelle.

DeThorne, L. S., Hart, S. A., Petrill, S. A., Deater-Deckard, K., Thompson, L. A., Schatschneider,

C., et al. (2006). Children's history of speech-language difficulties: Genetic influences and association with reading-related measures. *Journal of Speech, Language, and Hearing Research, 49,* 1280-1292.

Dodd, B. (1995). *Differential diagnosis and treatment of children with speech disorder.* San Diego, CA: Singular.

Dodd, B., Crosbie, S., McIntosh, B., Teitzel, T., & Ozanne, A. (2003). *Pre-reading inventory of phonological awareness.* San Antonio, TX: The Psychological Corporation.

Dodd, B., & Gillon, G. (2001). Exploring the relationship between phonological awareness, speech impairment and literacy. *Advances in Speech-Language Pathology, 3,* 139-147.

Dunn, L. M., & Dunn, L. M. (1997). *Peabody Picture Vocabulary Test-III.* Circle Pines, MN: American Guidance Service.

Felsenfeld, S., Broen, P. A., & McGue, M. (1994). A 28-year follow-up of adults with a history of moderate phonological disorder: Educational and occupational results. *Journal of Speech and Hearing Research, 37,* 1341-1353.

Fey, M., Cleave, P. L., Ravida, A. I., Long, S. H., Dejmal, A. E., & Easton, D. L. (1994). Effects of grammar facilitation on the phonological performance of children with speech and language impairments. *Journal of Speech and Hearing Research, 37,* 594-607.

Fey, M. E., & Stalker, C. H. (1986). A hypothesis-testing approach to treatment of a child with an idiosyncratic (morpho)phonological system. *Journal of Speech and Hearing Disorders, 51,* 324-336.

Fox, A. V., Dodd, B., & Howard, D. (2002). Risk factors for speech disorders in children. *International Journal of Language and Communication Disorders, 37,* 117-131.

Garrity, A. W., & Hoffman, P. (2005, November). *Cross-domain effect size: Phonological and language interventions.* Poster presented at the Annual Convention of the American Speech-Language-Hearing Association, San Diego, CA.

Gillam, R., Loeb, D., Friel-Patti, S., Hoffman, L., Brandel, J., & Champlin, C. (2005, November). *Comparing language intervention outcomes.*

Presented at the American Speech-Language-Hearing Association Annual Convention, San Diego, CA.

Gillon, G. (2000). The efficacy of phonological awareness intervention for children with spoken language impairment. *Language, Speech and Hearing Services in Schools, 31,* 126-141.

Gillon, G. (2002). Follow-up study investigating benefits of phonological awareness intervention for children with spoken language impairment. *International Journal of Language and Communication Disorders, 37,* 381-400.

Gillon, G. T. (2005). Facilitating phoneme awareness development in 3 and 4-year-old children with speech impairment. *Language, Speech, and Hearing Services in Schools, 36,* 308-324.

Girolametto, L., Pearce, P. S., & Weitzman, E. (1997). Effects of lexical intervention on the phonology of late talkers. *Journal of Speech, Language, and Hearing Research, 40,* 338-348.

Goldman, R., & Fristoe, M. (2000). *Goldman-Fristoe Test of Articulation-2.* Circle Pines, MN: American Guidance Service.

Harbers, H., Paden, E., & Halle, J. (1999). Phonological awareness and production: Changes during intervention. *Language, Speech, and Hearing Services in Schools, 30,* 50-60.

Haskill, A., Tyler, A., & Tolbert, L. (2001). *Months of morphemes.* Eau Claire, WI: Thinking Publications.

Hauner, K. K. Y., Shriberg, L. D., Kwiatkowski, J., & Allen, C. T. (2005). A subtype of speech delay associated with developmental psychosocial involvement. *Journal of Speech, Language, and Hearing Research, 48,* 635-650.

Hesketh, A., Adams, C., Nightingale, C., & Hall, R. (2000). Phonological awareness therapy and articulatory training approaches for children with phonological disorders: A comparative outcome study. *International Journal of Language and Communication Disorders, 35,* 337-354.

Jacoby, G. P., Lee, L., Kummer, A. W., Levin, L., & Creaghead, N. A. (2002). The number of individual treatment units necessary to facilitate functional communication improvements in the speech and language of young children.

American Journal of Speech-Language Pathology, 11, 570–580.

Johnson, C. J., Beitchman, J. H., Young, A., Escobar, M., Atkinson, L., Wilson, B., Brownlie, E. B., et al. (1999). Fourteen-year follow-up of children with and without speech/language impairments: Speech/language stability and outcomes. *Journal of Speech, Language, and Hearing Research, 42*, 744–760.

Kamhi, A., & Pollock, K. (2005). *Phonological disorders in children: Clinical decision making in assessment and intervention.* Baltimore: Brookes.

Karlsson, H. B., Shriberg, L. D., Flipsen, P., Jr., & McSweeny, J. L. (2002). Acoustic phenotypes for speech-genetics studies: Toward an acoustic marker for residual /s/ distortions. *Clinical Linguistics and Phonetics, 16*, 403–424.

Keogh, B. K. (1989). Applying temperament research to school. In G. A. Kohnstamm, J. E. Bates, & M. K. Rothbart (Eds.), *Temperament in childhood* (pp. 437–450). New York: Wiley.

Kwiatkowski, J., & Shriberg, L. D. (1998). Capability-focus treatment framework for child speech disorders. *American Journal of Speech-Language Pathology, 7*, 27–38.

Law, J., Garrett, Z., & Nye, C. (2004). The efficacy of treatment for children with developmental speech and language delay/disorders: A meta-analysis. *Journal of Speech, Language, Hearing Research, 47*, 924–943.

Lewis, B. A., O'Donnell, B., Freebairn, L. A., & Taylor, H. G. (2002). Spoken language and written expression—interplays of delays. *American Journal of Speech-Language Pathology, 7*, 66–73.

Lewis, B. A., Shriberg, L. D., Freebairn, L. A., Hansen, A. J., Stein, C. M., Taylor, H. G., et al. (2006). *Journal of Speech, Language, and Hearing Research, 49*, 1294–1312.

Marquardt, T., & Saxman, J. H. (1972). Language comprehension and auditory discrimination in articulation deficient kindergarten children. *Journal of Speech and Hearing Research, 15*, 382–389.

Martin, R. P. (1989a). Activity level, distractibility, and persistence: Critical characteristics in early schooling. In G. A. Kohnstamm, J. E. Bates, &

M. K. Rothbart (Eds.), *Temperament in childhood* (pp. 451–461). New York: Wiley.

Martin, R. P. (1989b). Temperament and education: Implications for under achievement and learning disabilities. In W. B. Carey & S. C. McDevitt (Eds.), *Clinical and educational applications of temperament research* (pp. 37–51). Amsterdam/Lisse: Swets & Zeitlinger.

Matheny, N., & Panagos, J. M. (1978). Comparing the effects of articulation and syntax programs on syntax and articulation improvement. *Language, Speech, and Hearing Services in Schools, 9*, 57–61.

McCauley, R. J., & Fey, M. E. (2006). *Treatment of language disorders in children.* Baltimore: Brookes.

Miller, J., & Chapman, R. (2000). *SALT: Systematic Analysis of Language Transcripts, Version 6.1.* Madison, WI: Language Analysis Laboratory, Waisman Center, University of Wisconsin.

Nathan, L., Stackhouse, J., Goulandris, N., & Snowling, M. J. (2004). The development of early literacy skills among children with speech difficulties: A test of the "critical age hypothesis." *Journal of Speech, Language, and Hearing Research, 47*, 377–391.

Norris, J. A., & Hoffman, P. R. (2005). Goals and targets: Facilitating the self-organizing nature of a neuro-network. In A. G. Kamhi & K. E. Pollock (Eds.), *Phonological disorders in children: Clinical decision making in assessment and intervention* (pp. 77–87). Baltimore: Brookes.

Raitano, N. A., Pennington, B. F., Tunick, R. A., Boada, R., & Shriberg, L. D. (2004). Preliteracy skills of subgroups of children with speech sound disorders. *Journal of Child Psychology and Psychiatry, 45*, 821–835.

Rapin, I., & Allen, D. A. (1983). Developmental language disorders: Nosalogic considerations. In U. Kirk (Ed.), *Neuropsychology of language reading, and spelling* (pp. 155–184). New York: Academic Press.

Robbins, J., & Klee, T. (1987). Clinical assessment of oropharyngeal motor development in young children. *Journal of Speech and Hearing Disorders, 52*, 271–277.

Rvachew, S., Chiang, P., & Evans, N. (2007). Characteristics of speech errors produced by children with and without delayed phonological awareness skills. *Language, Speech and Hearing Services in Schools, 38*, 60–71.

Rvachew, S., Ohberg, A., Grawburg, M., & Heyding, J. (2003). Phonological awareness and phonemic perception in 4-year-old children with delayed expressive phonology skills. *American Journal of Speech-Language Pathology, 12*, 463–471.

Shriberg, L. D. (2004). *Diagnostic classification of five subtypes of childhood speech sound disorders (SSD) of currently unknown origin.* Paper presented at the International Association of Logopedics and Phoniatrics, Brisbane, Queensland, Australia.

Shriberg, L. D. (April, 2007). *Puzzles and mysteries: Unraveling the origins of childhood speech sound disorders.* Presented at the University of Kansas.

Shriberg, L. D., & Austin, D. (1998). Comorbidity of speech-language disorders: Implications for a phenotype marker for speech delay. In R. Paul (Ed.), *Exploring the speech-language connection* (pp. 73–117). Baltimore: Paul H. Brookes.

Shriberg, L. D., Campbell, T. F., Karlsson, H. B., Brown, R. L., McSweeny, J. L., & Nadler, C. J. (2003). A diagnostic marker for childhood apraxia of speech: The lexical stress ratio. *Clinical Linguistics and Phonetics, 17*, 549–574.

Shriberg, L. D., Flipsen, P., Jr., Kwiatkowski, J., & McSweeny, J. L. (2003). A diagnostic marker for speech delay associated with otitis media with effusion: The intelligibility-speech gap. *Clinical Linguistics and Phonetics, 17*, 507–528.

Shriberg, L. D., Green, J. R., Campbell, T. F., McSweeny, J. L., & Scheer, A. (2003). A diagnostic marker for childhood apraxia of speech: The coefficient of variation ratio. *Clinical Linguistics and Phonetics, 17*, 575–595.

Shriberg, L. D., Kent, R. D., Karlsson, H. B., McSweeny, J. L., Nadler, C. J., & Brown, R. L. (2003). A diagnostic marker for speech delay associated with otitis media with effusion: Backing of obstruents. *Clinical Linguistics and Phonetics, 17*, 529–547.

Shriberg, L. D., & Kwiatkowski, J. (1982). Phonological disorders III: A procedure for assessing severity of involvement. *Journal of Speech and Hearing Disorders, 17*, 256–270.

Shriberg, L. D., Lewis, B.A., Tomblin, J. B., McSweeny, J. L., Karlsson, H. B., & Scheer, A. R. (2005). Toward diagnostic and phenotype markers for genetically transmitted speech delay. *Journal of Speech, Language, and Hearing Research, 48*, 834–852.

Snowling, M., Bishop, D. V. M., & Stothard, S. E. (2000). Is preschool language impairment a risk factor for dyslexia in adolescence? *Journal of Child Psychology and Psychiatry and Allied Disciplines, 41*, 587–600.

Stackhouse, J., & Wells, B. (1997). *Children's speech and literacy difficulties.* London: Whurr.

Stackhouse, J., Wells, B., Pascoe, M., & Rees, R. (2002). From phonological therapy to phonological awareness. *Seminars in Speech and Language, 23*, 27–42.

Sweat, L. (2003). *Comparing the effects of morphosyntax and phonology intervention on final consonant clusters in finite morphemes and final consonant inventories.* Unpublished masters' thesis, University of Nevada, Reno.

Tallal, P., Ross, R., & Curtiss, S. (1989). Familial aggregation in specific language impairment. *Journal of Speech and Hearing Disorders, 54*, 167–173.

Torgeson, J. K., Alexander, A. W., Wagner, R. K., Rashotte, C. A., Voeller, K. S., & Conway, T. (2001). Intensive remedial instruction for children with severe reading disabilities: Immediate and long-term outcomes from two instructional approaches. *Journal of Learning Disabilities, 34*, 33–58.

Tyler, A. A., Lewis, K. E., Haskill, A., & Tolbert L. C. (2002). Efficacy and cross-domain effects of a phonology and morphosyntax intervention. *Language, Speech, and Hearing Services in Schools, 33*, 52–66.

Tyler, A. A., Lewis, K. E., Haskill, A., & Tolbert L. C. (2003). Outcomes of different speech and language goal attack strategies. *Journal of Speech Language and Hearing Research, 46*, 1077–1094.

Tyler, A. A., & Sandoval, K. T. (1994). Preschoolers with phonological and language disorders: Treating different linguistic domains. *Language, Speech and Hearing Services in Schools, 25*, 215–234.

Tyler, A. A., & Watterson, K. H. (1991). Effects of phonological versus language intervention in preschoolers with both phonological and language impairment. *Child Language Teaching and Therapy, 7*, 141–160.

Van Daal, J., Verhoeven, L., & van Balkom (2004). Subtypes of severe speech and language impairments: Psychometric evidence from 4-year-old children in the Netherlands. *Journal of Speech, Language, and Hearing Research, 47*, 1411–1423.

Wiig, E. H., Secord, W. A., & Semel, E. (2004). *Clinical Evaluation of Language Fundamentals –Preschool 2.* San Antonio, TX: Psychological Corporation.

CHAPTER 5

Children's Speech Sound Disorders: An Acoustic Perspective

RAYMOND D. KENT, LUCIANA PAGAN-NEVES, KATHERINE C. HUSTAD, AND HAYDEE FISZBEIN WERTZNER

Introduction

Speech sound disorders are almost always identified and described by their auditory-perceptual properties, as determined by adult listeners. Given that auditory-perceptual properties are extracted from the acoustic signal of speech, it follows that acoustic methods should be highly suited to the study of these disorders. But the capability for doing something is not the same as the necessity or even desirability for doing so. What does acoustic analysis offer for the assessment, treatment, and understanding of developmental speech disorders? This chapter takes the view that acoustic analysis is a valuable complement and co-referent to perceptual analysis. The advantages that acoustic analysis offers to the understanding of children's speech sound disorders are primarily objectivity, quantification, and sensitivity. Each of

these advantages is discussed, with examples from the literature. Also included are suggestions to (a) improve the acoustic analysis of children's speech, and (b) apply acoustic methods to clinical assessment and treatment.

An Envisioned Future

A hopeful view of the future application of acoustic analysis to the clinical assessment and treatment of speech disorders includes the routine use of computer-based methods to record, display, analyze, and store information about speech sound patterns (also see Chapter 6). In fact, these functions have been available for some time, so this view of the future is not especially bold or revolutionary. But the operative word is "routine." Despite the general availability of computer-based acoustic analysis at relatively low cost, the use of such analysis tools is by no means routine. Are there real prospects for routine clinical application? And what needs to be done to bring these prospects to reality? This chapter addresses these questions and, in so doing, reviews major accomplishments in the acoustic analysis of speech disorders. The emphasis is on speech disorders in children, but occasional reference is made to disorders in adults as they help to reveal potential clinical tools for children's speech.

The pivotal technology is digital signal processing, which enables a user to record samples of speech as a digital file, display this file as a waveform or other pattern, select and edit parts of the saved file, conduct various types of analysis (e.g., waveform, spectrogram, spectrum, fundamental-frequency contour, intensity envelope, some of which are shown in Figure 5–1), play all or selected parts of the file, and save the results of analysis. The basic methods are found in several different systems that are available commercially at varying costs (Ingram, Bunta, & Ingram, 2004; Read, Buder, & Kent, 1990) or as free downloads (such as the computer analysis program *Praat* [Dutch for *talk*] developed by Paul Boersma and David Wee-

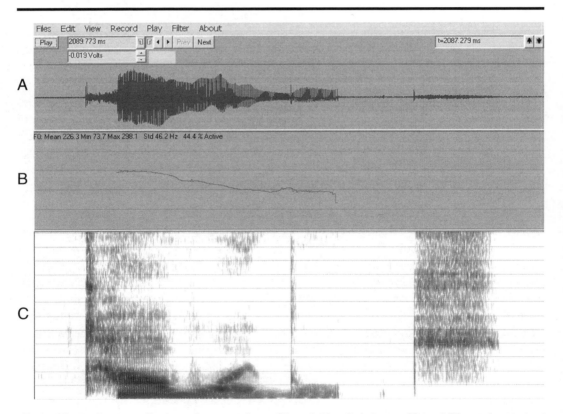

Figure 5–1. Screen display of a waveform (Panel A), pitch trace (Panel B), and spectrogram (Panel C) in TF32. Speech sample is from a three-year-old typically developing child producing the phrase "cowboy boots."

nink at the University of Amsterdam). Certainly, cost is not an obstacle to performing fairly sophisticated operations in the acoustic analysis and synthesis of speech. Perhaps a greater obstacle is a limited understanding of how these analyses can be used in the practice of speech-language pathology. Relevant discussions are available in articles and books explaining how these digital methods can be applied to speech and language disorders (Ingram et al., 2004; Kent & Read, 2002). Proficiency with acoustic methods may be the single most important factor that will lead to the increased use of these methods for clinical purposes. Acoustic analysis, like any laboratory tool, requires practice in its use (see Figure 5-1).

Speech Is More Than What Meets the Ear

The human auditory system is remarkable in its ability to segregate the speech signal from noise and to achieve a phonetic interpretation of that signal. The robustness of this process necessarily discards a fair amount of detail. A primary advantage of acoustic analysis is that it permits the detection of acoustic properties that may not be detected by auditory means. The ear is necessarily an informational filter that attends to certain aspects of sound and ignores others. Especially because of biases introduced through phonetic experience with a given language, human audition discards or neglects much of the acoustic signal of speech. Speech-language clinicians are taught to listen carefully to acoustic variations that the layperson may not hear at all. A recent study comparing the perception of correct and incorrect Brazilian Portuguese liquids /l/, /ɾ/, /ʎ/ by undergraduate and graduate students demonstrated a better performance of the under-

graduate students, indicating that sometimes expert listeners can be more influenced by their knowledge of the pathology than by what they are really listening to (Pagan & Wertzner, 2007a). Furthermore, even the experts' ears fail in comparison to acoustic analysis, which is free of phonetic biases and other influences that inevitably affect perception. This conclusion has been reached for several aspects of speech (Kent, 1996).

Toward a Pediatric Speech Science

Most of the literature on acoustic theory, methods of analysis, and acoustic databases pertains to normal adult speech, and especially to the speech of men. Gradually, theory, methods, and databases are becoming more comprehensive to include women and children, that is, the community of speakers. The analysis of children's speech, in particular, needs to take account of various factors that can complicate the analysis task. Some of the major factors are as follows:

1. Because children have shorter vocal tracts than adults, children's speech sounds (both vowels and consonants) have energy at higher frequencies than those observed for adults. One consequence is that the total frequency range of analysis may need to be extended for satisfactory results with children's speech. For example, the spectral energy associated with infants' fricatives may reach as high as 16 kHz (Kent & Read, 2002). Fortunately, most contemporary systems for recording and analyzing speech permit a total bandwidth of about 20 kHz. Increases in computer memory accommodate such extended bandwidths.

2. The precision of formant estimation varies with fundamental frequency (F_0). Voices with high F_0 (generally the case for children) are more challenging when it comes to estimating formant frequencies. The limitation is basically one of sampling. With higher F_0 values, the harmonics of the laryngeal source are farther apart, and this makes it more difficult to estimate the formant locations in the spectrum (Huggins, 1980: Kent & Read, 2002; Vorperian & Kent, 2007).

3. Children often are variable in their phonatory patterns, which may include transient or long-term features such as breathiness, roughness, pitch shift, and even register change (e.g., between chest and vocal fry registers). In contrast, adults tend to have fairly uniform phonatory patterns so that one set of analysis parameters generally is suitable for an entire utterance.

4. Velopharyngeal function may differ between children and adults. Although the precise maturational pattern is not well established, it appears that typically developing children may achieve speech-adequate control at about the same time as canonical babbling appears (Thom, Hoit, Hixon, & Smith, 2006). However, some children may show variable or unusual patterns of velopharyngeal function, which can complicate acoustic analysis.

5. Eccentric or idiosyncratic acoustic-phonetic patterns may appear. Because children are learning language, including its phonological and phonetic aspects, at the same time they are learning the motor skills of speech, they may exhibit behaviors that are seldom, if ever, observed in adult speech. Some of these behaviors may be highly transient, but others may persist over a substantial period of time.

6. The development of the vocal tract reflects a complicated interaction of the growth of its constituent structures, and this interaction is poorly understood (Kent & Hustad, 2009; Kent & Tilkens, 2007; Kent & Vorperian, 1995).

7. The acoustic database for children's speech is incomplete. The database is growing slowly, but it is not adequate for all purposes. Clinical interpretation depends critically on a secure knowledge of normative behavior.

These comments are not intended to discourage the use of acoustic analysis, but rather to forewarn those who attempt these analyses of the complications that lie in the path of discovery and application. Similar precautions could be issued on the use of phonetic transcription and physiologic analyses. These difficulties notwithstanding, there is no good reason why acoustics should not be a working partner with auditory-perceptual methods in the understanding of children's speech disorders.

Prosodic Patterns

Depending on the definition that is used, prosody can embrace a number of phenomena including intonation, tempo (pause and lengthening), vocal effort, and loudness. These are suprasegmental aspects of speech, meaning that their effects typically extend over two or more phonetic segments. It is not possible to offer an extensive review of prosody in this chapter, and the emphasis is on the tractability of an acoustic analysis of prosody in children. In one view of prosody that was designed expressly for application to language development (Gerken & McGregor, 1998), prosody was conceptualized as three general types of phenomena in language: phrasal stress, boundary cues, and meter. Each of these is elaborated in the following.

Phrasal Stress

Phrasal stress is the phenomenon of word prominence in a phrase. Stress is conveyed by adjustments of duration, fundamental frequency, and intensity. Children begin to regulate the acoustic cues of stress (fundamental frequency, amplitude, duration) as early as 18 to 30 months of age (Kehoe, Stoel-Gammon, & Buder, 1995). In a study of linguistic stress produced by 5 children with suspected developmental apraxia of speech (sDAS) and 5 children with phonological disorder, Munson, Bjorum, and Windsor (2003) reported that the children with sDAS were judged to be less successful than the children with phonological disorder in producing target stress contours. However, acoustic studies showed that the children with sDAS produced acoustic differences between stressed and unstressed syllables that apparently were not consistently detected by the listeners who made the stress judgments.

Boundary Cues

Boundary cues are pauses, adjustments in duration, or variations in pitch that mark the ends of language units. A well-known example of a boundary cue is phrase-final lengthening, in which a word or syllable that precedes the end of a major syntactic unit is lengthened. Phrase-final lengthening often is accompanied by a falling tone, and the two of these features are effective cues for a major constituent unit. Figure 5–2 illustrates both final syllable lengthening and falling tone. They also appear relatively early in speech-language development (Snow,

1994) and are robust in the face of speech or language disorder (Snow, 1998; Wang, Kent, Duffy, & Thomas, 2005). According to Snow's (1994) data on children aged 16 to 25 months, intonation is acquired earlier than final syllable timing. As Snow pointed out, one implication of this result is that final lengthening is a learned prosodic feature.

Meter or Rhythm

Meter (or rhythm) is the pattern of stressed and unstressed syllables for words and phrases. In American English, syllables usually have a strong-weak (SW) alternation, and this alternation defines the rhythm of the language. The SW pattern is linked to a stress unit called the foot, which is a SW syllable pair. Low, Grabe, and Nolan (2000) introduced a measure called the Pairwise Variability Index (PVI), which seems to be a useful measure of a speaker's adherence to the normal stressed-unstressed alternation in English. PVI is an index of changes in successive vowel length over an utterance, and it is not affected by speaking rate. It is computed as follows:

$$PVI = 100 \times [\Sigma \mid (d_k - d_{k-1})/d_k + d_{k-1})/2 \mid / (m-1)]$$

where m equals the number of vowels (or syllables) in an utterance and d is the duration of the kth vowel (syllable).

PVL has only recently been applied to the study of speech disorders (Henrich et al., 2006; Wang, Kent, Duffy, Thomas, & Fredericks, 2006), and, to our knowledge, has not been applied to the study of typical speech development.

The main conclusion is that acoustic correlates exist for prosodic constituents,

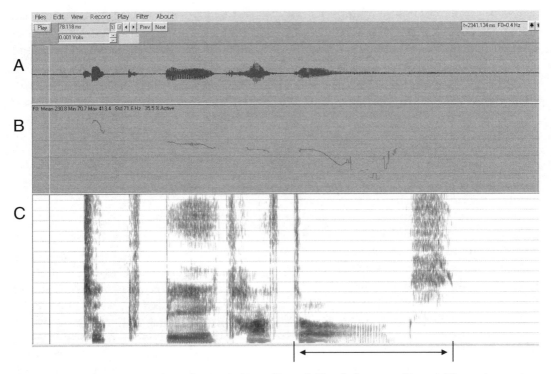

Figure 5–2. Screen display of a waveform (Panel A), pitch trace (Panel B), and spectrogram (Panel C) in TF32. Speech sample is from a three-year-old typically developing child producing the phrase "cook big hot dogs." Note the falling intonation pattern shown on the pitch trace (Panel B) and the syllable-final lengthening indicated by the arrow on the spectrogram (Panel C).

and these correlates are appropriate means for the study of speech and language development in children, or for disorders in development.

Segmental Analysis

Temporal Patterns

The temporal pattern of speech is determined by multiple influences, ranging from prosodic patterns (considered in the previous section) to intrinsic segment durations (Klatt, 1976). As children gain language proficiency and motor skill, the temporal pattern of their speech increasingly conforms to the adult standard in the language. At the segmental level, temporal measurement applies to the intrinsic duration of phonetic elements or to the effects of the immediate phonetic context. A number of generalizations have been established, including the following: (1) short or lax vowels have a briefer duration than long vowels; and (2) vowels preceding voiced consonants are longer than vowels before voiceless consonants. Other generalizations apply to segments in clusters or in word-sized units: (1) a singleton consonant has a longer duration than the same sound in a consonant cluster; (2) the base form of a word has a shorter duration as prefixes or suffixes are combined with it; and (3) new or novel words are produced with a longer duration than familiar words. These are regularities of American English, and children learn to incorporate them in their speech patterns. Their developmental appearance has clinical relevance. For example, Schwartz (1995) concluded that word familiarity is associated with shorter word duration, and he explained this outcome as evidence of word-specific motor maturation. An implication is that word duration can be used as a clinical index of familiarity or motor maturation.

Munson examined the mean duration of /s/ frication, and its variability in adults and in three groups of children (mean ages of 3;11; 5;04; and 8;04). Children had a larger temporal variability than adults. Weismer and Elbert (1982) studied the temporal characteristics of /s/ production in normally speaking adults, normal speaking children, and children with /s/ misarticulations. The /s/ durations of the misarticulating children were significantly more variable than those for the other two groups. This result was explained in terms of differences in speech motor control capabilities. It appears that temporal variability reflects both maturation and disorder (or perhaps only a single factor if it can be shown than disorder is equivalent to delayed maturation)

Figure 5–3 gives a comparison of typical and atypical (disordered) productions of a simple phrase. The atypical production is noticeably longer, with lengthening of phonetic segments and phrases.

One of the most frequently studied temporal features is the voicing contrast for word-initial stop consonants. These sounds are associated with a sequence of acoustic events, including a transient or burst (a pulse of energy that occurs with the initial release of the constriction), a frication interval (a period of turbulence noise generated as the constriction is progressively opened), and onset of voicing (the initiation of vocal fold vibration for the following vowel). An interval of aspiration typically occurs between the frication and the onset of voicing, so that word-initial voiceless stops in English are aspirated. The interval between the burst and the onset of voicing is called the voice onset time (VOT). VOT has a range of values that are often classified as voicing lead or prevoicing (voicing begins before the stop is released), simultaneous voicing (onset of voicing is simultaneous with the transient), short lag (onset of voicing begins shortly after the onset of voicing), and long lag (onset of voicing begins significantly after the onset of voicing. In short, VOT is a continuous variable on which various phonetic categories of voicing can be mapped, and these vary across languages. Perceptual studies have shown that listeners are generally oblivious to small differences within a voicing category. For example, a short-lag VOT of 5 msec cannot be distinguished from a short-lag VOT of 15 msec. As young children learn to control the production of VOT, they often begin with a preference for prevoicing or short-lag. Adults will tend to perceive both of these as voiced stops in American English. Macken and Barton (1980) reported that children produced small differences in VOT for voiced and voiceless cognates that were not perceived by adults. In an acoustic study of phonologically disordered children, Catts and Jensen (1983) concluded that some phonologically disordered children may have less mature speech timing control. A recent study with Brazilian Portuguese-speaking children aged between 6 and 10 years old (Gurgueira, 2006) demonstrated that voiced stops are always produced with prevoicing, which is also true

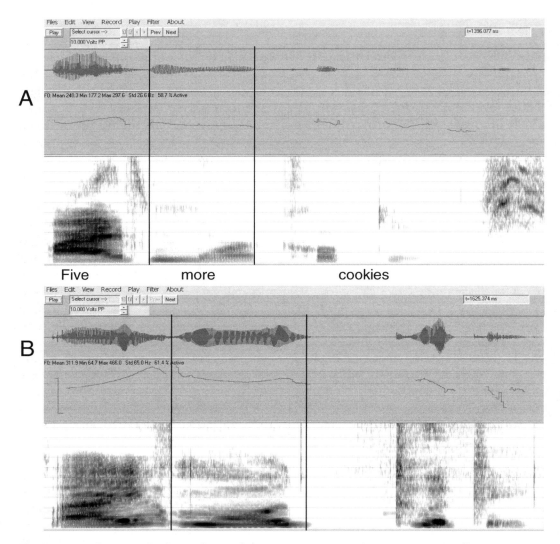

Five   more   cookies

Figure 5–3. Screen displays of waveform, pitch trace, and spectrogram in TF32. Panel A shows the speech of a 5-year-old boy who is typically developing. Panel B shows the speech of a 5-year-old boy with apraxia of speech and mild dysarthria. Both boys are producing the phrase "five more cookies." Note the overall duration difference for the two productions and the increased length of individual words and pauses for the child with the speech disorder (Panel B).

for Spanish, Italian, and French (Borden, Harris, & Raphael, 1994).

The differences in VOT that can be registered by acoustic means could have implications for treatment. Tyler, Edwards, and Saxman (1990) used both phonological and acoustic analyses to describe the speech of four children with a phonological disorder. The acoustic analyses indicated that three of the children produced significant, although frequently imperceptible, differences in VOT for a given stop when it represented different stops in adult speech. These small differences can be taken as evidence of productive phonological knowledge, and it was shown that such knowledge facilitated rapid generalization of correct production of the treated contrast. But when such knowledge was not evident in acoustic analysis, treatment over a longer period was needed to achieve production accuracy on the same treated contrast. But it should be noted that the voicing contrast can be based on several cues, not VOT alone. Forrest and Rockman (1988) suggested that a matrix of acoustic cues is needed to explain the perception of word-initial voicing in the speech of phonologically disordered children. In addition to VOT, these cues include fundamental frequency and F1 frequencies at the onset of voicing, and the amplitude of the burst and aspiration relative to the amplitude of the vowel onset.

Spectral Patterns

Formant descriptions (typically F1-F2 or F1-F2-F3, where Fn is a formant) are low-dimensional descriptions of vowel sounds. One advantage of a formant specification is that a fairly systematic relationship holds between formant pattern and vowel articulation (i.e., the acoustic-to-articulatory conversion). In the classic F1-F2 formant plot, the F1 and F2 frequencies are related principally to tongue height and advancement, respectively. Alternatively, the F2-F1 difference can be interpreted as tongue advancement/retraction. Formant patterns are readily observed in spectrograms or spectra and are among the most salient acoustic properties of speech.

The size of the vowel space, as typically displayed in an F1/F2 plot, is a potential index of the capacity for intelligible speech. Data on the acoustic vowel space in typically developing children have been summarized by Vorperian and Kent (2007). Data for children with speech disorders have been reported for several conditions including dysarthria (Higgins & Hodge, 2001; Liu, Tsao, & Kuhl, 2005), hearing loss (Kent, Osberger, Netsell, & Hustedde, 1987; Liker, Mildner, & Sindija, 2007; Rvachew, Slawinski, Williams, & Green, 1996; Schenk, Baumgartner, & Hamzavi, 2003), and various developmental disorders (Moura et al., 2008). Unusually small areas of the acoustic vowel space are correlated with reduced intelligibility, but it should be noted that some speakers maintain a fairly high level of intelligibility even with a compressed vowel space, so long as other acoustic cues are preserved. Furthermore, vowel-specific formant-frequency differences may have value in characterizing the vocal tract features of particular syndromes (Moura et al., 2008).

Among the most important noise events in speech are the bursts associated with stops and the frication intervals associated with fricatives and affricates. Generally, noise events in speech are characterized by diffuse spectra that possess varying degrees of resonant shaping. Without question, these events carry a great deal of phonetic information. What is less certain is how these acoustic intervals should be characterized. A valuable source of normative data for adults is the article by Jongman, Wayland, & Wong (2000). Some possibilities for the analysis of children's fricative sounds are considered next.

The earliest analyses used spectrograms and spectral analyses to characterize the noise energy in various /s/ distortions (Daniloff, Wilcox, & Stephens, 1986). One outcome of this work was recognition of the large inter- and intraspeaker variability for children who misarticulated the /s/ sound.

Daniloff et al. concluded that /s/ has a wide range of permissible acoustic allophonic variants, and that this sound accommodates a considerable variation in the upper and lower cutoff frequencies of the major noise energy, and the frequency and amplitude of major spectral peaks. An implication of this conclusion is that it may not be worthwhile to focus on fine spectral details for clinical purposes, but rather to emphasize major regions of noise energy. Taking together the results of the Daniloff et al. (1986), Weismer and Elbert (1980), and Munson (2004) studies reviewed earlier, it appears that both temporal and spectral variability are to be expected in children's misarticulated /s/. The variability is at once an interesting feature of misarticulated speech and a challenge to researchers and clinicians who would examine this sound.

Spectral moments were introduced as a speech analysis method by Forrest, Weismer, Milenkovic, and Dougall (1988) who treated FFTs as random probability distributions for which the first four moments (mean, variance, skewness, and kurtosis) were computed. The first spectral moment is the mean or center of gravity of the spectrum. The second moment is the distribution of energy around the mean, typically expressed as the variance or standard deviation. The third moment is skewness, which may appear as the degree of spectral tilt (although its exact meaning depends on the overall shape of the spectrum). The fourth moment is kurtosis, which is often defined as the degree of peakedness of the distribution or spectrum. Figure 5–4 illustrates the use of spectral moments for characterizing two fricatives produced by a child. It should be noted that these descriptions are most valid when the underlying distribution has the shape of the normal probability distribution. In fact, acoustic spectra rarely have that shape. The four moments are not uniform in their value in characterizing noise

spectra, and a major goal of the ensuing discussion is to identify the moments that hold particular value in spectral description.

Spectral moments have been used to describe fricatives in typically and atypically developing speech. Normative data on /s/ production were reported for 26 children aged 9 to 15 years by Flipsen, Shriberg, Weismer, Karlsson, and McSweeny (1999). It was concluded that /s/ can be characterized satisfactorily by data for the midpoint of the /s/ frication presented in a linear scale (as opposed to the Bark scale), with preference for the first and third spectral moments. In addition, the authors noted that the data should be referenced to individual linguistic-phonetic contexts. Rather different conclusions were reached by Nissen and Fox (2005), in a study of adults and children aged 3 to 6 years. Their results indicated that spectral slope and variance, usually neglected in earlier studies of child speech, contributed importantly to the differentiation and classification of the voiceless fricatives. The only measure that separated all for places of fricative articulation was spectral variance. Interestingly, it was also reported that /s/ and /ʃ/ were distinguished more sharply by adults than by children, with a remarkable change in several spectral parameters occurring at about 5 years of age. Munson (2004) compared spectral variability in /s/ production for adults and three groups of children (mean ages of 3;11; 5:04; and 8:04). Spectral variability was defined as changes in the spectral mean (first spectral moment) through the interval of frication noise. Adults produced the /s/ with less variability than the children's groups, who did not differ from one another. In view of the lack of effects of phonetic context on spectral variability, Munson concluded that that the differences between adults and children reflected a "subtle variability in place of articulation for /s/ in the children's productions (p. 58). It should also be noted that

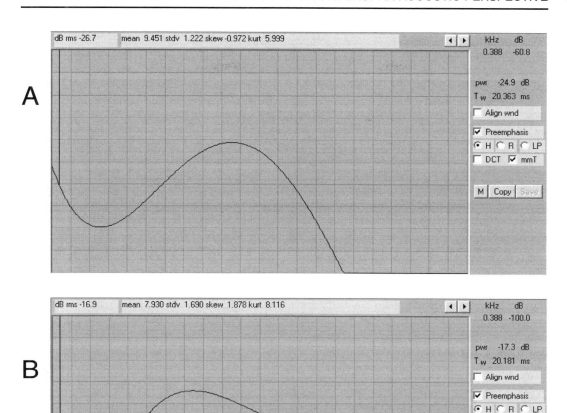

Figure 5–4. Spectral display and spectral moments analysis from a 4-year-old child, using a 20 msec window at the temporal midpoint of /s/ (Panel A) and /sh/ (Panel B). Note that the child's productions of both phonemes were characterized by developmental distortions. Spectral acoustic analyses, as shown here, provide a valuable tool for confirming perceptual impressions. This is seen in Panel B, where the spectrum for /sh/ resembles that for /s/, confirming the perceptual finding that /sh/ sounds somewhat like /s/ in this child's speech.

children's speech may differ from adults' speech in respect to the relative amplitude of its high-frequency components. Short-term spectra of children's speech sounds have been reported to have reduced amplitudes for /s/ and /ʃ/ and for vowel energy above kHz compared to the same speech sounds produced by adults (Pittman, Stelmachowicz, Lewis, & Hoover, 2003). These differences in relative amplitude are highly relevant to understanding the perception and transcription of children's speech.

Spectral analyses also have been reported for the burst of stop consonants, especially the voiceless stops /p t k/. In one of the earliest studies, spectral moments were calculated for word-initial /t/ and /k/ produced by both typically developing children and by children with phonological disorder (Forrest, Weismer, Hodge, Dinnsen, & Elbert, 1990). Using a discriminant function analysis, Forrest et al. achieved 82% correct classification of the two stops using the first, third and fourth moments. The discriminant function developed for the normally speaking children was applied to the phonologically disordered children, no distinction could be made between /t/ and /k/. Bunnell, Polikoff, and McNicholas (2004) compared spectral moments and Bark cepstral analyses for classification of children's word-initial voiceless stops. A better classification rate was achieved for the Bark cepstral analysis. For both types of analysis, four time frames that sampled the initial 40 msec of each burst was needed for the highest rates of correct classification. It is premature to recommend either spectral analysis or Bark cepstral analysis as the preferred method for inspecting stop bursts.

An example that demonstrates both clinical application and the sensitivity of acoustic analysis is for a common type of speech sound error in early speech development, omission or deletion of a segment. This is usually a conspicuous error, readily perceived by adult listeners. However, Weismer (1984) reported that in some cases of an ostensible deletion, acoustic analyses showed that the supposedly deleted consonant had formant transitions appropriate to its phonetic properties. The acoustic cue was not detected by listeners. In another study of apparent omission of word-final stops (Weismer, Dinnsen, & Elbert, 1981), it was shown that two of three children with the omission pattern produced vowel duration differences that were suited to the voicing characteristic of the omitted stop (i.e.,

longer vowels before voiced stops). Apparently, these two children preserved the stop-voicing feature in their speech, even though listeners judged the stop to be deleted. According to data reported by Krause (1982), the vowel duration cue for voicing appears at least by the age of 3 years. She described the early pattern of development as involving both exaggerated vowel lengthening (before voiced stops) and exaggerated vowel shortening (before voiceless stops).

Spectrotemporal Patterns for Liquids and Glides

The liquids in American English are the lateral /l/ and the rhotic /r/, both of which can be problematic for children acquiring speech. Acoustically, liquids are characterized especially by their formant pattern (/r/) or formant-antiformant pattern (/l/). Acoustic analyses for /r/ are illustrated in Figure 5–5. The glides in American English are the palatal /j/ and the labiovelar /w/ (and its voiceless allophone, which may not be used by all speakers. The glides are associated with a relatively gradual formant transition into the following vowel. Acoustic data on correctly produced /w, r, l/ in both children and adults were reported by Dalston (1975). Chaney (1988) studied three groups of children: a group that correctly produced /w, r, l, j/, a group with developmental w/r and w/l substitutions, and a group of articulation-impaired children who had w/r and w/l substitutions. The children with /w, r/ errors produced the glide /j/ with acoustic properties similar to those seen in the control group, but neither of the groups with errors differentiated among /w, r, l/ by either formant frequencies or transition rate. Interestingly, the /w/ produced for target /w/ and in substitution for /r/ and /l/ by some of the children with errors did not

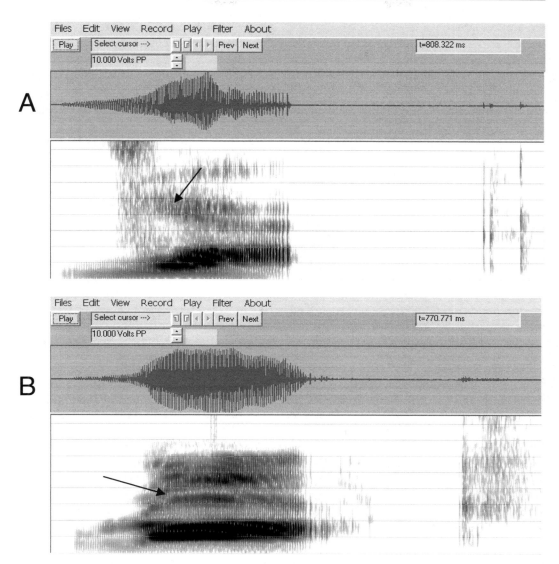

Figure 5–5. Screen display of a waveform and spectrogram in TF32. Panel A shows a production of the word "rock" from a three-year-old typically developing child, where the /r/ phoneme is distorted. Panel B shows a production of the same word by a 6-year-old typically developing child, where the /r/ phoneme is produced appropriately. Note the difference in the 3rd formant frequency (as indicated by the arrows in each panel).

match the acoustic pattern of /w/ as produced by the children without errors. Shuster (1996) showed how speech resynthesis based on linear prediction coding (LPC) can be used to modify disordered productions of /r/ so that they approximate correct productions. Flipsen et al. (2001) suggested that speech-genetics research would be enhanced by the availability of acoustic phenotypes, such as residual distortions of rhotic sounds.

Pagan and Wertzner (2007b) studied the acoustic patterns of two of the three Brazilian Portuguese liquids (/r/, a voiced alveolar tap, and /l/, a voiced alveolar lateral) as produced by typically developing children and by children with a phonological disorder who had r/l substitutions. It was found that the /l/ produced as a substitution for /r/ was different from both the /l/ correctly produced by the phonologically disordered children and the /l/ produced by the control group. The /l/ substituting for /r/ had a longer duration, different steady-state values, and a smaller formant slope. This result is another example of an acoustic differentiation for sounds that are judged to be the same by listeners

Coarticulation

Coarticulation, or the simultaneous adjustment of the articulators to two or more phones, is a basic characteristic of competent adult speech. In forward or anticipatory coarticulation, a phonetic property of a given phone is assumed earlier in the phonetic string. For example, lip rounding for the vowel in the word appears during the initial consonant /s/. In backward or retentive coarticulation, a phonetic property of a given phone is retained to a later position in the phonetic string. An example is the nasalization of the vowel in the word *no*. The development of coarticulation is not well understood, and rather different conclusions have been reached from research on children's speech. In several studies, young children were observed to show more extensive coarticulation than adults (Nittrouer, Studdert-Kennedy, & McGowan, 1989; Nittrouer, Studdert-Kennedy, & Neely, 1996;

Siren & Wilcox, 1995), whereas other studies showed no developmental difference, variable patterns across sounds, or greater coarticulation in adults than children (Flege, 1988; Katz, Kripke, & Tallal, 1991; Kent, 1983; Kuijpers, 1993; Repp, 1986; Sereno, Baum, Marean, & Lieberman, 1987; Sussman, et al., 1996; Turnbaugh, Hoffman, Daniloff, & Absher, 1985). The different results probably can be explained by reference to the different methods of analysis, and the phonetic properties of the speech material interacting with the maturational status of the child. It appears that there is no single maturational pattern of coarticulation for various sounds, and that a child seeks to balance coarticulatory adjustments against contrastive distinctiveness (Gibson & Ohde, 2007; Nittrouer, 1993; Sussman, Duder, Dalston, & Cacciatore, 1999; Sussman, Hoemeke, & McCaffrey, 1992).

Acoustic Correlates of Speaker Intelligibility

A long-term goal in the application of acoustics is to determine the acoustic correlates of intelligibility (see also Chapter 10). Research on this topic is hindered by the potentially large number of acoustic features that can be considered, and also by the fact that speakers can deploy acoustic cues in various combinations to achieve a satisfactory degree of intelligibility. It seems safe to conclude on the basis of available evidence that the same general acoustic properties are relevant to both adult and child speech (Hazen & Markham, 2004).

Research on "clear" versus "conversational" speech holds value in understanding the acoustic bases of speech intelligibility (Picheny et al., 1985, 1986, 1989). Acoustic analyses of the two forms of speech have shown consistent differences, thereby laying a foundation for a general understanding of the acoustic correlates of intelligibility (Picheny et al., 1985, 1986, 1989). As compared to "clear" speech, "conversational" speech tends to have modified or reduced vowels, nonreleased word-final stops, and reduced intensities for obstruents. Although "clear" speech typically is slower than "conversational" speech, it is important to note that enhancements of intelligibility can be achieved even at rapid speaking rates (Krause & Braida, 1995). The acoustic differences between "clear" and "conversational" speech may explain intrinsic intelligibility differences among individual speakers. Bond and Moore (1994) studied the acoustic-phonetic differences between a talker with relatively high intelligibility and two talkers with relatively low intelligibility. The high-intelligibility talker had many acoustic-phonetic properties similar to those described for "clear" speech. In a similar study of individual differences in intelligibility, Bradlow, Torretta, & Pisoni (1996) concluded that global characteristics (e.g., speaking rate and mean F_0 level) did not correlate strongly with intelligibility, but the fine-grained characteristics (F_0 and F_1 variation, formant frequency range for vowels, intersegmental timing) did correlate. The profile of a highly intelligible speaker was one who produced sentences with a relatively wide range of F_0, a relatively expanded vowel space that includes a substantial F_1 variation, precise articulation of the point vowels, and a high precision of intersegmental timing. Therefore, there is an important linkage between two general approaches to the study of intelligibility differences in normal speakers.

Similar results can be seen in studies of dysarthric and deaf speakers that have established fine-grained acoustic characteristics relating to differences in speaker intelligibility (Kent et al., 1989; Metz et al., 1985;

Monsen, 1976; Weismer & Martin, 1992). In the main, the results from dysarthric and deaf speech agree with the results reviewed above for normal speech. That is, the differences in intelligibility appear to be rooted in a common set of fine-grained acoustic measures including vowel formant frequencies and intersegmental timing.

If these results can be generalized to speech development and to developmental speech disorders, then the implication is that fine-grained acoustic properties are the key to understanding differences in speech intelligibility.

Variability as an Index of Precision and Maturation

As earlier sections of this chapter make clear, variability has been a particular focus of research on both typical and atypical speech development. Across motor skills, it is generally presumed that increasing accuracy is a characteristic of skill maturation. One way of gauging accuracy is to determine the variability in a motor response, or, in the case of speech, the acoustic consequences of that motor response. In one of the earliest studies to address this issue, Eguchi and Hirsh (1969) reported that there were nearly continuous decreases in the variability of both F1 and F2 frequencies from 3 to 11 years of age in typically developing children. One interpretation is that motor skill for speech improves with age, and acoustic measures of formant structure reflect this improvement up until the age of puberty. But other acoustic data point to a different conclusion. Nittrouer (1993) reported that the variability in F1 frequency was minimal by the age of 3 years whereas variability in F2 frequency continued to decrease beyond that age. The early accuracy in F1 frequency was related to an early maturation of jaw movement control, given that jaw movement has a strong effect on F1 frequency. In fact, the maturation of motor control over different oral structures is open to discussion. Although it has been reported that children's jaw movements are less variable than lip movements (Green, Moore, & Reilly, 2002; Walsh & Smith, 2002), it also has been shown that there are parallel decreases in the variability of jaw and lip movements with maturation (Walsh & Smith, 2002).

Variability in the temporal patterns of speech also has been examined. The general conclusion is that variability declines with age until late childhood, puberty, or adolescence (Kent & Forner, 1978; Lee, Potamianos, & Narayanan, 1999; Lehman & Sharf, 1989; Munson, 2004; Smith & Kenney, 1999). However, changes in variability are not necessarily uniform across different segments (Kent & Forner, 1978; Smith & Kenney, 1999).

Variability is actually relevant to several developmental issues, including the following:

(a) Estimates of the variability of either spectral or temporal features have been proposed as an index of the maturation of speech motor control, as noted above. Variability, commonly expressed as a standard deviation, is considered as an estimate of precision of articulation. This approach requires analysis of multiple tokens of a given speech target. It is assumed that the speaker is able to create a stable representation of the target behavior from which motor commands to the articulators can be formulated.

(b) In general, the variability in temporal segments is related to speaking rate, such that a slow rate is associated with greater variability. Because children typically have a slower rate of speech than adults, speaking rate is confounded with the maturational factor mentioned in (a) above (Kent & Forner, 1978). Children with a speech-language disorder may have even slower speaking rates than typically developing children. This slow rate may be related to the combined effects of development and disorder.

(c) Variability may be a gauge of category breadth or coarticulatory range. For example, as children add elements to their vowel systems, the allowable range for any one vowel may be adjusted to accommodate the insertion of new vowel sounds. Similarly, variability in producing a particular word may be related to the lexical density for that word. Presumably, a word with a high neighborhood density would be produced more accurately than a word with a low neighborhood density.

(d) Variability in a spectral or temporal feature (or a spectrotemporal property) may be an indication of destabilizing forces. In a dynamic systems perspective, periods of destabilization may be optimum times for intervention.

(e) Measures of temporal pattern are not as sensitive to age and gender variables as are measures of formant or general spectral pattern. Reliability estimates of temporal measures are reviewed in Kent and Read (2002).

Obviously, a simple interpretation of variability is not likely to be correct unless this list can be pruned to one or two applicable alternatives. Unfortunately, many developmental studies were not designed to address each of these factors in an empirical fashion that allows their separation.

The clinical implication is not necessarily that a clinician will record ten or more tokens of a sound pattern and then calculate standard deviations for a selected measurement. Such a procedure may be forbiddingly tedious for both the child and the clinician. Rather, the object is more likely to be to ascertain the stability of production in relation to a clinical objective. Say, for example, that the objective is treatment of a speech sound disorder. Frequently, clinicians want to establish a degree of stability in production of a certain sound pattern before introducing a change of some kind, such as working on another target sound, changing the phonetic context of sound production, or varying prosodic features such as speaking rate or stress.

Sensitivity

Acoustic analysis is capable of resolving fine differences in the timing and spectra of speech sounds. Differences that are not detected by the ear can be detected by suitable acoustic analyses that are performed in the time domain (waveform), frequency domain (FFT or LPC spectrum, cepstrum, or other analysis), or the time-frequency domain (spectrogram or other running spectral display). The issue here is not necessarily quantification, as important as that may be, but identifying the shear presence or absence of an acoustic property. Examples from the literature are discussed below to illustrate the concept for both segmental and suprasegmental aspects of speech.

The sensitivity of acoustic analysis does not necessarily depend on quantification. Sometimes, simply observing the presence or absence of an acoustic phenomenon is sufficient. In some examples given earlier in this chapter, measurements were not always needed. Rather, the person performing the analysis used acoustics as a kind of alternative visual display—a highly sensitive one—to the analysis performed by the ear. This approach made it possible to detect (a) acoustic differences between stressed and unstressed syllables that were not consistently perceived by adults (Munson, Bjo-rum, & Windsor, 2003), (b) small differences in VOT even for stimuli that were not distinguished by adult listeners (Macken & Barton, 1980; Tyler, Edwards, & Saxman (1990), and (c) acoustic evidence of a phonetic feature of a speech sound that was supposedly omitted (Weismer, 1984; Weismer, Dinnsen, & Elbert, 1981).

This "look and listen" strategy can be quite powerful, as it enables the observer (e.g., clinician, researcher) to observe the visual display of speech and to reconcile it with what is heard. Qualitative analysis has much to recommend it. As noted by Liss and Weismer (1992), "traditional acoustic measures of temporal and spectral characteristics of normal speech may not necessarily reveal the inherently 'important' aspects of disordered speech production" (p. 2984). This is not to assert that quantitative analyses are irrelevant to the study of disordered speech, but rather to say that qualitative analyses are a valuable complement to quantitative methods. For additional discussion of this issue, see Weismer and Liss (1991).

Each individual clinician must ask herself or himself whether acoustic tools will make for better clinical services. Technology is only as useful as the use to which it is put. The dramatic progress in speech technology (automatic speech recognition, speech synthesis, no-cost or low-cost speech analysis software) presents a powerful set of tools for the future practice of speech-language pathology.

Conclusion

The first author was a long-term faculty colleague of Larry Shriberg at the University of Wisconsin-Madison. We co-authored a text, *Clinical Phonetics*, now in its third edition.

In preparing the text and the accompanying audiotapes, we accomplished a kind of mutual calibration of our "phonetic" ears as we listened (repeatedly) to samples of children's speech disorders. Our labors began in the pre-DSP days, which meant that speech samples existed physically as pieces of audiotape (analog recordings). I recall seeing strips of tape hanging around the room where we worked. These were eventually assembled by tape-splicing methods into tapes for auditory exercises for phonetic transcription. If we undertook that effort today, it would be very different. We would use digital signal processing to record, store, and analyze the samples. Rather than compare notes strictly on our respective auditory impressions (which differed now and then) of each sample, we would examine visual displays of acoustic information. Would this information be helpful? I have no doubt that it would.

References

Boersma, P., & Weenink, D. (2008). PRAAT (computer program). University of Amsterdam; available at http://www.fon.hum.uva.nl/praat .

Bond, Z. S., & Moore, T. J. (1994). A note on the acoustic-phonetic characteristics of inadvertently clear speech. *Speech Communication, 14,* 325-337.

Borden, S. J., Harris, K. S., & Raphael, L. J. (1994). *Speech science primer: Physiology, acoustics and perception of speech.* Baltimore: Williams & Wilkins.

Bradlow, A. R., Torretta, G. M., & Pisoni, D. B. (1996). Intelligibility of normal speech. I. Global and fine-grained acoustic-phonetic talker characteristics. *Speech Communication, 20,* 255-272.

Bunnell, H. T., Polikoff, J., & McNicholas, J. (2004). *Spectral moment vs. Bark cepstral analysis of children's word-initial voiceless*

stops. Available at http://www.asel.udel.edu/speech/reports/icslp04/ICSLP04_paper.pdf .

Catts, H. W., & Jensen, P. J. (1983). Speech timing of phonologically disordered children: Voicing contrast of initial and final stop consonants. *Journal of Speech and Hearing Research, 26,* 501-510.

Chaney, C. (1988). Acoustic analysis of correct and misarticulated semivowels. *Journal of Speech and Hearing Research, 31,* 275-287.

Dalston, R. M. (1975). Acoustic characteristics of English /w, r, l/ spoken correctly by young children and adults. *Journal of the Acoustical Society of America, 57,* 462-469.

Daniloff, R. G., Wilcox, K., & Stephens, M. I. (1980). An acoustic-articulatory description of children's defective /s/ productions. *Journal of Communication Disorders, 13,* 347-363.

Eguchi, S., & Hirsh, I. J. (1969). Development of speech sounds in children. *Acta Otolaryngologica, Supplementum, 257,* 1-51.

Flege, J. E. (1988). Anticipatory and carry-over nasal coarticulation in the speech of children and adults. *Journal of Speech and Hearing Research, 31,* 525-536.

Flipsen, P., Jr., Shriberg, L., Weismer, G., Karlsson, H., & McSweeny, J. (1999). Acoustic characteristics of /s/ in adolescents. *Journal of Speech, Language, and Hearing Research, 42,* 663-677.

Flipsen, P., Jr., Shriberg, L., Weismer, G., Karlsson, H., & McSweeny, J. (2001). Acoustic phenotypes for speech-genetics studies: Reference data for residual /Er/ distortion. *Clinical Linguistics and Phonetics, 15,* 603-630.

Forrest, K., & Rockman, B. K. (1988). Acoustic and perceptual analysis of word-initial stop consonants in phonologically disordered children. *Journal of Speech, Language, and Hearing Research, 31,* 449-459.

Forrest, K., Weismer, G., Hodge, M., Dinnsen, D. A., & Elbert, M. (1990). Statistical analysis of word-initial K and T produced by normal and phonologically disordered children. *Clinical Linguistics and Phonetics, 4,* 327-340.

Forrest, K., Weismer, G., Milenkovic, P., & Dougal, R. N. (1988). Statistical analysis of word-initial voiceless obstruents: Preliminary data.

Journal of the Acoustical Society of America, *84*, 115–123.

Gerken, L., & McGregor, K. (1998). An overview of prosody and its role in normal and disordered child language. *American Journal of Speech-Language Pathology*, *7*, 38–48.

Gibson, T., & Ohde, R. N. (2007). F2 locus equations: Phonetic descriptors of coarticulation in 17- to 22-month-old children. *Journal of Speech, Language, and Hearing Research*, *50*, 97–108.

Green, J. R., Moore, C. A., & Reilly, K. U. (2002). The sequential development of jaw and lip control in speech. *Journal of Speech, Language, and Hearing Research*, *45*, 66–79.

Gurgueira, A. L. (2006). *Estudo acústico dos fonemas surdos e sonoros do português do Brasil, em crianças com distúrbio fonológico apresentando o processo fonológico de ensurdecimento* [Acoustic study of the voice onset time (vot) and the vowel duration for the distinctiion of voicing of the stop sounds of the Brazilian Portuguese in children with typical development and with phonological disorders]. Doctoral dissertation. Department of Linguistics of the Faculty of Philosophy, Sciences and Literature and Languages from the University of São Paulo, Brazil.

Hazen, V., & Markham, D. (2004). Acoustic-phonetic correlates of talker intelligibility for adults and children. *Journal of the Acoustical Society of America*, *116*, 3108–3118.

Henrich, J., Lowit, A., Schalling, E., & Mennen, I. (2006). Rhythmic disturbances in ataxic dysarthria: A comparison of different measures and speech tasks. *Journal of Medical Speech-Language Pathology*, *14*, 291–296.

Higgins, C. M., & Hodge, M. M. (2001). F2/F1 vowel quadrilateral area in young children with and without dysarthria. *Canadian Acoustics*, *29*, 66–68.

Huggins, A. W. F. (1980). Better spectrograms from children's speech: A research note. *Journal of Speech and Hearing Research*, *23*, 19–27.

Ingram, K., Bunta, F., & Ingram, D. (2004). Digital data collection and analysis. *Language,*

Speech, and Hearing Services in Schools, *35*, 112–121.

Jongman, A., Wayland, R., & Wong, S. (2000). Acoustic characteristics of English fricatives. *Journal of the Acoustical Society of America*, *108*, 1252–1263.

Katz, W. F., Kripke, C., & Tallal, P. (1991). Anticipatory coarticulation in the speech of adults and young children. *Journal of Speech and Hearing Research*, *34*, 1222–1232.

Kehoe, M., Stoel-Gammon, C., & Buder, E. H. (1995). Acoustic correlates of stress in young children's speech. *Journal of Speech and Hearing Research*, *38*, 338–350.

Kent, R. D. (1976). Anatomical and neuromuscular maturation of the speech mechanism: Evidence from acoustic studies. *Journal of Speech and Hearing Research*, *19*, 421–447.

Kent, R. D. (1983). Segmental organization of speech. In P. F. MacNeilage (Ed.), *The production of speech*. New York: Springer-Verlag.

Kent, R. D. (1996). Hearing and believing: Some limits to the auditory-perceptual assessment of speech and voice disorders. *American Journal of Speech-Language Pathology*, *7*, 7–23.

Kent, R. D., & Forner, L. L. (1980). Speech segment durations in sentence recitations by children and adults. *Journal of Phonetics*, *8*, 157–168.

Kent, R. D., & Hustad, K. C. (2009). Speech production, development. In L. Squire, T. Albright, F. Bloom, F. Gage, & N. Spitzer (Eds.), *New encyclopedia of neuroscience*. Oxford: Elsevier.

Kent, R. D., & Murray, A. D. (1982). Acoustic features of infant vocalic utterances. *Journal of the Acoustical Society of America*, *72*, 353–365.

Kent, R. D., Osberger, M. J., Netsell, R., & Hustedde, C. G. (1987). Phonetic development in twins who differ in auditory function. *Journal of Speech and Hearing Disorders*, *52*, 64–75.

Kent, R. D., & Read, C. (2002). *The acoustic analysis of speech* (2nd ed.). Albany, NY: Singular/Thomson Learning.

Kent, R. D., & Tilkens, C. (2007). Oral motor foundations of speech. In S. McLeod (Ed.), *The international guide to speech acquisition.* Albany, NY: Delmar.

Kent, R. D., & Vorperian, H. K. (1995). Anatomic development of the craniofacial-oral-laryngeal systems: A review. *Journal of Medical Speech-Language Pathology, 3,* 145–190. (Also published as a monograph (1995) San Diego, CA: Singular.).

Kent, R. D., Weismer, G., Kent, J. F., & Rosenbek, J. C. (1989). Toward phonetic intelligibility testing in dysarthria. *Journal of Speech and Hearing Disorders, 54,* 482–499.

Klatt, D. H. (1976). Linguistic uses of segmental duration in English: Acoustic and perceptual evidence. *Journal of the Acoustical Society of America, 59,* 1208–1221.

Krause, J. C., & Braida, L. D. (1995). The effects of speaking rate on the intelligibility of speech for various speaking modes. *Journal of the Acoustical Society of America, 98,* 2982.

Krause, S. E. (1982). Developmental use of vowel duration as a cue to postvocalic stop consonant voicing. *Journal of Speech and Hearing Research, 25,* 388–393.

Kuijpers, C. (1993). Temporal aspects of the voiced-voiceless distinction in speech development of young Dutch children. *Journal of Phonetics, 21,* 313–327.

Lee, S., Potamianos, A., & Narayanan, S. (1999). Acoustics of children's speech: Developmental changes of temporal and spectral parameters. *Journal of the Acoustical Society of America, 105,* 1455–1468.

Lehman, M. E., & Sharf, D. J. (1989). Perception/production relationships in the development of the vowel duration cue to final consonant voicing. *Journal of Speech and Hearing Research, 32,* 803–815.

Liker, M., Mildner, V., & Sindija, B. (2007). Acoustic analysis of the speech of children with cochlear implants: A longitudinal study. *Clinical Linguistics and Phonetics, 21,* 1–11.

Liss, J. M., & Weismer, G. (1992). Qualitative acoustic analysis in the study of motor speech disorders. *Journal of the Acoustical Society of America, 92,* 2984–2987.

Liu, H. M., Tsao, F. M., & Kuhl, P. K. (2005). The effect of reduced vowel working space on speech intelligibility in Mandarin-speaking young adults with cerebral palsy. *Journal of the Acoustical Society of America, 117,* 3879–3889.

Low, E. L., Grabe, E., & Nolan, F. (2000). Quantitative characterizations of speech rhythm: Syllable-timing in Singapore English. *Language and Speech, 43,* 377–401.

Macken, M. A., & Barton, D. (1980). The acquisition of the voicing contrast in English: Study of voice onset time in word-initial stop consonants. *Journal of Child Language, 7,* 41–74.

Metz, D., Samar, V., Schiavetti, N., Sitler, R., & Whitehead, R. (1985). Acoustic dimensions of hearing-impaired speakers' intelligibility. *Journal of Speech and Hearing Research, 28,* 345–355.

Monsen, R. B. (1976). Normal and reduced phonological space: The productions of English vowels by deaf adolescents. *Journal of Phonetics, 4,* 189–198.

Moura, C. P., Cunha, L. M., Vilarinho, H., Cunha, M. J., Freitas, D., Palha, M., et al. (2008). Voice parameters in children with Down syndrome. *Journal of Voice, 22,* 34–42.

Munson, B. (2004). Variability in /s/ production in children and adults: Evidence from dynamic measures of spectral mean. *Journal of Speech, Language, and Hearing Research, 47,* 58–69.

Munson, B., Bjorum, E. M., & Windsor, J. (2003). Acoustic and perceptual correlates of stress in nonwords produced by children with suspected developmental apraxia of speech and children with phonological disorder. *Journal of Speech, Language, and Hearing Research, 46,* 189–202.

Nissen, S. L., & Fox, R. A. (2005). Acoustic and spectral characteristics of young children's fricative productions: A developmental perspective. *Journal of the Acoustical Society of America, 118,* 2570–2578.

Nittrouer, S. (1993). The emergence of mature gestural patterns is not uniform: Evidence from an acoustic study. *Journal of Speech and Hearing Research, 36,* 959–972.

Nittrouer, S., Studdert-Kennedy, M., & McGowan, R. S. (1989). The emergence of phonetic segments: Evidence from the spectral structure of fricative-vowel syllables spoken by children and adults. *Journal of Speech and Hearing Research, 32,* 120–132.

Nittrouer, S., Studdert-Kennedy, M., & Neely, S. (1996). Howe children learn to organize their speech gestures: Further evidence from fricative-vowel syllables. *Journal of Speech and Hearing Research, 39,* 379–389.

Pagan, L. O., & Wertzner, H. F. (2007a). *Perceptual analysis of the three Brazilian Portuguese liquid sounds.* Poster presented at the 27th World Congress of the International Association of Logopedics and Phoniatrics, Copenhagen, Denmark.

Pagan, L. O., & Wertzner, H. F. (2007b). *Description of the acoustic characteristics of the liquid sounds /l/ and /r/ in phonologically disordered children.* Poster presented at the 2nd International Association of Logopedics and Phoniatrics Composium, Sao Paulo, Brazil, March 24–25.

Picheny, M. A., Durlach, N. I., & Braida, L. D. (1985). Speaking clearly for the hard of hearing I: Intelligibility differences between clear and conversational speech. *Journal of Speech and Hearing Research, 28,* 96–103.

Picheny, M. A., Durlach, N. I., & Braida, L. D. (1986). Speaking clearly for the hard of hearing II: Acoustic characteristics of clear and conversational speech. *Journal of Speech and Hearing Research, 29,* 434–446.

Picheny, M. A., Durlach, N. I., & Braida, L. D. (1989). Speaking clearly for the hard of hearing III: An attempt to determine the contribution of speaking rate to difference in intelligibility between clear and conversational speech. *Journal of Speech and Hearing Research, 32,* 600–603.

Pittman, A. L., Stelmachowicz, P. G., Lewis, D. E., & Hoover, B. M. (2003). Spectral characteristics of speech at the ear. *Journal of Speech, Language, and Hearing Research, 46,* 649–657.

Read, C., Buder, E., & Kent, R. D. (1990). Speech analysis systems: A survey. *Journal of Speech and Hearing Research, 33,* 363–374.

Repp, B. (1986). Some observations on the development of anticipatory coarticulation. *Journal of the Acoustical Society of America, 79,* 1616–1619.

Rvachew, S., Slawinski, E. G., Williams, M., & Green, C. L. (1996). Formant Frequencies of vowels produced by infants with and without early onset ititis media. *Canadian Acoustics/ Acoustique Canadienne, 24,* 19–28.

Schenk, B. S., Baumgartner, W. D., & Hamzavi, J. S. (2003). Changes in vowel quality after cochlear implantation. *ORL Journal of Otorhinolaryngology and Related Specialties, 65,* 184–188.

Schwartz, G. R. (1995). Effect of familiarity on word duration in children's speech: A preliminary investigation. *Journal of Speech and Hearing Research, 38,* 76–84.

Sereno, J. A., Baum, S. R., Marean, G. C., & Lieberman, P. (1987). Acoustic analyses and perceptual data on anticipatory coarticulation in adults and children. *Journal of the Acoustical Society of America, 81,* 512–519.

Shuster, L. I. (1996). Linear predictive coding parameter manipulation/synthesis of incorrectly produced /r/. *Journal of Speech and Hearing Research, 39,* 827–832.

Siren, K. A., & Wilcox, K. A. (1995). Effects of lexical meaning and practiced productions on coarticulation in children's and adults' speech. *Journal of Speech and Hearing Research, 38,* 351–359.

Smith, B. L., & Kenney, M. K. (1999). A longitudinal study of the development of temporal properties of speech production: Data from 4 children. *Phonetica, 56,* 73–102.

Snow, D. (1994). Phrase-final syllable lengthening and intonation in early child speech. *Journal of Speech, Language, and Hearing Research, 37,* 831–840.

Snow, D. (1998). Prosodic markers of syntactic boundaries in the speech of 4-year-old children with normal and disordered language development. *Journal of Speech, Language, and Hearing Research, 41,* 1158–1170.

Sussman, H. M., Duder, C., Dalston, E., & Cacciatore, A. (1999). An acoustic analysis of the development of CV coarticulation. *Journal of Speech, Language, and Hearing Research*, *42*, 1080–1096.

Sussman, H. M., Hoemeke, K. A., & McCaffrey, H. A. (1992). Locus equations as index of coarticulation for place of articulation distinctions in children. *Journal of Speech and Hearing Research*, *35*, 769–781.

Sussman, H. M., Minifie, F. D., Buder, E. H., Stoel-Gammon, C., & Smith, J. (1996). Consonant-vowel interdependencies in babbling and early words. *Journal of Speech and Hearing Research*, *39*, 424–433.

Thom, S., Hoit, J., Hixon, T., & Smith, A. (2005). Velopharyngeal function during vocalization in infants. *The Cleft Palate-Craniofacial Journal* [published online 15 November; doi: 10.1597/05-113].

Turnbaugh, K., Hoffman, P., Daniloff, R. G., & Absher, R. (1985). Stop-vowel coarticulation in 3-year-olds, 5-year-olds, and adults. *Journal of the Acoustical Society of America*, *77*, 1256–1258.

Tyler, A. A., Edwards, M. L., & Saxman, J. H. (1990). Acoustic validation of phonological knowledge and its relationship to treatment. *Journal of Speech and Hearing Disorders*, *55*, 251–261

Vorperian, H. K., & Kent, R. D. (2007). Vowel acoustic space development in children: A synthesis of acoustic and anatomic data. *Journal of Speech, Language, and Hearing Research*, *50*, 1510–1545.

Walsh, B., & Smith, A. (2002). Articulatory movements in adolescents: Evidence for protracted development of speech motor control processes. *Journal of Speech, Language, and Hearing Research*, *45*, 1119–1133.

Wang, Y.-T., Kent, R. D., Duffy, J. R., & Thomas, J. E. (2005). Dysarthria in traumatic brain injury: A breath group and intonational analysis. *Folia Phoniatrica et Logopaedica*, *57*, 59–89.

Wang, Y.-T., Kent, R. D., Duffy, J. R., Thomas, J. E., & Fredericks, G. V. (2006). Dysarthria following cerebellar mutism secondary to resection of a fourth ventricle medulloblastoma: A case study. *Journal of Medical Speech-Language Pathology*, *14*, 109–122.

Weismer, G. 1984). Acoustic analysis strategies for the refinement of phonological analyses. In M. Elbert, D. A. Dinnsen, & G. Weismer (Eds.), *Phonological theory and the misarticulation child* (pp. 30–52). *ASHA Monographs* (No. 22). Rockville, MD: American Speech-Language-Hearing Association.

Weismer, G., Dinnsen, D., & Elbert, M. (1981). A study of the voicing distinction associated with omitted, word-final stops. *Journal of Speech and Hearing Disorders*, *46*, 320–328.

Weismer, G., & Elbert, M. (1982). Temporal characteristics of "functionally" misarticulated /s/ in 4- to 6-years-old children. *Journal of Speech and Hearing Research*, *25*, 275–287.

Weismer, G., & Liss, J. M. (1991). Acoustic/perceptual taxonomies of disordered speech. In C. Moore, K. Yorkston, & D. Beukelman (Eds.), *Dysarthria and apraxia of speech: Perspectives on management* (pp. 245–270). Baltimore: Brookes.

Weismer, G., & Martin, R. (1992). Acoustic and perceptual approaches to the study of intelligibility. In R. Kent (Ed.), *Intelligibility in speech disorders* (pp. 67–118). Philadelphia: John Benjamins.

CHAPTER 6

Computer Processing for Analysis of Speech Disorders

JOHN-PAUL HOSOM

Motivation for Computer-Based Speech Processing

Computers for Assisting Humans

Over the past 65 years, the computer has been an effective assistant to humans on a wide range of tasks. The development of the modern computer began with the need to quickly compute mathematical tables (Weik, 1961). Since then, the number of applications has grown immensely, and the computer is now widely used to assist humans with tasks as varied as composing letters, driving cars, and taking photographs.

The computer has several strengths that enable it to effectively complement human decision-making. First, the computer can perform many mathematical computations very quickly. This may eliminate drudgery from tedious tasks, and it also enables tasks that would simply not be possible at human rates of computation. Second, the computer makes almost no errors in its computations.

(The errors that a computer does make are typically a result of poor programming design by a human, which is effectively a human error rather than a computer error.) This lack of error results in an extremely high level of consistency. Third, computers are now both compact and cost effective, allowing their widespread use in almost any location.

Because software that runs on a computer is continually evolving, this chapter presents a "snapshot" of the current algorithms and use of computers for speech processing and the analysis of speech disorders. The use of computers has become much more prevalent within the last decade, and yet a number of significant improvements still lie ahead.

Reliability of Measurements

Whereas humans excel at reasoning and adapting to new environments, computers provide precise and repeatable measurement and computation of signals. If a human estimates the strength or quality of a signal without a clear, objective basis for measurement, the same person may give different results at different times. Two people may yield even larger measurement differences under these circumstances. As an example, consider the task of locating the boundary between a voiced fricative and a vowel in a waveform or spectrogram. If one person is given the same task and the same recording every day for one week, the results will probably be slightly different from day to day. This *intralabeler agreement* may be consistent within a threshold of 10 msec, but vary considerably within that threshold. If ten people with the same technical background are given the same task and the same recording, results will likely have even more variance. This *interlabeler agreement* may be consistent within a larger threshold of, say, 30 msec, with different people using criteria that are different in subtle ways. The reason for this variability is that speech is a complex, context-dependent, environment-dependent, and speaker-dependent signal, even for a given phoneme sequence. There are a large number of ways in which the speech signal can be affected, including background noise, speaker characteristics such as age, gender, and accent, and within-speaker variability due to prosodic or emotional factors. The guidelines that humans use to measure and quantify the speech signal, such as determining phoneme identity, phoneme boundaries, or formant locations, are not numerous or precise enough for perfect repeatability of all measures in all cases. In the case of phonetic labeling, interlabeler agreement of American English phoneme identity has been measured at 71% using a set of 55 phonemes (Cole, Oshika, Noel, Lander, & Fanty, 1994), and average interlabeler agreement of phoneme boundaries has been measured at 93.8% within a 20-msec threshold (Hosom, 2009).

A computer, on the other hand, despite being unable to generalize well to new situations, will always produce the same result when given the same input and when using the same software. Although a human is limited to being in one place at one time, identical computer software can be used on a large number of different computers. This duplication of software enables the same decision process to be used at many remote locations. Thus, the computer has not only greater consistency than an individual human in repeated measurements, but also greater consistency than a group of humans when there is a large-scale, geographically diverse study or application. This consistency has the potential to improve the collection, measurement, and analysis of speech data, providing reliable and repeatable data measures.

Strengths and Weaknesses of Computer-Based Speech Processing

Computers have been applied to speech processing almost since the development of the modern computer (Levinson, 2005, p. 1). Computers have a number of strengths when applied to speech-processing tasks. For data collection, computers can record high-quality audio directly to the computer's hard drive, reducing noise from the recording process, automatically segmenting recordings into manageable units, and automatically naming audio files for easy reference (e.g., Shobaki, Hosom, & Cole, 2000). For data analysis and visualization, computers can perform complicated mathematical operations, such as computing the Fourier Transform to display spectrograms. Some kinds of analysis can only be done in practice by computer, such as digital removal of formant resonances from a vowel in order to estimate the airflow characteristics at the glottis (Kent & Read, 2002, p. 100). As we will see in this chapter, computers can also be used to compute the probabilities of different speech events (e.g., the probabilities of different phonemes), and select the most-likely event as a final result. These probabilities can be used to provide a ranked list of likely events, in order of decreasing probability. Finally, computers can process many kinds of information much faster than humans, often generating results nearly instantaneously.

Computers, however, have a number of weaknesses. One primary disadvantage of computer analysis of speech is that the computer does not process speech in the same way that the human brain processes speech. This difference in methods results in the computer making decisions that are obviously incorrect to a human. Computers are only as good as the models they use, and current computational models for speech processing are much simpler than human speech processing. These relatively simplistic models sometimes have difficulty in tasks that humans consider quite basic, such as identifying formant locations in a spectrum, identifying pitch periods (the region from the beginning of one glottal pulse to the next glottal pulse), and distinguishing between phoneme types such as labial stop and alveolar stop.

A second weakness is that computers generally will provide the same kind of output regardless of the quality of the input signal. If an utterance is inappropriate for a particular analysis, due to issues such as excessive background noise or incorrect phoneme sequence, a human may easily identify the utterance as data that should be excluded from analysis. A computer is not always programmed to decide between acceptable and unacceptable speech data, due to the wide variety of forms that unacceptable data can take. The computer will then process this signal and generate a result, even though this result should not be utilized. There is then the risk that final results from analysis will be negatively impacted. This risk may be alleviated by automated verification during data collection and human verification of speech input or computer output, but human verification can be time consuming and in some cases impractical.

Considerations for Computer Processing of Speech Signals

As pointed out by Kent, Pagan-Neves, Hustad, and Fiszbein Wertzner (Chapter 5), the computer has become a useful tool in the field of speech processing, and the potential use of computers for speech processing is even greater. The computer's consistency, widespread use, and processing speed are obvious advantages. In addition, the computer can analyze the speech signal at a level of detail not possible by humans. However, computers are only as good as the models they use, and current models do not provide the flexibility and accuracy of a human expert. Therefore, computers have had notable success in some areas of speech processing, especially data collection and verification, while not yet being commonly used for more difficult tasks such as recognizing conversational speech from young children. It is important to ensure that as the difficulty of a task increases, the computer is provided sufficient constraints when developing computational models. As research progresses and computational models become more powerful, computers are expected to take on increasingly difficult tasks. In this chapter we discuss current techniques and models, and describe how they are applied to the analysis of speech disorders.

Computer-Based Data Collection and Analysis

Computer-Based Data Collection

In computer-based data collection, the computer presents the user with explanatory messages and instructions, prompts the subject, and records their response. Messages and prompts can be presented in a number of modalities: video only (in which a picture is presented on the computer screen instead of in a booklet (Shriberg, Kwiatkowski, & Snyder 1986)), audio only (e.g., the recorded verbal request, "Repeat after me: 'helicopter'"), audio with an accompanying picture on the screen (e.g., the verbal request "What is this?," with a picture of a chicken on the screen), written text on the screen with no audio (e.g., the written instruction "Please say 'hammer'"), or audio with an accompanying video (e.g., a video of a human examiner or a computer-generated "animated agent" (Cole et al., 1999; Shobaki, Hosom, & Cole, 2000). The recording can start immediately after (or sometimes just before) the end of the prompt, and recording ends either when the person stops speaking or after a predetermined time limit. Recordings can be of audio, video, or input from a touch-sensitive screen (e.g., Coulston, Klabbers, de Villiers, & Hosom, 2007). The collection software may, when necessary, allow the user to pause in order to take a break, repeat a prompt when errors are detected in the data (e.g., detecting only

silence when a word is expected), or resume a partially completed data collection at a later date. It has been found that, in comparison with booklet-based data collection that does not use a computer, computer-based collection can be equally effective, efficient, and engaging (Shriberg, Kwiatkowski, & Snyder, 1989). Although data collection without a computer may be more effective for children who require frequent eye contact, computer-based collection may be more effective for some children due to a greater level of engagement (Shriberg, Kwiatkowski, & Snyder, 1989).

The collection of audio and/or video data by computer has a number of advantages over more traditional techniques. The computer presents the same protocol in exactly the same way to all subjects, practically eliminating variability in the elicitation of data. Each utterance from each subject is stored individually in its own file on the computer, so segmentation of a long recording session into relevant utterances is not necessary. Problems during recording, such as data clipping (when the input sound is too loud or the recording level is too sensitive, and the recorded sound becomes distorted), excessive background noise, or lack of response to a prompt, can be automatically detected. The subject can then be reprompted for these utterances, either immediately or at the end of the recording session. As noted previously, the same software can be used at numerous sites, allowing large-scale data collection with minimal human oversight. Finally, because a subject's utterances are recorded and saved indefinitely, the subject responses can be reviewed and interpreted later by more than one human expert. Playback of specific regions of the speech signal is typically easier by computer than by analog tape. If there are any questions about a subject's response, it is easy to go back to the original data to have those questions answered.

The reliability and validity of transcription and scoring from analog recordings, as compared to live transcription and scoring, has been confirmed (Shriberg & Kent, 2003). The transcription of computer-based recordings has been shown to have a somewhat (not statistically significant) smaller time requirement than transcription of analog data (Shriberg et al., 2005). Data transcribed from computer-based recordings show reliability and validity comparable with analog recordings at the group level, although differences between recording types may affect transcription at the level of individual samples (Shriberg et al., 2005). As noted in Shriberg et al. (2005),

> . . . transcribers appeared to favor the digital system for glossing, transcription, and prosody-voice coding. In comparison to the analog system, the digital system was perceived as having a higher quality signal and more efficient operational features. Transcribers reported that, in comparison to the analog system, the digital system allowed them to find the speech sample much more easily and rapidly among other recorded tasks in the assessment protocol.

Data Collection Requirements

Because of the unique requirements of each data collection, computer-based data collection software must be tailored to each new project. As a result, the development of such software is time-consuming, and a high-quality collection is often achieved only after several iterations of testing on the expected user population.

A number of factors must be kept in mind when designing data-collection software. First, is the protocol going to be copied from an existing human-interviewer protocol? If so, are there limitations that must be considered? For example, if the protocol specifies that the examiner continues testing until a subject makes two errors in a row, this will require real-time analysis of the data. If this analysis is to be performed by the computer, then there are subsequent questions about the accuracy of the computer's analysis. If the analysis is to be performed by a human attendant, then the software must have an interface for both the subject and the attendant, and the subject should, ideally, not see the attendant's interface or responses.

A second factor that must be considered is how the data are expected to be used, and how the data might be used in the future by other researchers. (It is assumed here that the collection of any human-subjects data has met with approval from the appropriate Institutional Review Board, and that permission has been given to retain the data indefinitely, transfer the data to other research sites, and allow data to be used in future studies.) For example, although high-quality audio recordings may be required, it may not be necessary to sample the data at 44.1 kHz, the standard sampling rate for audio CDs. A sampling rate of 16 kHz will capture all of the speech-related information for adult speakers and consume less storage space. As a result, 16 kHz has become a standard sampling rate for computer processing of speech. However, a sampling rate of 25 kHz or higher may be required to capture the high-frequency energy in strong fricatives of very young children (Kent & Read, 2002, p. 197). In some cases, a head-mounted microphone may be advantageous, as it keeps the microphone a constant distance from the user's mouth. In other cases, getting the user to wear such a microphone may be impractical, and a desktop microphone may be required (Shriberg & Kent, 2003, p. 382). The type of microphone is also an important consideration, whether it should be dynamic or condenser, with a cardioid pattern or omnidirectional (Chial, 2003, p. 3). If the fundamental frequency (F_0) may be information of interest, either for the proposed study or in the future, it can be important to ensure that frequencies as low as 50 Hz are captured by the microphone. Some headset microphones have a low-frequency cutoff of 200 Hz, recording only frequencies above 200 Hz. Although recordings made with such microphones are suitable for many speech-related purposes, and although F_0 can often be reconstructed from higher frequency harmonics, the fundamental frequency itself will be missing from the data for all but the highest pitched voices. If exact determination of F_0 is required, or if characteristics of the glottal source are to be analyzed, microphone characteristics can be an important consideration.

A review of computer-based data collection and a detailed list of important considerations for computer-based recording is given by Ingram, Bunta, and Ingram (2004).

Data Analysis

After recording by computer, data can be transcribed manually using a software interface, and these transcriptions can then be analyzed by computer software. Two programs for computer analysis of transcriptions are SALT (Systematic Analysis of Language Transcripts) and PEPPER (Programs to Examine Phonetic and Phonologic Evaluation Records) (Weston, Shriberg, & Miller, 1989). SALT analysis includes pause and timing statistics, frequency of items such as topic change, and morphological analysis. Pepper

analysis includes analysis of phoneme errors, phonemic feature analysis, and the Percentage Consonants Correct (PCC) metric (Shriberg, Austin, Lewis, McSweeny, & Wilson, 1997).

Computer systems can also provide spectrograms, estimate fundamental frequency (F_0), estimate formant frequencies and bandwidths, and estimate the probabilities of certain speech events (e.g., Kent & Read, 2002; Rabiner & Juang, 1993). For example, a commonly used software package, Praat (Boersma & Weenink, 2008), provides F_0, spectrum, formant, glottal-closure instant, jitter, shimmer, voice break, and intensity analysis. These analysis functions have parameters that can be used to "tune" the system to the characteristics of the data being analyzed, for greater accuracy. Data can be saved in text or binary format. Phoneme labels and other annotations can be created and saved in text files. In addition, a sequence of operations can be specified and then easily repeated any number of times. Another software package, Wavesurfer (Beskow & Sjölander, 2000), also provides many of the same functions as Praat, although using different algorithms and parameters for F_0, formant, and other parameter estimation. Other software includes MultiSpeech (KayPENTAX, 2008), SpeechView (Carmell, Hosom, & Cole, 1999), Speech Filing System (Huckvale, 2008), and Speech Studio (SpeechStudio, 2008), with a total of over 30 software packages currently available. Each software package has been designed with specific needs and end users in mind, and each tends to have certain advantages and disadvantages for a particular application. When selecting a system for use, one must consider not only of the accuracy of analysis, but also the easy and flexibility of recording and playback, the number of data channels available, editing functions, documentation, compatibility of data formants, and processing time and memory requirements (Read, Buder, & Kent, 1992).

Automatic Measurement of Features of the Speech Signal

The Speech Signal

The speech signal can be analyzed and described in a number of different ways, including the signal's energy, durations, spectrum, formants, fundamental frequency, and glottal source (see also Kent et al., Chapter 5, for additional discussion of these terms). We now discuss methods for measuring each of these descriptions, or features, using a computer. Most of the explanations here will serve only as an introduction to the topic. The references describe methods in more detail, if actual implementation is desired.

First, we assume that the waveform has been digitally sampled, and is notated $x(t)$ for discrete time samples $t = 0 \ldots T$, where 0 is the beginning of a recording and T is the end of a recording. The values of x measure the amplitude of this signal as it varies over time. In an analog signal, the amplitude is measured in units of micropascals; in a digital signal, the amplitude is a unitless number that has a maximum range from -32768 to $+32767$. (Although one can calibrate a digital signal so that, for example, an amplitude value of 64 corresponds to 20 micropascals, in most computer systems such calibration is not performed. The digital amplitude values therefore are relative to an unknown scale, and are hence considered unitless.) The time points at which the signal is measured depend on the *sampling frequency*, or the number of measurements obtained every second.

Energy

The energy of the speech signal is a measurement of the strength of the signal. The normalized energy, E, of a signal x at a point in time t can be computed by

$$E(t) = \frac{\sum_{p=t-W/2}^{t+W/2} x^2(p)}{W} \tag{1}$$

where W is the size of the analysis window, in samples (Rabiner & Schafer, 1978, p. 119). This computation is illustrated in Figure 6–1. The total energy is given in the numerator, and the normalized energy, E, is the total energy divided by the length of the analysis window, W. Normalizing by W allows comparison of energy values computed with different window lengths. This measure of energy can be better correlated with the human perception of loudness by expressing energy on the logarithm scale. The unit of bels can be used to measure energy, with

$$E_{bel}(t) = \log(E_1(t)/E_0) \tag{2}$$

where $E_1(t)$ is the linear energy of the signal at time t (computed using Eqn (1)) and E_0 is a reference-level energy. A typical value for E_0 in an analog signal is 20 micropascals, which is close to the average absolute threshold of human hearing for a 1000-Hz sinusoid (Moore, 1997, p. 10). In a digital signal, because the amplitude values are unitless, the reference value E_0 can be any arbitrary number, and for convenience a value of 1.0 is chosen. For speech, the units of bels tend to be in a smaller range than one would prefer to work with, and so a more common scale is decibels, or dB, obtained by multiplying the bel scale by a factor of 10. For a digital signal, where $E_0 = 1$, this becomes:

$$E_{dB}(t) = 10 \cdot \log(E_1(t)) \tag{3}$$

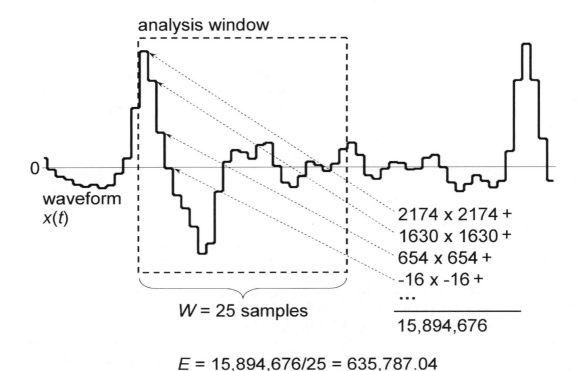

Figure 6–1. Computation of energy of a speech signal, using 25 samples.

Spectrum and Cepstrum

The *power spectrum* of a speech signal at time t graphs the energy in the signal as a function of frequency. The Fourier transform, which is used to compute the power spectrum, represents a signal at time t in terms of amplitude and phase as a function of frequency. For a digital signal, the Discrete Fourier transform (DFT) is used (e.g., Rabiner & Schafer, 1978, p. 16; Read & Kent, 2002, p. 83). The energy in the Fourier Transform of a signal is computed, as in the energy of the time-domain signal, by computing the sum of the squared magnitudes of the DFT. This result is called the power spectrum. The energy given by the power spectrum is usually converted to the deci-

bel scale by taking the logarithm and multiplying by a factor of 10. (As before, the reference intensity is assumed to have a value of 1.0). The power spectrum on the decibel scale is called the log power spectrum.

Given a voiced region of speech and an analysis window that is at least several times the length of a single pitch period, *harmonics*, or evenly-spaced energy peaks in the log power spectrum, can be seen, as illustrated in Figure 6–2. These harmonics occur at the fundamental frequency (F_0) and at all multiples of F_0. For example, if F_0 is 100 Hz and the upper frequency limit is 8000 Hz, then there will be harmonics in the log power spectrum at 100, 200, 300, ... 7900, 8000 Hz. In Figure 6–2, the fundamental frequency is 91 Hz, and so the first

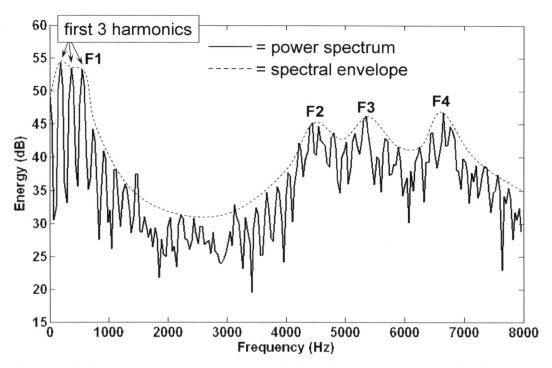

Figure 6–2. The power spectrum of a vowel /i/, showing spectral envelope (*dashed line*), harmonics, and approximate locations of the first four formants.

three harmonics occur at 91 Hz, 182 Hz, and 273 Hz. If harmonics are not present at some of these frequencies, then the periodic nature of the signal has been obscured by noise at these frequencies. Such noise may come from background sounds, breathiness of the speaker, or other nonvoiced sounds produced by the speaker. Voiced fricatives such as /z/ may show harmonics at lower frequencies as well as strong frication noise at higher frequencies. Figure 6–2 also shows the spectral envelope of the log power spectrum, indicated by a dashed line, and the approximate locations of the first four formants, F1 through F4.

The *cepstrum* is a frequency analysis of the log power spectrum (e.g., Read & Kent, 2002, p. 94; Rabiner & Schafer, 1978,

p. 365). (The word "cepstrum" is derived from the letters of the word "spectrum.") As such, it is readily computed by taking the Fourier Transform (or DFT) of the log power spectrum. The cepstral representation of the log power spectrum from Figure 6–2 is shown in Figure 6–3. This brings up two questions: How can one interpret the information in the cepstrum, and why is it a useful representation? If the spectrum in Figure 6–2 is interpreted as a time-domain waveform, it can be seen that there is a strong high-frequency component corresponding to the evenly spaced harmonics. Therefore, in a frequency analysis of this spectrum, we can expect a strong component located at the pitch period, due to the evenly spaced harmonics. In Figure 6–3,

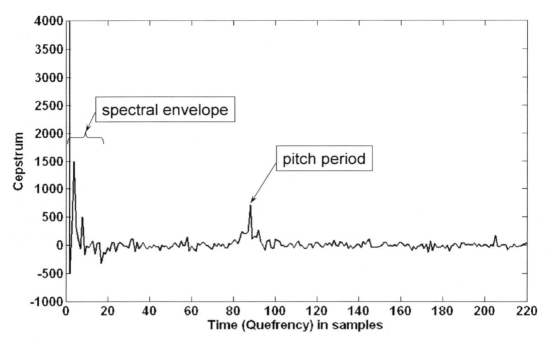

Figure 6–3. The cepstrum of a vowel /i/, showing lower cepstral values representing the spectral envelope and a peak in the cepstrum at the location of the pitch period.

this strong component can be seen at sample 88. If we convert from samples to frequency (using the equation *frequency = sampling frequency / samples*), this corresponds to 91 Hz, which is the F_0 value at this time *t*. If we continue to view Figure 6–2 as a time-domain waveform, and ignore the harmonics, then it can be seen that there are several low-frequency components to the spectral envelope, including the spectral tilt and formants. Therefore, we can expect large values within the first few cepstral indices, corresponding to the dominant aspects of the spectral envelope. In Figure 6–3, it can be seen that the cepstral values at lower indices (sample 0 to around sample 18) have greater intensity than at higher indices, except for the region corresponding to the fundamental period.

This leads us to answer the second question, why the cepstrum is a useful representation of speech. There are several answers to this: First, we can remove any information about the fundamental frequency from the cepstrum simply by ignoring values at higher indices. As pitch is not conventionally considered to be an important feature in the recognition of languages such as English, removing the higher indices removes superfluous information and leaves a feature set that is more focused on relevant characteristics of English phonemes. (Note, however, that removal of fundamental frequency information may not be suitable for tonal languages such as Mandarin or Vietnamese. In addition, F_0 has been shown to play a role in vowel perception in English (Bunton, 2006; Ryalls & Lieberman, 1981), indicating that even for English, F_0 and phoneme identity are not entirely independent.) A second reason for the cepstrum being a useful feature is that most of the information relevant to the spectral envelope is usually captured within the first 10 or 15 values of the cepstrum. Therefore, we can represent the spectral envelope with a very compact feature set, with 15 values instead of the typically hundreds of values used to represent the log power spectrum. A third reason is that the cepstral values tend to not be strongly correlated with each other, at least less so than spectral values. This reduced correlation between cepstral values simplifies the mathematics of Gaussian Mixture Models that are used in automatic speech recognition.

Linear Predictive Coefficients (LPC)

Linear predictive coefficients, or LPC features, are a set of numbers that, like the lower cepstral indices, provide a compact representation of the spectral envelope (Rabiner & Juang, 1993). The speech signal can be modeled using LPC by predicting the value at time t from the previous p waveform values. In this case, the following linear model is used:

$$s(t) \approx \hat{s}(t) = a_1 \cdot s(t-1) + a_2 \cdot s(t-2) \quad (4)$$
$$+ \cdots a_p \cdot s(t-p)$$

where $s(t)$ is the signal being modeled, $\hat{s}(t)$ is the model's approximation of $s(t)$, and the model describes $s(t)$ by the values $a_1 \ldots a_p$ and the previous p values of the signal. A convenient property of LPC coefficients is that as p increases, the amount of detail in the spectral envelope increases; a typical value of p is in the range of 10 to 16 (Chen, 1988, p. 542). When p is in this range, these LPC coefficients, or values of a, model the general trend of the speech signal but not the fine details or pitch period. Therefore, they provide a representation of the spec-

tral *envelope* of the signal that is useful in speech processing and recognition. LPC coefficients are a useful representation of the speech signal because, like cepstral coefficients, they represent phonetic information using a small number of parameters and remove information about F_0. Although LPC coefficients have greater correlation with each other than cepstral coefficients, an advantage of LPC over cepstral coefficients is the ability to estimate formant frequencies and bandwidths directly from the values of $a_1 \ldots a_p$, as mentioned below. LPC coefficients are often used in speech processing programs to estimate formants, and a variant of LPC coefficients, called perceptual linear prediction (PLP) coefficients (Hermansky, 1990), are commonly used in automatic speech recognition as features that represent the speech signal.

Formants

LPC coefficients can be converted into a representation of the speech signal's spectral envelope. There are several methods of determining formant frequencies from the peaks in this LPC spectral envelope, including (a) simple peak-picking and (b) solving for the roots of the polynomial represented by the LPC coefficients (Rabiner & Schafer, 1972, p. 442) to obtain a list of resonant frequencies and bandwidths in the spectral envelope, and then selecting those resonances with the smallest bandwidths. Although LPC analysis is the most common method for formant estimation, analysis-by-synthesis (Bell, Fujisaki, Heinz, Stevens, & House, 1961) is another technique.

Formants are widely used when studying characteristics of speech and speech disorders. However, formants are not widely used in computer processing of speech; instead, computer speech-processing systems tend to rely on representations of the spectral envelope, such as cepstral or LPC coefficients. The reason for formants not being more widely used in computer-based speech processing is that errors in computer-estimated formants make them not sufficiently reliable for most tasks. The power spectrum may have a number of nonformant peaks, such as the "glottal formant" (Bozkurt, Doval, D'Alessandro, & Dutoit, 2004) or resonances and antiresonances from the nasal cavity or subglottal cavity (Stevens, 2000, p. 300). Two formants may also be so close in frequency as to appear as a single peak. These sources of variability make reliable, automatic formant estimation a still unsolved problem. Errors in analysis at one time, t, may be partially corrected by estimating formant values at 10-msec intervals throughout an entire voiced segment, and then removing or smoothing outlier values. This process of *formant tracking* provides some robustness, but even so, manual correction is often required and computer-estimated formants are not widely used in fully-automated systems.

A formant can be described as a resonance, or region of increased energy at one region of the spectrum. Digital filters also increase or decrease energy at certain frequencies of a spectrum, and so the characteristics of a formant resonance can be implemented using a digital filter. The type of filter used to implement formant-style resonance is called an infinite-impulse response, or IIR, filter, and it computes a value of the filtered signal $y(t)$ from the input signal $x(t)$ and the previous two values of y, namely $y(t-1)$ and $y(t-2)$:

$$y(t) = a_2 x(t) + a_0 y(t-1) + a_1 y(t-2) \qquad (5)$$

where a_0, a_1, and a_2 are filter coefficients that can be computed from the formant's frequency and bandwidth (Klatt, 1980). Given a glottal-source waveform, one can construct a speech signal by filtering this source with three or more formant frequencies according to Equation (5). The vowel identity of the resulting speech signal depends, of course, on the formant frequencies used in filtering.

Glottal Source

Once the formants in a speech signal have been identified, the remaining two components of the signal are the airflow at the glottis (called the glottal source) and the acoustic effect of sound radiating from the lips. (The topic of poles and zeros, or resonances and antiresonances that are not caused by the shape of the vocal tract but are due to the nasal cavity or subglottal cavity, is not covered here.) The effect of sound radiating from the small opening of the lips is approximately the same as the effect of sound radiating from a single point, which can be mathematically described as applying a filter that increases 6 dB with every octave (doubling of frequency). This filter, a +6 dB/octave filter, can be implemented by taking the derivative of the time-domain signal, and is known as pre-emphasis.

The effect of formants can be *removed* from a speech signal by "inverse filtering." The remaining signal contains, according to the source-filter theory (e.g., Kent & Read, 2002) an estimate of the glottal source and radiation characteristic. (A typical filter can be thought of as *emphasizing* energy at different frequencies, with a certain shape of energy enhancement as a function of frequency. For a formant-type filter, the energy peak is at the formant's center frequency. An inverse filter *attenuates* energy in a complementary way, with an energy minimum at the formant's center frequency.) By further filtering this signal with a −6 dB/octave filter to cancel the effects of sound radiation from the lips, the waveform representing airflow at the glottis can be estimated. The accuracy of this estimated glottal airflow depends on a number of factors, but especially on the accuracy of the first-formant frequency and bandwidth (Hosom & Yamaguchi, 1994).

Fundamental Frequency

Pitch is a perceptual quality that is usually highly correlated with the fundamental frequency, or F_0. Because the correlation is quite good, and because F_0 is a feature that can be measured objectively, the terms pitch and F_0 are sometimes used interchangeably, especially when referring to a "pitch period." F_0 is a measurement of the rate of vibration of the vocal folds during voiced speech; its inverse, pitch period length, is the length of time for one glottal pulse. A single F_0 measurement is the fundamental frequency at one time point, and a sequence of F_0 values over time is called the F_0 contour or F_0 trajectory. There are numerous ways of computing F_0 using a computer, although most techniques are based on one or more of the following four techniques: (1) autocorrelation analysis, (2) cepstral analysis, (3) inverse filtering, and (4) harmonic sieve analysis. In this section, we will discuss the computation of F_0 at a single time point.

In the autocorrelation technique (e.g., Rabiner & Schafer, p. 150), W comparisons are made, with each comparison measuring the similarity of two regions of the time-domain signal. The correct value of the pitch period length is selected from the results of these W comparisons. In each comparison, the waveform in the region of the beginning of the analysis window (w_1) is compared with the waveform at an offset from the beginning of the window. Each comparison yields a single autocorrelation value,

and uses only multiplication and addition of waveform values:

$$AC(p) = \sum_{m=w_1}^{w_2-p} x(m) \cdot x(m+p) \quad 0 \le p \le W \quad (6)$$

where $AC(p)$ is the autocorrelation value for offset p, and $x(m)$ is the speech signal at time m. If we consider a waveform that is periodic, then AC will often have a locally maximum value at the index corresponding to the pitch period. The autocorrelation of a speech signal is shown in Figure 6–4. The pitch period length can then be determined by locating the first local maximum of $AC(p)$ with p greater than 20 (representing an F_0 maximum of 400 Hz). If we denote the value of p associated with this first local maximum as p_{max}, then F_0 is computed as (*sampling frequency* / p_{max}), or 91 Hz in this example. A strength of the autocorrelation method is that no assumptions are made about the presence or locations of harmonics in the signal; this technique works equally well for a pure sine wave as for a complex (but periodic) speech wave. One limitation of this technique is that when formants or amplitude change quickly (especially during the coarticulation between a vowel and a consonant), two consecutive pitch periods may have dissimilar waveforms, yielding a low autocorrelation peak at the pitch period. Another limitation is that a very strong second harmonic can result in a peak in the autocorrelation values at half the pitch period, causing an F_0 doubling error. A variant of the autocorrelation method is used in the Praat software package (Boersma & Weenink, 2008).

In the cepstral technique (Noll, 1967), first the cepstrum is computed as described above and as illustrated in Figure 6–3. The range of F_0 is then determined, based on the age range and/or gender(s) of the speakers being analyzed. For an adult male,

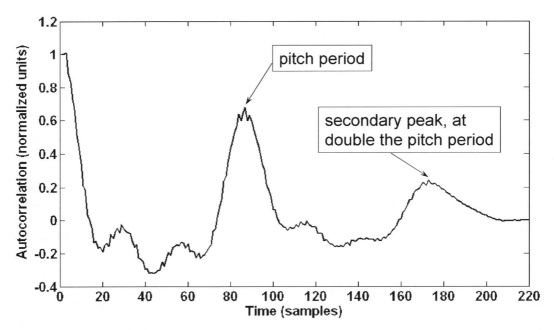

Figure 6–4. Autocorrelation plot of a vowel /i/, showing the first local maximum above 20 samples occurring at the pitch period, as well as a secondary peak occurring at twice the pitch period.

F_0 may range from around 50 to 250 Hz. For a young child, the mean F_0 may be as high as 400 Hz (Kent & Read, 2002, p. 196). These limits on F_0 are converted to samples, and the cepstrum is then searched between those sample limits for a local maximum. In Figure 6–3, with speech from an adult male, the search range may be from sample 32 (250 Hz) to 160 (50 Hz), and the peak within those limits, p_{max}, is located at sample 88. The F_0 value is then computed as (*sampling frequency / p_{max}*), or 91 Hz in this example. An advantage of the cepstral technique is that it is less sensitive to formant changes and strong harmonics than the autocorrelation technique. However, the cepstral technique does not work as well on sounds, such as nasals or the phoneme /w/, that may contain only a few harmonics. The cepstral technique is available in the PitchWorks software package (Scion R&D, 2008).

In the inverse-filtering technique, formants are estimated using a method such as solving for the roots of the LPC polynomial. The estimated formants are then removed from the signal using inverse filtering. The pitch period length and F_0 of the estimated glottal source, instead of the original speech waveform, is then determined using a technique such as autocorrelation. The advantage of removing the formants from the signal before autocorrelation is that a low first-formant frequency can cause a large increase in energy in the second or third harmonics. If the energy in these harmonics is too strong, then the autocorrelation method may estimate the F_0 value as being at the frequencies of one of these harmonics, which is double or triple the correct F_0 value. Removing the formants in this inverse-filtering technique reduces these pitch-doubling or pitch-halving errors. However, when removing the formant information, it is possible to inadvertently remove glottal-source information as well, yielding a signal that has had all harmonics removed. This risk is especially great in telephone-channel speech, in which all information below 300 Hz has already been removed. It is then impossible to determine the correct F_0 value of such an inverse-filtered signal. The inverse-filtering technique is the basis for the well-known Simplified Inverse Filter Tracking (SIFT) method of F_0 estimation (Markel, 1972). A variant of this method is used in the Wavesurfer (Beskow & Sjölander, 2000) software package.

In implementation of the harmonic sieve theory of pitch perception (Goldstein, 1973), an analysis window long enough to include at least several pitch periods is used in computing a log power spectrum of the signal. Such a power spectrum is illustrated in Figure 6–2. This log power spectrum will, if the signal is periodic, contain harmonics at the fundamental frequency and at multiples of F_0. One method for estimating F_0 is to hypothesize a range of F_0 values, and for each hypothesized F_0 value, compute the sum of energy at the hypothesized fundamental frequency and at all multiples of the hypothesized F_0. When the hypothesized F_0 value is the correct value, the total energy at all of these frequencies is expected to be maximum, because the harmonics are local energy peaks in the power spectrum. Although this method is straightforward in theory, in practice care must be taken to properly normalize the total energy by the number of hypothesized harmonics. Although the harmonic sieve method is not commonly used in current speech analysis software, it is an important technique with a direct relationship to theories of human pitch perception.

The examples presented here have illustrated cases in which estimating F_0 is relatively easy. In many cases, F_0 estimation is complicated by the signal not being perfectly periodic, a strong first formant, rapidly changing amplitudes, and other factors. Because no one measure of F_0 always produces reliable results, the gold standard for measuring F_0 is to visually inspect the waveform and locate "anchor points," or instants of local maxima, local minima, or zero crossing that are judged to be related to the fundamental frequency. If two such anchor points are measured in msec from the beginning of one pitch period (t_1) to the beginning of the next period (t_2), then F_0 (in Hz) is computed as $1000/(t_2-t_1)$, where the factor of 1000 converts between msec and seconds.

A comparison of different F_0-estimation algorithms on both normal and pathological voices was conducted by Parsa and Jamieson (1999). They found that each of the evaluated methods had different strengths and weaknesses, although the most successful method was a modified form of autocorrelation used in the CSpeech software package (Milenkovic & Read, 1992). In general, when using F_0-estimation software, one should be aware of the potential for common errors, such as pitch halving or doubling errors. Many software packages have parameters that can be changed to reduce certain types of observed errors, although the default parameters have been selected to optimize for overall performance.

Computer Models for Speech Classification and Recognition

The Challenge of Computer Speech Recognition

When one first considers the task of computer-based classification and recognition of speech, it may seem to be a relatively straightforward problem. For example, speech is a one-dimensional, time-varying signal, and there are many existing mathematical techniques for processing such signals. Speech is a well-structured communication process, and the speech signal depends on known and repeated physical movements. The building blocks of speech, that is, phonemes, are relatively small in number and, by definition, distinct from one another. Finally, in a communication environment in which there is significant background noise, a speaker will modify speaking style in order to maximize intelligibility for the listener.

Although these statements are true, there are a number of other factors that make computer speech recognition, or automatic speech recognition (ASR), a challenging problem. The foremost difficulty in ASR is the challenge of identifying the underlying structure of the speech signal given the large amount of variability present in speech. Sources of variability include different speakers having different acoustic and prosodic characteristics, the rate of speech possibly varying greatly from one sentence to the next, the fundamental frequency being high, low, or absent (in whispered speech), and the types of background noise being unpredictable and almost infinite in number. In addition, while there is a small set of phonemes, there are often no distinct acoustic boundaries between successive phonemes (e.g., a glide to a vowel, or a vowel to a liquid), and the acoustics of a phoneme are usually modified by the characteristics of the phonemes that precede and follow it. Phoneme durations and formant patterns will change in relatively complex ways, depending on speaking rate and speaking style. The number of words that may need to be recognized can be in the tens or hundreds of thousands, and the pronunciation of a word may vary greatly depending on accent, speaking rate, and

speaking style. Children's speech has even more variability than adult speech (e.g., Koenig, 2001), making analysis of children's speech an even more challenging task. These sources of variability make automatic classification of speech a difficult problem, even with advanced techniques from the fields of statistics, signal processing, and machine learning. As a result, it is important to constrain a particular task to remove or isolate as many sources of variability as possible. If one wants to identify prosodic or phonemic characteristics of children with a suspected speech disorder, it will not be possible to simply take an "off the shelf" speech recognition system, recognize the words, and identify the speech patterns of interest. Instead, a system must be developed that, for example, accounts for the specific types of background noise in the data, the age range of the children, expected pronunciation variations, and other factors.

The need to focus on the important characteristics of the signal being recognized is the primary reason that speech recognition systems use cepstral or LPC features for classification, discarding information about F_0, harmonics, and fine spectral detail. Although formants are directly related to phonetic identity and vary in predictable ways as a function of age and gender, formant frequencies are usually not used in automatic speech recognition systems because errors in formant analysis cause more errors in word recognition than a cepstral or LPC-based representation of the spectral envelope. Therefore, automatic speech recognition uses a simplistic representation of the spectral envelope for phoneme or word recognition, and other sources of information, such as F_0 contour or formant frequency, can be analyzed independently for specific issues such as monopitch, vowel neutralization, or articulatory difficulties.

Current Approach to Computer Speech Recognition: Hidden Markov Models

The dominant method for performing automatic speech recognition is called a Hidden Markov Model (HMM). This model uses a statistical representation, or template, of speech sounds. These statistical templates are developed from training data, and characterize the spectral features during a phoneme in terms of mean and variance. An HMM performs recognition of a test utterance by determining the sequence of (phoneme) templates that has the highest probability of matching the input speech. The templates are mapped directly to phonemes and words, yielding a word-level recognition result.

The process of computer speech recognition follows the four steps described here (Rabiner & Juang, 1993, Chapter 6):

STEP 1: Before analyzing a speech signal, each word in the recognizer's vocabulary is assigned a pronunciation, using letter-to-sound rules or a pronunciation dictionary. For each word, a model is constructed from a sequence of *states*, which contain statistical templates; each state and template is associated with one phoneme or a subphonemic unit. States are used to relate known characteristics of phonemes to observed acoustic data; for a speech signal at time t, a state's template is used compute the probability of this signal at time t given this template. The higher the probability, the better the signal at time t matches this state template. States (which are generally associated with phonemes or subphonemic units) are connected in sequence, so that the word "tip," composed of the phonemes /t ɪ p/, has a word model containing a "t" state followed by an "ɪ" state, followed by a "p" state. Each state is connected to the next phoneme in the word and to itself. Each connection has a probability of occurrence,

called a state transition probability; the sum of all state transition probabilities leaving any state is 1.0. HMM models of the words "tip" and "pit" are shown in Figure 6–5. In large-vocabulary systems, the end state of each word is then connected to the beginning state of all other words, so that the model allows any word to follow any other word. In small-vocabulary systems, the system designer usually constrains the sequence of allowable words to isolated words or phrases that are expected in the test data. In this case, the words "stop recording" may be a valid phrase, and so the "p" state in "stop" is connected to the "r" state in "recording," but "recording stop" may not be a valid phrase, and so the "ŋ" state in "recording" is not connected to the "s" state in "stop."

STEP 2: The speech signal to be recognized is converted into a representation that is compact and emphasizes the phonetic (rather than pitch or noise) qualities of the signal. This representation is typically based on the cepstrum or LPC coefficients, in order to simplify the mathematics of the probability estimation (described in Step 3). The speech signal is first divided into frames, or uniform-length segments, with 10 msec per frame. Each frame can be thought of as a "snapshot" of the speech signal at times $t = 0$ msec, 10 msec, 20 msec, and so forth, until the utterance end time, T. At each frame, the waveform is converted to a cepstral-domain representation, often using a somewhat longer analysis window of 16 msec. The higher cepstral values are discarded, in order to represent only the spectral envelope; usually only the first 13 cepstral values are used. This results in a vector of 13 cepstral values at every 10 msec of the signal. These cepstral values are weighted to roughly approximate some of the characteristics of human auditory processing, for example, with conversion from a linear frequency scale to a Bark or Mel

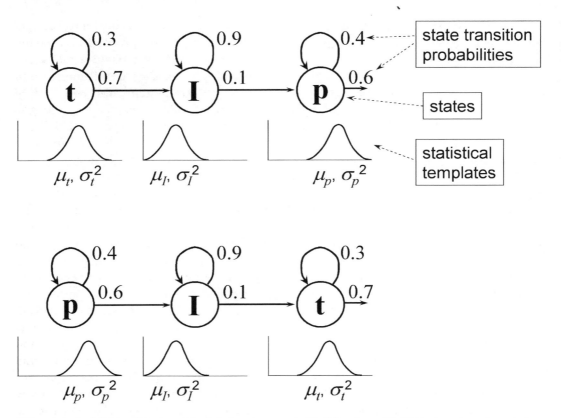

Figure 6–5. Hidden Markov Models for the words "tip" (*top*) and "pit" (*bottom*), using states with phoneme-level statistical templates. State transition probabilities are indicated next to state transition arcs, and statistical templates are located below each corresponding state.

scale. This vector of 13 cepstral values may be appended with other information, derived from the cepstrum, that indicates the degree of change at this time t, resulting in a final vector of 26 or 39 values.

STEP 3: The data at each frame is passed to all states in the HMM. At each state, a Gaussian Mixture Model (GMM) is used to compute the probability of this cepstral vector given this state, using the statistical template. This probability is usually denoted $b_j(o_t)$, where j is a state, o_t is an "observation" or cepstral vector at time t, and b is the probability of o_t given state j. In the simplest case, a GMM models the

probability density function (p.d.f.) of a single Gaussian, or Normal, distribution. In this case, it is said that the GMM has only one "component." This p.d.f. of observations for a given state can be estimated from training data; one simple estimation method fits a Normal distribution to a histogram of observations of a given state. In speech it is common to use more than one component (Normal distribution) in the GMM, as the cepstral features are often not Normally distributed due to gender differences and contextual differences.

STEP 4: An algorithm called a *Viterbi search* finds the sequence of states specified in the vocabulary that has the highest cumulative probability when considering all cepstral vectors from time 1 to time T. The probability of a state sequence from time 1 to time T depends on the probability values estimated by the GMM for each state and observation at time t, and also on the probabilities of transitioning from one state to another. The output of the Viterbi search contains this maximum probability, the states that yielded this maximum probability, and the word or word sequence that yielded this maximum probability.

It should be noted that this approach does *not* first identify where phonemes are located, then classify the phoneme identities, and finally construct words from the identified phonemes. The primary difficulty with such an approach is that phoneme boundaries are not easily identified by computer. In some cases, phoneme boundaries are characterized by gradual spectral change (e.g., the transition from a /w/ to an /e/), which makes automatic determination of phoneme boundaries from local spectral information a challenging task. The HMM approach addresses this problem by *simultaneously* solving for both phoneme locations and phoneme identities. This advantage in simultaneously solving for both location (i.e., duration) and identity aspects means, however, that sophisticated duration and prosodic models are difficult to apply within the HMM framework.

The HMM approach also makes it difficult to identify words that are not specified in the recognizer's vocabulary. One method for addressing this problem is called "garbage modeling" (e.g., Hosom, Cole, & Cosi, 1998). To implement garbage modeling, the classifier identifies the probability that a frame contains an unknown event, for example, a nonspeech event or a phonemic event that does not correspond to a known vocabulary word. Then a "word" with identity

"garbage" is created and added to the recognizer's vocabulary. This special word contains one or more consecutive frames of this garbage event. When the search for the most likely word is performed using the Viterbi algorithm, the garbage word may have a higher score than other words in the vocabulary if the acoustics in a region correspond to nonspeech noise or an out-of-vocabulary word.

One reason why HMMs are not more widely used in tasks that could potentially be automated with speech recognition is that the probability estimates are not, given the current state of the art, sufficiently reliable to allow identification of words with the same level of accuracy as humans. The difficulty of reliably estimating these probabilities can be appreciated when one considers how coarticulation, duration, and speaker differences impact acoustics, and how the Gaussian Mixture Model estimates phoneme probabilities from a single 10-msec region of the signal without knowledge of phoneme boundaries. Obtaining more reliable probability estimates is an area of active research, and it involves techniques such as speaker adaptation and discriminative training.

Although HMMs have proven to be the most successful method so far for automatic speech recognition, this technique rests on a number of requirements. First, one must know all possible states and state connections in advance, which means that one must know the vocabulary that might be spoken and how each word in that vocabulary is pronounced. Second, a number of mathematical assumptions are made, such as statistical independence between 10-msec observations or independence between features, and these assumptions may not conform well to observed speech signals. Third, medium- and long-range dependencies (such as the impact of speaking rate, degree of articulation, and phoneme identity on a neighboring phoneme's duration) and not specifically modeled, and so speech that has a high degree of variation in these factors tends to not be recognized as robustly as speech that is more regular.

Measuring Accuracy

The accuracy of a speech-processing system can be measured in various ways, depending on the task. In the most simple case, the presence and location of a word or phoneme is known, and the task is simply to classify that region of the speech signal into one of several categories. This task is known as *classification*. For phoneme classification, a set of 39 phonemes has become standard in the ASR literature (beginning with Lee & Hon, 1989). For word classification, the set of words depends entirely on the task. Accuracy is reported as the number of words or phonemes in a test sample that have been correctly classified, divided by the total number of test samples, multiplied by 100 (to obtain percent classification accuracy). (Note that the number of categories is independent of the number of test samples; a 1000-word vocabulary may be evaluated on a test set of 50 words, or a 39-phoneme set may be evaluated on a test set of thousands of phonemes.)

A more difficult task is *recognition*. In recognition, the same categories (phonemes or words) may be used, but the number and location of these categories within a test utterance is not known in advance. Therefore, the system must identify the presence of phonemes or words, in addition to classifying those phonemes or words. The types of errors that can be made in recognition are substitution, insertion, and deletion errors. A substitution error is a classification error; for example, recognizing the word

"for" when the correct word was "or." An insertion error occurs when the system recognizes a word that wasn't present in the speech signal. Insertion errors are common when there is background noise in the signal and when one long word is recognized as two shorter words (which becomes one substitution error and one insertion error). A deletion error occurs when the system fails to recognize as word that was present in the signal. Deletion errors are common for short and poorly-articulated words. The recognition accuracy is computed as $100 \times (1 - ((sub + ins + del)/total))$, where *sub* is the number of substitution errors in the test set, *ins* is the number of insertion errors in the test set, *del* is the number of deletion errors in the test set, and *total* is the total number of words in the test set.

When the task is to locate known phonemes or words within a test utterance, then a speech recognition system can still be used. In this case, the system is constrained to recognize only the known phonemes or words, and determine the phoneme or word boundaries. Because an ASR system solves for identity and location simultaneously, the output of this system contains the locations of the known speech units. Using an ASR system in this way is called "forced alignment" (e.g., Hosom, 2009), and this process can be used to identify phoneme durations, CV boundaries, voice-onset time, and other features useful in speech processing. To measure the accuracy of a forced alignment system, there must be a "correct" alignment, which is typically created by one or more human experts. The accuracy of the forced alignment system is then measured in terms of the percentage of boundaries that are correctly placed within a specified threshold. For example, if a forced-alignment system has 92.5% accuracy with a threshold of 20 msec, that means that 92.5% of all boundaries are within 20 msec of the correct boundaries. Accuracy of 100% with a 20-msec threshold can not be expected, because the agreement between two humans on phoneme-boundary placement has been measured to be a fairly consistent 93.78% on average (standard deviation 1.14%), with maximum reported agreement of 96% within 20 msec (Hosom, 2009). As the threshold increases, accuracy of both computer and interlabeler agreement increases; two humans can have greater than 98% agreement within a threshold of 40 msec (Hosom, 2009).

It is important to be aware of the larger context when accuracy of an ASR system is reported. Generally, an ASR system is trained and evaluated on data from a group of speakers that have some common characteristics (e.g., adult Americans, children between the ages of 7 and 12, or adult men over the age of 50 from the greater Boston area). The speakers in the corpus tend to be focused on the same verbal task, such as making an airplane reservation, listing all the animals they can think of, or saying nonsense words such as "doif." The characteristics of the recordings are also generally consistent, in that they often have the same background-noise conditions, type of microphone, and recording procedure. In addition, systems are trained and evaluated with a predetermined vocabulary and set of pronunciation models. Accuracy of a system is reported on a particular corpus, task, and vocabulary, and because ASR systems are sensitive to all of these parameters, the level of accuracy under these conditions does not usually extend to corpora, tasks, or vocabularies that the system has not been trained on. As a corollary to this, better performance is expected with more specific characteristics and a better match between training and testing conditions. As the characteristics become more generic (e.g., all Americans, instead of males from Boston), or as the mismatch between training and testing conditions becomes greater, the performance will become worse.

Applying Computers to Processing of Speech Disorders

Motivation for Computer Processing of Speech Disorders

Application of computer processing to speech disorders is motivated by a number of factors. First, as pointed out by Kent et al. (Chapter 5) there is the potential for improved accuracy of diagnosis. This improved accuracy may be realized by reducing errors caused by human fatigue or human variability. Improved accuracy may also result from collecting and analyzing more data than would be possible with human diagnosis alone, with the greater amount of data improving the consistency of measurements. Finally, improved accuracy of diagnosis may be made possible by computer processing that measures aspects of the speech signal that can not be accurately quantified without a computer, such as phoneme timing, pause duration, voice onset time, glottal source qualities, or degree of vowel reduction.

A second motivation for computer speech processing is to enable a decrease in analysis time or an increase in scale of use. For example, automated hearing tests that involve the subject repeating a word heard over headphones with noise can be scored by automatic speech recognition. The subject's hearing-test score can be provided immediately after testing, and testing can be performed at many sites on large numbers of subjects without human fatigue. A third motivation is to enable better communication for people with speech-production difficulties; an assistive device may, for example, recognize or improve the intelligibility of a dysarthric person's speech. Finally, the computer can be used as a tool for data collection, data visualization, and training. The remainder of this section describes some specific applications of computer speech processing.

The Coefficient of Variation Ratio Applied to Childhood Apraxia of Speech

One characteristic of one subtype of child speech disorder, childhood apraxia of speech (CAS), is isochrony, with related constructs including "scanning speech, robotic speech, staccato-like speech, and more generally, abnormal speech timing." (Shriberg, Green, Campbell, McSweeny, & Scheer, 2003). In a study by Shriberg et al. (2003), speech timing characteristics of children with childhood apraxia of speech were quantified using a Matlab-based software package. This software, called the Speech Pause Algorithm (SPA), implemented a measurement of the coefficient of variation ratio (CVR). The CVR measures the amount of variation in pause events relative to the amount of variation in speech events. Children diagnosed with CAS have been found to have a higher CVR value, due to the isochrony of their speech. In this study, the coefficient of variation (CV) of speech was computed as the standard deviation of the duration of the speech events in an utterance divided by the mean duration of the speech events in that utterance. The CV of pause was computed similarly for pause events. The CVR was then computed as the average CV for pause divided by the average CV for speech. Speech and pause events were first identified by means of amplitude- and duration-based thresholds using an interactive Matlab-based algorithm. Prior to computing the CVR, pauses less than

100 msec were eliminated from the data set to minimize the effect of intra-phoneme pauses (e.g., stop closure) on pause event variability estimates. Speech events less than 100 msec were also eliminated from the data set to minimize the effect of transient acoustic events, such as voiceless bursts or lip smacks, on speech event variability estimates. The diagnostic accuracy of SPA was evaluated on speech samples from 30 children with typical speech acquisition (TS), 30 children with speech delay of unknown origin (SD), and 15 children suspected to have speech motor involvement (SMI), which includes childhood apraxia of speech and speech delay consistent with dysarthria. A comparison of the results from the SMI group with the TS and SD groups yielded effect sizes (ES) of 0.72 and 0.71, respectively, reflecting the ability of this technique to discriminate children with SMI from children with TS and SD. An implementation of the SPA using ASR techniques (Hosom, Shriberg, & Green, 2006) has recently shown comparable effect sizes.

Hidden Markov Models for Detecting /r/ Pronunciation Errors in Children

A study by Bunnell, Yarrington, and Polikoff (2000) investigated the use of HMMs in an articulation-training software system for children. In this system, an interactive speech-enabled video game is used, in which the child "teaches" aliens to understand spoken words. The words become successively more complicated as the game progresses. Bunnell, Yarrington, and Polikoff (2000) focused on detecting /r/ errors in children who were asked to say the name "Rhonda" in a simulation of the video game that was controlled by a speech-language pathologist. The most common type of error was a /w/

substitution resulting in the name "Wanda." A total of 56 acceptable samples were collected, being recorded directly to hard drive with a sampling frequency of 22.05 kHz. Fifty listeners rated the stimuli on a five-point scale, resulting in 31 acceptable /r/ tokens (each token having an average score of at least 4.0) and 25 unacceptable tokens (each token having an average score less than or equal to 2.5). The HMM in this study was trained on a different corpus of children's speech, the CMU Kids Corpus (Eskenazi, Mostow, & Graff, 1997). The HMM determined the locations and probability scores of each phoneme in the assumed word "Rhonda" using a forced-alignment procedure. Probability scores were converted into likelihood ratios. The likelihood ratios of the phonemes /w/ and /l/ were also computed as substitutes of the /r/ phoneme. The probability difference between the correct /r/ likelihood ratio and incorrect /w/ or /l/ likelihood ratio was computed for each word. These differences were then compared with the average listener scores for each word sample. Results showed that the HMM scores accounted for 60% of the variance in the human scores. A model of the HMM scores of only the unacceptable tokens accounted for 80% of the variance in the unacceptable tokens, while there was poor correlation between the HMM scores and acceptable tokens.

Improving the Intelligibility of Dysarthric Speech

In a study by van Santen, Hosom, and Kain, the intelligibility of a dysarthric speaker's vowels was improved using a speaker-transformation technique (Kain et al., 2007). A speaker transformation system learns the short-term spectral characteristics of two speakers, A and B, and determines a function that maps from these spectral features of A to those of B. As a result, speech input from speaker A is transformed to sound more like speaker B (Kain, 2001). In this study, a speaker with Friedrich's Ataxia had vowel intelligibility of 48% in an isolated Consonant-Vowel-Consonant (CVC) context. A system was first trained to map from her vowel space to the vowel space of a non-dysarthric speaker using the first three formants and vowel duration as features. (The formants were automatically extracted using the ESPS Waves+ software package and not manually corrected.) Then, during evaluation, the system took her recorded speech, automatically extracted F_1, F_2, F_3, and duration, and used the mapping function to determine new values for these parameters. A formant-based speech synthesizer was then used to synthesize the vowel with the new parameters, while the consonant regions of the CVC were copied and not modified. Results from 24 listeners without experience in listening to dysarthric speech showed vowel intelligibility of 54% for the modified speech, which was a significant (p <0.05) improvement over the non-modified speech.

Summary

In this chapter, we have looked at motivations for applying computer processing to the analysis of speech disorders, computer use in data collection, measurement of speech features by computer, computer models for speech classification and recognition, and applications of computers to processing speech from children or adults with a speech disorder. Work in this area is ongoing, with current topics of research including diagnosis of autism, diagnosis of childhood apraxia of speech, and the development of assistive devices using automatic speech recognition for people with dysarthria.

References

Bell, C. G., Fujisaki, H., Heinz, J. M., Stevens, K. N., & House, A. S. (1961). Reduction of speech spectra by analysis-by-synthesis techniques. *Journal of the Acoustical Society of America, 33*, 1725-1736.

Beskow, J., & Sjölander, K. (2000). WaveSurfer— a public domain speech tool. *Proceedings of the International Conference on Spoken Language Processing, 4*, 464-467.

Boersma, P., & Weenink, D. (2008). PRAAT: Doing phonetics by computer (Version 5.0.05) [Computer program]. Retrieved January 30, 2008, from http://www.praat.org/

Bozkurt, B., Doval, B., D'Alessandro, C., & Dutoit, T. (2004). A method for glottal formant frequency estimation. *Proceedings of the 8th International Conference of Spoken Language Processing*, pp. 2417-2420.

Bunnell, H. T., Yarrington, D. M., & Polikoff, J. B. (2000). STAR: Articulation training for young children. *Proceedings of the International Conference on Spoken Language Processing, 4*, 85-88.

Bunton, K. (2006). Fundamental frequency as a perceptual cue for vowel identification in speakers with Parkinson's disease. *Folia Phoniatrica et Logopaedica, 58*(5), 323-339.

Carmell, T., Hosom, J.-P., & Cole, R. (1999). A computer-based course in spectrogram reading. *Proceedings of ESCA/SOCRATES Workshop on Method and Tool Innovations for Speech Science Education*, London, UK.

Chen, C. H. (1998). *Signal processing handbook*. New York: Dekker.

Chial, M. R. (2003). *Suggestions for computer-based audio recording of speech samples for perceptual and acoustic analyses* (Tech. Rep. No. 13). Phonology Project, Waisman Center, University of Wisconsin–Madison. Retrieved November 14, 2007, from http://www.waisman.wisc.edu/phonology/TREP13.PDF

Cole, R., Massaro, D. W., Rundle, B., Shobaki, K., Wouters, J., Cohen, M., et al. (1999). New tools for interactive speech and language training: Using animated conversational agents in the classrooms of profoundly deaf children. *Proceedings of ESCA/SOCRATES Workshop on Method and Tool Innovations for Speech Science Education*.

Cole, R., Oshika, B. T., Noel, M., Lander, T., & Fanty, M. (1994). Labeler agreement in phonetic labeling of continuous speech. *Proceedings of the International Conference on Spoken Language Processing*, pp. 2131-2134.

Coulston, R., Klabbers, E., de Villiers, J., & Hosom, J. P. (2007). application of speech technology in a home based assessment kiosk for early detection of Alzheimer's disease. *Proceedings of InterSpeech 2007*.

Eskenazi, M., Mostow, J., & Graff, D. (1997). *The CMU KIDS speech corpus*. Linguistic Data Consortium, University of Pennsylvania. August, 1997. LDC Cat, LDC97S63, ISBN 1-58563-120-5. Retrieved November 14, 2007, from http://www.ldc.upenn.edu/Catalog/CatalogEntry.jsp?catalogId=LDC97S63

Goldstein, J. L. (1973). An optimum processor for the central formation of pitch of complex tones. *Journal of the Acoustical Society of America, 54*, 1496-1516.

Hermansky, H. (1990). Perceptual linear predictive (PLP) analysis of speech. *Journal of the Acoustic Society of America, 87*, 1738-1752.

Hosom, J. P. (2009). Speaker-independent phoneme alignment using transition-dependent states. *Speech Communication, 51*, 352-368.

Hosom, J. P., Cole, R. A., & Cosi, P. (1998). Improvements in neural-network training and search techniques for continuous digit recognition. *Australian Journal of Intelligent Information Processing Systems, 5*(4), 277-284.

Hosom, J. P., Shriberg, L., & Green, J. R. (2006). The coefficient of variation ratio determined using automatic speech recognition. *Stem-, Spraak- en Taalpathologie, 14*(Supp.), 88.

Hosom, J. P., & Yamaguchi, M. (1994). Proposal and evaluation of a method for accurate analysis of glottal source parameters. *The Institute of Electronics, Information and Communication Engineers (IEICE) Transactions on Information and Systems*, E77-D(10), 1130-1141.

Huckvale, M. (2008). Speech filing system: Tools for speech research [Computer program]. Retrieved January 30, 2008, from http://www.phon.ucl.ac.uk/resource/sfs/

Ingram, K., Bunta, F., & Ingram, D. (2004). Digital data collection and analysis: Application for clinical practice. *Language, Speech, and Hearing Services in Schools, 35,* 112–121.

Kain, A. (2001). *High resolution voice transformation.* Ph.D. thesis, Oregon Health and Science University, OGI School of Science and Engineering.

Kain, A., Hosom, J. P., Niu, X., van Santen, J., Fried-Oken, M., & Staehely, J. (2007). Improving the intelligibility of dysarthric speech. *Speech Communication, 49,* 743–759.

KayPENTAX (2008). Multispeech, Model 3700 [Computer program]. Retrieved January 30, 2008, from http://www.praat.org/

Kent, R. D., & Read, C. (2002). *The acoustic analysis of speech* (2nd ed.). Albany, NY: Singular, Thompson Learning.

Klatt, D. H. (1980). Software for a cascade/parallel formant synthesizer. *Journal of the Acoustical Society of America, 67*(3), 971–995.

Koenig, L. L. (2001). Distributional characteristics of VOT in children's voiceless aspirated stops and interpretation of developmental trends. *Journal of Speech, Language, and Hearing Research, 44*(5), 1058–1068.

Lee, K. F., & Hon, H. W. (1989). Speaker-independent phone recognition using hidden markov models. *IEEE Transactions on Acoustics, Speech, and Signal Processing, 37*(11), 1641–1648.

Levinson, S. E. (2005). *Mathematical models for speech technology.* Hoboken, NJ: John Wiley & Sons.

Markel, J. D. (1972). The SIFT algorithm for fundamental frequency estimation. *IEEE Transactions on Audio Electroacoustics, AU-20,* 367–377.

Milenkovic, P., & Read, C. (1992). *CSpeech 4.0, Laboratory version* [Computer program], Department of Electrical and Computer Engineering, University of Wisconsin, Madison, WI.

Moore, B. C. J. (1997). *An introduction to the psychology of hearing* (4th ed.). San Diego, CA: Academic Press.

Noll, A. M. (1967). Cepstrum pitch determination. *Journal of the Acoustical Society of America, 41,* 293–309.

Parsa, V., & Jamieson, D. G. (1999). A comparison of high precision F0 extraction algorithms for sustained vowels. *Journal of Speech, Language, and Hearing Research, 42*(1), 112–126.

Rabiner, L. R., & Juang, B. H. (1993). *Fundamentals of speech recognition.* Englewood Cliffs, NJ: Prentice-Hall.

Rabiner, L. R., & Schafer, R. W. (1978). *Digital processing of speech signals.* Englewood Cliffs, NJ: Prentice-Hall.

Read, C., Buder, E. H., & Kent, R. D. (1992). Speech analysis systems: An evaluation. *Journal of Speech and Hearing Research, 35,* 314–332.

Ryalls, J. H., & Lieberman, P. (1981). Fundamental frequency and vowel perception. *Journal of the Acoustical Society of America, 70*(S1), S96.

Scion R&D. (2008). *PitchWorks for Mac and PC* [Computer program]. Retrieved January 30, 2008, from http://www.sciconrd.com/pitchworks.html

Shobaki, K., Hosom, J. P., & Cole, R. A. (2000). The OGI Kids speech corpus and recognizers. *Proceedings of the Sixth International Conference on Spoken Language Processing, 4,* 258–261.

Shriberg, L. D., Austin, D., Lewis, B. A., McSweeny, J. L., & Wilson, D. L. (1997). The percentage of consonants correct (PCC) metric: Extensions and reliability data. *Journal of Speech, Language, and Hearing Research, 40,* 708–722.

Shriberg, L. D., Green, J. R., Campbell, T. F., McSweeny, J. L., & Scheer, A. R. (2003). A diagnostic marker for childhood apraxia of speech: The coefficient of variation ratio. *Special Issue: Diagnostic Markers for Child Speech-Sound Disorders, Clinical Linguistics and Phonetics, 17*(7), 575–595.

Shriberg, L. D., & Kent, R. D. (2003). *Clinical phonetics* (3rd ed.). Boston: Allyn & Bacon.

Shriberg, L. D., Kwiatkowski, J., & Snyder, T. (1989). Tabletop versus microcomputer-assisted speech management: Stabilization phase. *Journal of Speech and Hearing Disorders, 54,* 233–248.

Shriberg, L. D., McSweeny, J. L., Anderson, B. E., Campbell, T. F., Chial, M. R., Green, J. R., et al. (2005). Transitioning from analog to digital audio recording in childhood speech sound disorders. *Clinical Linguistics and Phonetics*, *19*(4), 335–359.

SpeechStudio. (2008). Speech Studio: Speech-Studio Suite [Computer program]. Retrieved January 30, 2008, from http://www.speech studio.com/

Stevens, K. (2000). *Acoustic phonetics*. Cambridge, MA: The MIT Press.

Weik, M. H. (1961). The ENIAC story, *ORDNANCE*, US Army Ordnance Corps Association, Jan-Feb. Retrieved November, 14, 2007, from http://ftp.arl.army.mil/~mike/comphist/eniac-story.html

Weston, A. D., Shriberg, L. D., & Miller, J. F. (1989). Analysis of language-speech samples with salt and pepper. *Journal of Speech and Hearing Research*, *32*, 755–766.

CHAPTER 7

Motor Speech Disorders in Children with Autism

SHELLEY L. VELLEMAN, MARY V. ANDRIANOPOULOS,
MARCIL J. BOUCHER, JENNIFER J. PERKINS, KEREN E.
AVERBACK, ALYSSA R. CURRIER, MICHAEL J. MARSELLO,
COURTNEY E. LIPPE, AND RICHARD VAN EMMERIK

Introduction: Oral Motor and Motor Speech Deficits in Autism

Communication deficits are key to a diagnosis of autism (DSM-IV-TR, 2000). Until recently, 40 to 50% of people with autism spectrum disorder (ASD, a term we use to include pervasive developmental disorder and Asperger disorder as well as autism) were unable to communicate orally (Seal & Bonvillian, 1997), although the proportion of nonverbal children with ASD is decreasing with the advent of earlier identification and intervention (Tager-Flusberg, Paul, & Lord, 2005). The speech deficits found in this population generally are thought to reside primarily in the pragmatic areas of language (Tager-Flusberg et al., 2005), such as a lack of adaptation to the speech patterns of peers (Baron-Cohen & Staunton, 1994; Paul, Bianchi, Augustyn, & Volkmar, 2008). But recent research has suggested there may be motorically based differences, as well (see review below). Until recently, the latter have received little attention in the research literature. In this chapter, that small literature is reviewed and some newer preliminary interpretations of findings relating to the nature of the speech deficits of children with ASD are presented.

Motor Deficits in Children with ASD

General motor deficits in children with ASD have been reported (DeMyer, 1976; Ghaziuddin, Butler, Tsai, & Ghaziuddin, 1994; Klin, Volkmar, Cichetti, & Rourke, 1995; Manjiviona & Prior, 1995; Noterdaeme et al., 2002; Page & Boucher, 1998; Wing, 1981). Repetitive and stereotypical movements are common. In addition, both Ornitz, Guthrie, and

Farley (1977) and Johnson, Siddons, Frith, and Morton (1992) found that many children with autism exhibit delays in gross motor development that are already evident, and increasing, within the first 12 to 18 months of life. Berkeley, Zittel, Pitney, and Nichols (2001) administered the Test of Gross Motor Development (TGMD) to 15 children with autism; 73% fell within the poor to very poor categories on locomotor and object control skills. Unusual postures, clumsiness, and motor planning problems have also been reported, even in children without cognitive delays (Watson, Baranket, & DiLavore, 2003). Diamond, Dobson, and Boucher (1998) found motor abnormalities, especially with respect to organization and sequencing of movements, in a case study of a child with autism, including clapping imitations of rhythms. Specific difficulties with the preparation phases for movement patterns have also been identified in children with both autism and Asperger's disorder (Rinehart, Bradshaw, Brereton, & Tonge, 2001). Overall, children with ASD appear to have more general motor deficits than control subjects at the same developmental level (DeMyer, 1976; Ghaziuddin et al., 1994; Klin et al., 1995; Manjiviona & Prior, 1995; Noterdaeme, Mildenberger, Minow, & Amorosa, 2002; Page & Boucher, 1998; Wing 1981), although this finding has not been universal (cf. Chawarska, Klin, Paul, & Volkmar, 2007, who found gross motor skills to be a relative strength).

One possible source of these motor differences is a deficit in imitation, which has been reported by many authors (see Williams, Whiten, & Singh, 2004 for an overview), although, again, not universally (cf. Hamilton, Brindley, & Frith, 2007, who found no differences in imitation between children with ASD and verbal mental age-matched controls). It has been proposed that this deficit could be associated with a (currently theoretical) impairment in the mirror neuron system (Williams, Whiten, Suddendorf, & Perrett, 2001 but see Hamilton et al., 2007). Others have hypothesized that these motor deficits and differences result from abnormalities in the brainstem and/or the cerebellum (Rodier, 2000). Allen (2006) proposes that one of the principal functions of the cerebellum is to detect or predict temporal patterns and to anticipate and prepare appropriate responses. A deficit in such a system would reduce "rapid and efficient processing or production of coordinated sequences of events or actions" (p. 202), whether they be social, motor, or cognitive, with the possible consequence of a strong preference for predictability and sameness, including motor repetition. One research group, Mostofsky, Goldberg, Landa, and Denckla (2000), has further hypothesized that such cerebellar abnormalities may underlie deficits in procedural learning —learning of rule-based processes for combining elements sequentially or hierarchically into more complex patterns (Ullman, 2004)—that they have identified in children with autism.

Prizant (1996) proposed that motor speech limitations, as well as cognitive or pragmatic limitations, may be important factors in the relative lack of oral communication found among children with ASD. His justifications for this hypothesis include the fact that many children who do not communicate orally make more (though often limited) progress in communicating using augmentative communication systems, thus demonstrating that they have the cognitive and social capacity to do so. He cited anecdotal evidence that those with ASD often demonstrate symptoms of motor speech disorders, including feeding difficulties, drooling, low facial muscle tone, and difficulty moving the articulators independently. Some demonstrate specific features of childhood apraxia of speech, in Prizant's view: limited use of consonants, difficulty with longer or more complex sequences of sounds (multisyllabic words or longer utterances), and differences between their ability to produce automatic speech versus volitional speech, with automatic speech being superior. Szypulski (2003) echoed Prizant, stating that "the prevalence of motor functioning deficits are [sic] widely recognized as impairments affecting the acquisition and development of speech, language, and manual forms of communication in children with [autism]" (p. 9). She added that "motor dysfunction in praxis and imitation in children with [autism spectrum disorder] impair [sic] their ability to coordinate sequential movement[s] for social affective, reciprocal, exchange" (p. 9).

What are the bases for Prizant's (1996) and Szypulski's (2003) hypotheses that children with ASD have motor speech disorders? Several studies, mostly of children with Asperger's disorder and high functioning autism (HFA), have documented phonetic deficits, such as atypical vocalizations (Amoroso, 1992; Sheinkopf, Mundy, Oller, & Steffens, 2000; Wetherby, Yonclas, & Bryan, 1989), unexpected phonetic repertoires (Wolk & Edwards, 1993; Wolk & Giesen, 2000), deficits in syllable production (Wetherby, Yonclas, & Bryan, 1989; see also Amoroso, 1992; Sheinkopf et al., 2000), persistent articulation errors (Shriberg, Paul, McSweeny, Klin, Cohen, & Volkmar, 2001; see also Kjelgaard & Tager-Flusberg, 2001; Boucher, 1976), atypical ranges of prosodic features (frequency, intonation contour, terminal fall, etc.; Baltaxe, 1984; Eisenmajer et al., 1996), and high levels of variability (Velleman, 1996). Phonological differences have also been reported, such as unusual patterns of phonological development (Bartolucci, Pierce, Streiner, & Eppel, 1976; Velleman, 1996; Wolk & Edwards, 1993; Wolk & Giesen,

2000), restricted use of phonological contrasts necessary to signal meaning differences (Foreman, 2001; Wolk & Edwards, 1993) including deficits in producing contrastive stress (Baltaxe 1984, Foreman, 2001), deviant phonological processes (Gibbon, McCann, Peppe, O'Hare, & Rutherford, submitted), prosodic differences (Shriberg et al., 2001) and developmental asynchronies (Wolk & Edwards, 1993; Wolk & Giesen, 2000). Estimates of the prevalence of persistent phonological/articulation deficits, primarily distortions, in HFA are higher (Gibbon et al., submitted: 20%; Shriberg et al., 2001: 33%) than those in the general population (2–3%; Kirkpatrick & Ward, 1984), although Paul et al. (2008) suggest that the subtle differences in such high-functioning children may be due to a lack of social emulation, rather than to motor deficits. However, it is important to note that some of these studies have included few participants (Velleman, 1996; Wolk & Edwards, 1993; Wolk & Giesen, 2000). Furthermore, some contradictory findings have been reported (Wetherby et al., 1989, vs. Amoroso, 1992, and Sheinkopf et al., 2000, re: syllable production; Shriberg et al., 2001, vs. Kjelgaard & Tager-Flusberg, 2001, and Boucher, 1976 re: articulation errors).

Even more importantly, researchers have not carefully distinguished motor speech from other speech sound disorders (e.g., phonological disorders), and few have focused specifically on oro-motor skills in children with ASD. A few researchers have identified characteristics of oral apraxia (Page & Boucher, 1998; Rogers, Bennetto, McEvoy, & Pennington, 1996), with praxis skills correlated with vocabulary (Seal & Bonvillian, 1997). Some researchers have attributed communication and social deficits to praxis deficits; others hypothesize causality in the other direction, ascribing speech imitation difficulties among children with

ASD to impaired representational abilities (Smith & Bryson, 1994) or to decreased motivation for social emulation (Paul et al., 2008). No studies have attempted to differentiate childhood apraxia of speech versus dysarthria symptoms in children with ASD.

Motor Speech Disorders

Dysarthria and apraxia of speech are neurologically based motor speech disorders thought to be caused by disturbances or disruptions within the central and peripheral nervous systems underlying oral communication. Motor speech processes typically affected include motor planning, motor programming and neuromuscular execution. Darley, Aronson, and Brown (1969a, 1969b) carefully documented and correlated motor speech behaviors and acoustic features in neurologically impaired adults to differentially diagnose and categorize acquired motor speech disorders (dysarthria and apraxia of speech). These landmark studies established a systematic classification metric to allow differential diagnosis of various subtypes of acquired motor speech disturbances in adults. Darley et al. (1996a, 1996b) identified subtypes of speech disturbances associated with approximately seven discrete neurologic groups. They demonstrated that each set of associated symptoms correlated with the location of a specific lesion site within the central and/or peripheral nervous systems. Within this classification system, specific subtypes of dysarthria result when motor speech execution is impaired in executing the precise strength, speed, precision, timing, coordination, and feedback necessary for speech communication. Acquired apraxia of speech, in this classification scheme, is an impairment in the capacity to plan or program sensorimotor commands necessary for facilitating phono-

tactic and prosodic aspects of oral communication. Apraxia of speech as an entity is defined in the absence of motor execution problems (i.e., dysarthria) and cognitive-linguistic problems (i.e., aphasia). Although Darley et al.'s (1996a, 1996b) findings were based on the adult model and generalization to developing children with communication disorders is inappropriate, their work laid the foundation for the diagnosis of motor speech disorders.

Whiteside and Varley (1998) have proposed a different perspective on apraxia of speech. Their argument focuses on the distinction between "direct" phonetic encoding (p. 222), during which relatively stereotyped, stored motor representations or "movement synergies" (p. 223) of high frequency linguistic units are rapidly retrieved and implemented, and "indirect . . . on-line subsyllabic" (p. 222) phonetic encoding, used more slowly and with more effort in novel contexts. They propose that, in apraxia, the direct route is either disrupted or inaccessible, resulting in inconsistent, segregated speech production with reduced coarticulation and increased timing errors as each unit (consonant, vowel, or syllable) is planned anew for each use. These symptoms, along with vowel deviations and decreased syllable stress contrast, are hallmarks of childhood apraxia of speech. This distinction between direct and indirect phonetic encoding recalls the symptoms of cerebellar impairment in autism proposed by Allen (2006) and the autism-related deficits in procedural learning hypothesized by Mostofsky et al. (2000). In fact, Rogers, Hepburn, Stackhouse and Wehner (2003) have suggested a similar impairment of direct encoding as the source of the imitation deficit they identified in children with ASD: " . . . perhaps children with autism use the second, [intentional], apprenticeship imitation system, but without the benefit of the first [automatic system], resulting in imitations that are more effortful, less exact" (p. 777).

With respect to dysarthria and its associated sensorimotor and acoustic correlates of speech in children, there is a surprising lack of published literature. Of the literature published, there exists much variability amongst studies and their chosen populations. This is due, in part, to the multiple and varied subtypes of dysarthria. Tomik (1999) specifically noted that the hypoglossal motor neurons, the neurons that provide motor information to the tongue, are affected differently than other motor neurons in either the face or the jaw. Chen and Stevens (2001) also stated that in childhood dysarthria a commonly affected articulator is the tongue, along with respiration and phonation processes which both play a supporting role in the production of speech. Such articulatory, phonatory, resonatory, and respiratory deficits are the cause of the slower than normal speech rate that is frequently seen within individuals who have dysarthria (Tjaden, Rivera, Wilding, & Turner, 2005). Individuals with dysarthria frequently present with slower or irregular speech rates and lower than normal intelligibility ratings (Laures & Weismer, 1999).

The prevalence of dysarthria in the pediatric population is indeterminate to date; however, developmental and acquired dysarthria in children is certainly not rare (van Mourik, Catsman-Berrevoets, Pacquier, Yousef-Bak, & van Dongen, 1997). Despite this, children are infrequently diagnosed with dysarthria. Our hypotheses regarding the underdiagnosis of dysarthria in children are three-fold: (1) the application of the adult model and classification system for the differential diagnosis of dysarthria in children has not been validated; (2) few clinicians diagnose dysarthria or specific subtypes of dysarthria in the pediatric population in that children with congenital or develop-

mental abnormalities are typically diagnosed by syndrome or disorder and not by speech and/or language impairment; and (3) children with motor speech disorders may not always exhibit the same constellation of symptoms as adults with acquired motor speech disorders due to the beneficial effects of neurodevelopment and neuroplasticity in children. We speculate that a more efficient approach to specifically study dysarthria in the pediatric population is to investigate or find those children with specific developmental or acquired childhood disorders that most likely result in coexisting motor speech disorders.

Nonetheless, congenital forms of dysarthria have been reported as deficits associated with various developmental, genetic and chromosomal childhood disorders. Children born with spina bifida with hydrocephalus (SBH) exhibit dysarthria. The cluster of speech- and voice-related features associated with SBH due to underlying neurodevelopmental abnormalities to both the central and peripheral nervous systems include: articulatory inaccuracies, phonatory-prosodic insufficiency, prosodic excess, monoloudness, monopitch, harsh vocal quality, vowel distortions, imprecise consonants, and repetitive movements leading to breakdowns in articulation (Huber-Okraine, Dennis, Brettschneider, & Spiegler, 2002).

Some genetic disorders, such as fragile X syndrome and Prader-Willi syndrome, present with symptomatology consistent with both dyspraxia and dysarthria. Speech characteristics noted in fragile X syndrome include articulatory distortions and substitutions, and voice and resonatory abnormalities. Children with fragile X syndrome may also exhibit telegraphic- and echolalic-like speech and jargon (Shprintzen, 2000). Speech symptomatology associated with Prader-Willi syndrome due to hypotonia include reduced speech intelligibility, hypernasality, and articulatory inaccuracies (Stark, 2006). Children with congenital chromosomal abnormalities associated with Down syndrome exhibit dysarthric speech characteristics, due to low muscle tone and possible structural-anatomic abnormalities of the speech mechanism. These include low pitch, hypernasality, breathiness, and speech inaccuracies (Shprintzen, 2000).

Developmental disabilities associated with cerebral palsy primarily include three to four forms of underlying neuromuscular problems: (1) spasticity (rigidity); (2) hyperkinesis (athetosis and dyskinesis); (3) ataxia (cereballar form); and (4) mixed presentations (Bax et al., 2005). Depending on the degree of neurologic involvement, children with cerebral palsy may demonstrate mild to severe forms of dysarthria and anarthria, a total inability to speak, requiring alternative or augmentative forms of communication.

Infants and children of all ages can also acquire dysarthria due to surgical resection or treatment of cerebral, basal ganglia, cerebellar, and brainstem tumors, lesions, or strokes. Most reported cases of children with acquired dysarthria are documented single subject studies. In a retrospective study by van Mourik et al. (1997), children with acquired dysarthria did not always exhibit the same constellation of perceptual and articulatory features as those found in adults using the classification system by Darley et al. (1969a, 1969b).

From a diagnostic standpoint, four tasks are especially sensitive to changes resulting from dysarthric-like sensorimotor disruption to the speech mechanism: vowel phonation; Alternating Motion Rates (AMRs); Sequential Motor Rates (SMRs); and Maximum Phonation Time (MPT). Numerous studies have reported that adults with dysarthria have impaired AMR rates (Kent, Weismer, Kent, Vorperian, & Duffy, 1999; Nishio, 2006; Portnoy, 1982; Wit & Maassen, 1993; Ziegler,

2002), possibly caused by prolongation of syllables and of inter-syllabic pauses (Kent, Kent, Duffy, Thomas, Weismer, & Stuntebeck, 2000). Among the three syllables most commonly used to obtain AMR rates, /pə/ is frequently produced the fastest, followed by /tə/ and /kə/ (Ziegler, 2002). There exists some variability among individuals with different forms of dysarthria, in that adults with Parkinson's disease have AMR rates resembling those seen in people with apraxia of speech with respect to festinating or dysfluent-like repetitions produced with reduced range of movement, both of which are faster in rate than in other types of dysarthria (Ziegler, 2002).

Dysarthria can affect neuromotor systems on one or several levels including articulation, phonation, resonation, and respiration. Due to the multidimensional nature of dysarthria, it is a difficult disorder to diagnose based solely on singular acoustic measures of speech. For this reason, various acoustic analysis software programs enable investigators to study the spectral characteristics of both isolated sounds and connected speech. Kent, Vorperian, Kent, and Duffy (2003) suggest that such technologies provide a wide range of measures better suited to accurately assessing motor speech disorders through acoustic means. Chapters 5 and 6 discuss these technologies in more detail. In addition, a thorough neuromotor examination of central and peripheral nervous systems that underlie speech is crucial to the differential diagnosis of dysarthria from other types of motor speech and linguistically based problems.

With respect to Childhood Apraxia of Speech (CAS), whether acquired or developmental in nature, the specific neurologic basis of this disorder has not been discovered with any certainty. However, some possible genetic base for some subtypes of CAS have been identified (see Chapter 1).

Some theories about the developmental form of childhood motor speech disorders have been proposed based on the symptomatology associated with the acquired adult counterpart (e.g., Caruso & Strand, 1999); others have been based solely on the characteristics of CAS itself (e.g., Nijland, Maassen, & van der Meulen, 2003). It is the view of the latter that, although similar, CAS and the adult-acquired form of apraxia of speech (AOS) are separate disorders. Both are characterized by inability or difficulty planning or programming the movements of the musculature of the speech mechanism for communication purposes (Caruso & Strand, 1999), but children with CAS typically do not have identifiable neurologic differences from their peers; nor do they have the automatic speech movement synergies of a lifetime to rely upon for routine communications. Children with a pure form of CAS do not exhibit any visible weakness or paralysis of the speech mechanism, although a dysarthria may coexist in some of them. All children with CAS exhibit incorrect sequencing and placement of articulators when attempting to produce voluntary speech.

There is much debate regarding the underlying cause of CAS. It has often been theorized that the "location of the causal factor . . . [is] found somewhere in the transition from a phonological code into articulomotor and signal output; that is, [in] phonetic planning, motor programming, or motor execution." (Nijland et al., 2003, p. 438). The uncertainty regarding the diagnostic criteria and symptomatology associated with this childhood motor speech disorder makes the differential diagnosis very difficult. There is a lack of agreement as to the core deficits of CAS (Nijland, Maassen, van der Meulen, Gabreëls, Kraaimaat, & Schreuder, 2002). Aram (1984) and others purport that it is important to acknowledge CAS as a "symptom complex," which implies

that not all characteristics will be present in any one individual. Furthermore, symptoms among those with CAS have been found to change over time due to factors associated with development and neuroplasticity, so the same characteristics will not be present in the same individual over the entire course of that person's life or even childhood (Lewis, Freebairn, Hansen, Iyengar, & Taylot, 2004; Shriberg, Campbell, Karlsson, Brown, McSweeney, & Nadler, 2003; Skinder, Connaghan, Strand, & Betz, 2000).

Recently the American Speech-Language-Hearing Association released a Position Statement and Technical Report (ASHA 2007a, 2007b) on the possible etiologies, clinical and behavioral symptomatology, underlying neuropathologic mechanisms, and treatment approaches for Childhood Apraxia of Speech using an evidence-based practice approach. According to the ASHA (2007a) position statement:

There is no validated list of diagnostic features of CAS that differentiates this symptom complex from other types of childhood speech sound disorders, including those primarily due to phonological-level delay or neuromuscular disorder (dysarthria). Three segmental and suprasegmental features that are consistent with a deficit in the planning and programming of movements for speech have gained some consensus among investigators in apraxia of speech in children: (a) inconsistent errors on consonants and vowels in repeated productions of syllables or words, (b) lengthened and disrupted co-articulatory transitions between sounds and syllables, and (c) inappropriate prosody, especially in the realization of lexical or phrasal stress. Importantly, these three features are not proposed to be the necessary and sufficient signs of CAS.

Acoustic Investigations of CAS

Although some investigations have examined specific acoustic characteristics of speech in CAS, there has yet to be a comprehensive acoustic profile of a single sample population of children with CAS compared to a matched sample of children with typically developing (TD) speech. The majority of studies conducted on apraxia have focused on adult-acquired apraxia of speech (AOS) and not CAS. This statement also holds true with respect to acoustic investigations of this disorder (Nijland et al., 2002). Of those studies that have focused on the speech production characteristics of CAS, intelligibility and perceptual studies are more commonly reported than acoustic investigations (Ansel & Kent, 1992; Nijland et al., 2002;). The findings of such studies have highlighted articulatory, syllabic, and prosodic differences: vowel distortions, difficulty achieving and maintaining correct articulatory formations, substitutions, timing errors, omissions, ordering errors, and stress differences (Caruso & Strand, 1999; Davis, Jakielski, & Marquardt, 1998; McCabe, Rosenthal, & McLeod, 1998; Nijland et al., 2002; Shriberg, Aram, & Kwiatkowski, 1997b; Shriberg, Campbell et al., 2003; Whiteside & Varley, 1998). A problem associated with perceptual investigations of speech and voice is the lack of consistency and reliability of human listeners in identifying speech and vocal disturbances in human speech and voice samples (Kreiman, Gerratt, & Precoda, 1990; Rabinov, Kreiman, Gerratt, & Bielamowicz, 1995). Further investigations regarding the acoustic features associated with CAS are needed to determine if there are specific acoustic differences that may be unique to CAS.

With respect to those investigations that have examined the acoustic characteristics of CAS, there has been little agreement and very few significant findings. This lack of conclusiveness is due to several factors that include (1) the variety of methods and sampling procedures in different investigations, (2) the fact that each individual investigation has used only a few acoustic measures, and (3) a lack of comparison between CAS speech profiles and age- and gender-matched speech-delayed (SD) or TD controls. The interested reader is also referred to Chapter 8.

Strand and McNeil (1996) found that those with CAS displayed increased vowel durations and longer pause durations between word segments than those without CAS. Munson, Bjorum, and Windsor (2003) examined stress characteristics of CAS in nonsense words and reported no group differences between CAS and TD controls based on vowel duration, fundamental frequency of vowels, timing of peak formant frequency relative to vowel onset, and intensity of the vowel at midpoint. However, during the same year, Shriberg, Campbell, et al., (2003) developed a composite "lexical stress ratio" score (LSR) to investigate previous findings by Shriberg and others (e.g., Shriberg, Aram, & Kwiatkowski, 1997a, 1997b, 1997c; Velleman & Shriberg, 1999) that children with apraxia produce "excessive/equal stress"; that is, there is less difference in their speech between stressed versus unstressed syllables. In the Shriberg, Campbell, et al. (2003) study, 11 children with suspected CAS ("sAOS," here henceforth notated as sCAS) between the ages of 3;3 and 10;10 and 24 children with speech delay (SD) between the ages of 3;4 and 12;0 were recorded repeating 8 familiar trochaic (first syllable stressed) nouns. Frequency area, amplitude area, and duration were calculated for each stressed and unstressed syllable. Lexical stress ratios (LSR) were calculated as follows:

> . . . factor regression scores were obtained
> on [these] three significant variables, and

the composite score for each speaker was defined as the Lexical Stress Ratio (LSR). The LSR for each individual was defined as $LSR_i = C_1S_{1i} + C_2S_{2i} + C_3S_{3i}$, where C1, C2 and C3 were the factor regression scores for the three acoustic measures (frequency area = 0.490, amplitude area = 0.507 and duration = 0.303), and S was the averaged [stressed/unstressed] ratio score for individual (i) for each acoustic measure. (p. 562)

Both children with SD and children with sCAS had lexical stress ratios with group averages near 1.0 (0.94 for children with SD, range 0.65 to 1.14; 0.99 for children with sCAS, range 0.65 to 1.65), indicating that the difference between stressed and unstressed syllables is very subtle if measured in this manner. However, they also found that children with suspected CAS were responsible for five of the six most extreme LSR values. The children with SD appeared to have less, not more, contrast between stressed and unstressed syllables, with a standard deviation of 0.131 in comparison to a standard deviation of 0.296 for the children with sCAS. Shriberg, Campbell, et al. (2003) concluded that those with suspected apraxia had more extremely high LSR's (up to 1.65), and a higher proportion of low LSR's (including one case of 0.65 and one case of 0.71, whereas the lowest values for children with SD were 0.65 and 0.72). The authors therefore hypothesized that extreme lexical stress ratios are a symptom of CAS. No explanation was given for how this accords with the perception of excessive/*equal* stress in children with sCAS.

Several studies have suggested that variability is a main feature of CAS. Nijland et al. (2002) investigated the second formant frequency of vowels within nonsense repetitions, as well as anticipatory coarticulatory behaviors in individuals with CAS. The

authors found that second formant values and anticipatory coarticulation of CAS varied greatly; however, both control groups, composed of normally speaking children and adult women, also demonstrated variability on the same tasks. Similarly, Maassen, Nijland, and Van der Meulen (2001) reported acoustic variability in children with CAS as one of their findings.

Shriberg, Green, Campbell, McSweeney, and Scheer (2003) explored timing variation in 15 children labeled in the study as having "sAOS" (henceforth referred to as "sCAS"), although 8 of them reportedly had more symptoms of dysarthria than apraxia. These sCAS participants (aged 3–14 years; mean age 6;11; 87% male) were selected because they sometimes produced speech characterized by "syllable segregation." They included three members of the KE family (a British family in which members with symptoms of CAS have been found to have a specific genetic difference, known as "FoxP2"; see Chapter 1). Other subjects included 30 children with SD (aged 3–5 years; 50% male) and 30 TD children (aged 3–5 years; 50% male). Using 24 utterances each from spontaneous speech samples, they calculated the groups'/participants' "coefficient of variation ratios" by dividing the standard deviation for pause durations by the mean for pause durations (= pause coefficient of variation, or CoV), then doing the same for speech (= speech CoV). Next, the resulting pause CoV was divided by the resulting speech CoV to determine the CoV ratio (= CVR). Typically developing children had the most variation in their speech, followed by children with speech delays (SD). Children with sCAS had the most isochrynous (regularly timed) speech, in keeping with the percept of "excessive/equal stress" and many past research reports of segregated syllables in the speech of children with this disorder. In contrast, their pause durations were not more variable (i.e., pause CoV's were higher) than those of the TD children; the children with SD had less variable pauses than the other groups. These patterns, when divided, yielded high CVR's for the children with sCAS (mean CVR 1.26; TD mean CVR 1.08; SD mean CVR 1.06). The authors concluded that children with sCAS produce less varied speech durations than TD children and children with SD, yielding high CVR's and indicating that speech timing may be a core deficit in CAS. They note that pause timing variability in this group presents a challenge to their model, however, because their hypothesis was that the speech of the children with sCAS would be less variable in all respects. A further important limitation to this research is that, given that spontaneous samples were used, the reduced variation in the speech of the children with CAS could result from these children's use of simpler word shapes (e.g., words composed of open monosyllables rather than multisyllabic words encompassing consonant clusters) and/or of simpler sentence structure, resulting in less variation in the form of the "speech events" (e.g., more single word speech events; fewer phrases uninterrupted by pauses of 100 msec or more).

In addition to spectral characteristics of speech, maximum phonation time (MPT) is one norm-referenced method frequently employed clinically to assess the integrity of the respiratory and vocal mechanisms for speech purposes. According to published normative data, a typically developing child between the ages of 6 and 10 years can sustain the isolated vowel [a] prolongation for a period of nine seconds (Haynes & Pindzola, 2004). Maximum prolongation time of fricatives, such as [f], in individuals with certain motor speech disorders has also proved revealing. Nijland et al. (2003) reported that CAS speakers have a decreased ability to prolong this specific fricative sound compared to controls.

Additional research is needed to confirm and strengthen the acoustic profile consistent with CAS by measuring a set of acoustic variables from the speech of the same group of children with verified CAS as compared to gender- and age-matched TD children. Such acoustic research should clarify the appropriateness of various hypotheses concerning the underlying basis for CAS with respect to the acoustic features of this symptom complex.

The acoustic, motoric, and phonological aspects of speech among individuals with childhood apraxia speech (CAS) and autism spectrum disorders are currently under investigation by our group. The purpose of our research program is to verify the acoustic characteristics associated with CAS and to explore the nature and extent of motor speech disorders in children with ASD. It is our hope that these studies will shed light onto those diagnostic markers that enable clinicians to diagnose childhood apraxia of speech and dysarthria in all populations, especially those with ASD, more efficiently and effectively.

Our Studies

Parent Survey

Marili, Andrianopoulos, Velleman, and Foreman (2004) used an in-depth parent survey to identify comorbid speech-related behaviors in 40 individuals with ASD. The group mean age among the 40 participants was 8.05 years, with a range of 22 months to 22 years and a standard deviation of 55.3 months. With respect to gender, there were 34 (85%) males and six (15%) females. The results of this survey study provide support and evidence that young individuals on the autism spectrum do indeed exhibit behaviors suggestive of a neuromotor speech impairment. Results indicated a probable underlying motor-related problem consistent with apraxia of speech and/or dysarthria in a subset of individuals with ASD. In this investigation, parental reports indicated symptoms that could be associated with motor speech impairment in 60% of the participants, with 12.5% of the participants demonstrating symptoms of apraxia of speech only, 10% demonstrating dysarthric symptoms only, and coexisting symptoms that could be associated with both apraxia and dysarthria in 37.5%.

In this investigation (Marili et al., 2004), we teased out motoric-related impairments by comparing the participants on 10 discrete variables most consistent with child and/or adult dysarthric symptomatology to 14 discrete variables most consistent with child/adult apraxia of speech. The 10 variables most consistent with dysarthric symptoms included: rough vocal quality; breathy vocal quality; strained vocal quality; generally distorted speech; problems with mouth or lips; problems with tongue; problems with velum; muscular weakness of the speech mechanism; abnormal oral motor postures during speech; and production of unclear consonants. The 14 variables most consistent with apraxic symptoms included: unclear vowels; poorer articulation as word or phrase complexity increases; inconsistent pronunciation; speech worse under social pressure; history of learning words then losing them; struggle to make sounds for communication purposes; struggle to make words; struggle to make sentences; clumsiness of oral speech mechanism; difficulty with AMRs; sounds out of order in words; sounds out of order in sentences; problems sequencing activities of daily living; and normal posture during speech.

Motor speech impairments were not suspected in approximately 40% of the participants in the investigation as the parents/guardians of participants reported very few or no symptoms consistent with either childhood apraxia of speech or childhood dysarthria. The variables vocal features, general motor weakness, and general postures did not neatly divide survey participants into groups (apraxic, dysarthric or both) in this study. The most useful variables gleaned from parent/guardian report among the 228 items surveyed appear to be clarity of consonants and presence of distorted speech in those with dysarthric-like symptoms, and evidence of struggle for those with apraxic symptoms. Moreover, the authors found a statistically significant correlation between the number of dysarthria symptoms and the number of apraxia symptoms that coexisted in participants. Thus, rather than defining distinct subgroups of children on the autism spectrum, apraxic and dysarthric symptoms appear more often to co-occur in this population.

The results of this study support Prizant's (1996) theory that oral motor problems affecting motor planning, motor programming and motor speech may be a factor in the speech and language deficits of individuals with autism spectrum disorder. Participants demonstrated many behaviors that support the presence of an underlying speech motor processing problem, especially poorer articulation as word or phrase complexity increases, drooling, deletion of consonants, and sequencing difficulties. In addition, participants diagnosed with autism, PDD-NOS and PDD+ Other syndromes were found to have greater difficulty on most measures than those clinically diagnosed with Asperger's disorder. Among the 10 children (25%) with Asperger's disorder in this study, only one participant was reported to have problems with their oral mechanism with respect to their lips, face, and velum. Two of the 10 participants (20%) with Asperger's disorder exhibited clumsiness of the oral mechanism and drooling and only one of these two participants exhibited difficulty moving food in their mouth or muscular weakness of the speech mechanism. Among the 40 participants surveyed, 20 children (50%) were reported to have general clumsiness of extremities performing tasks. Of the 20 children, six of the 10 participants (15%) with Asperger's; 10 of the 17 (25%) with Autism; two of the seven (5%) with PDD-NOS; and two of the six (5%) with PDD-Other exhibited general clumsiness of extremities when performing tasks. With re-spect to perceptual features of speech, only one of the 10 participants (10%) with Asperger's exhibited strained phonation and another one (10%) exhibited breathy phonation. None of the participants with Asperger's disorder exhibited difficulty or struggle to make sounds, words or sentences. These findings are consistent with published literature and diagnostic criteria utilized for differential diagnosis of autism and Asperger's Disorder (Reid & Collier, 2002; DSM IV, 1994).

Acoustic Investigation of Childhood Apraxia of Speech

sCAS and TD Participants

Before acoustically investigating the nature and extent of motor speech disorders in children with ASD, it was deemed necessary to verify the acoustic characteristics associated with CAS in children without ASD, while also establishing and validating protocols and procedures for the assessment of these characteristics within our laboratory. For this purpose, Andrianopoulos, Velleman, Perkins, Boucher, and Van Emmerik (2007) studied 16 participants ranging in age from 5;0 years to 8;11 years (mean age 7;8) behaviorally and acoustically. Eight of these children had previous diagnoses of CAS given by their local speech-language pathologists. The other eight were typically devel-

oping children matched for age (within two months) and gender with the first eight. Five pairs were male and three female. Potential participants were initially screened over the phone to confirm eligibility. Inclusionary criteria, including diagnosis of CAS by an ASHA-certified SLP for the sCAS group, included: (1) documented receptive language within normal limits; (2) absence of craniofacial or structural differences; (3) absence of uncorrected visual or auditory deficits; (4) absence of other known physical, sensory, neurologic, or cognitive deficits; and (5) expected progress within an age-appropriate school placement. Parents of participants with sCAS were asked to forward a copy of the most recent speech-language evaluation to confirm diagnosis and provide results of previous testing. Table 7-1 provides further information regarding participants in this study of the acoustic features of CAS.

Diagnoses of CAS were verified via calculation of the Focal Oral Motor (FOM) and Sequencing (SEQ) subscores of the Verbal Motor Production Assessment for Children (VMPAC; Hayden & Square, 1999). The tasks included in these subscores involve elicited and imitated productions of speech and non-speech actions, ranging from isolated postures or vowels to phrases and sentences (e.g., Stick out your tongue, Say [a], Say [a-m-u], Say "Dad sat on a mat," Count to 10, Tell me what's happening in this picture). The VMPAC was administered to all participants. Scores on these and the Speech Characteristics subtests are given in Table 7-1. sCAS FOM scores ranged from 54% to 96% correct (mean = 77), whereas TD scores ranged from 96% to 100% correct (mean = 98). sCAS SEQ scores ranged from 50 to 100% correct (mean = 76); TD SEQ scores ranged from 98 to 100% correct (mean = 100). The TD child with the lowest FOM score had 100% correct on SEQ. Those with sCAS scored significantly lower than

Table 7–1. CAS and TD Participants

Participant Number	Age	VMPAC Focal Oral Motor Score	VMPAC Sequencing Score	VMPAC Speech Characteristics
CASM1	6;10	96	87	100
CASM2	6;9	54	72	71
CASM3	7;5	86	93	71
CASM4	5;5	71	54	100
CASM5	6;8	60	52	71
CASF1	8;1	89	98	71
CASF2	5;0	65	50	29
CASF3	7;0	96	100	100
CAS Mean	**6;8**	**77**	**76**	**77**
TDM1	7;0	100	100	100
TDM2	6;9	99	98	100
TDM3	7;6	99	100	100
TDM4	5;5	97	100	100
TDM5	6;9	96	100	100
TDF1	8;3	99	100	100
TDF2	5;2	97	100	100
TDF3	7;1	100	100	100
TD Mean	**6;8**	**98**	**100**	**100**

CASM = Male with diagnosis of CAS; CASF = Female with diagnosis of CAS; TDM = Male typically developing; TDF = Female typically developing.

those who were TD on the FOM and SEQ subtests ($p = .006$, $p = .016$, respectively; paired t-tests).

The VMPAC Speech Characteristics score also differentiated the sCAS and TD groups; some of the children with a diagnosis of sCAS had noticeable voice differences (rate, resonance, intensity, etc.). None of those who were typically developing triggered any concerns with respect to any of these aspects of their speech. Interestingly,

the sCAS children's scores on the FOM and SEQ subtests were bimodal: FOM scores ranged from 54 to 71% correct for four children with a diagnosis of sCAS and 89 to 96% correct for the other four with the same diagnosis. The SEQ scores for the same two groups also clustered into scores of 50 to 72% versus 87 to 100% correct.

Diagnoses of CAS were further verified/ investigated by having one research assistant create a set of video clips for each child with CAS (8 total) and for four TD children in the middle of the age range. These sets of clips included the sequential motor rates (SMR) task from the VMPAC, counting to 10 or reciting the alphabet, and approximately 3 minutes of spontaneous speech. These sets of clips were randomized by the research assistant and then given to the two first authors and to two CAS clinical specialists who were otherwise completely uninvolved in the study. All four of these raters were blind to the subjects' group assignments, test scores, etc. Each one rated each of these participants, based on their clips, on a seven-point scale where 1 = "definitely has CAS" and 7 = "definitely doesn't have CAS." Ratings for the TD children ranged from 6.13 to 6.88 (very unlikely/definitely does not have CAS); ratings for children with a diagnosis of CAS ranged from 1.53 (definitely/very likely has CAS) to 5.63 (unlikely/very unlikely to have CAS). Thus, there was a gap between the range of ratings for the TD children and those with a CAS diagnosis. The experts' video rating judgments correlated highly with the participants' VMPAC FOM and SEQ scores (p <.01 for both comparisons), suggesting that these subscores of the VMPAC correspond well with specialist clinicians' judgments of the disorder.

As noted above, the experts had rated some of the children who had been given the diagnosis elsewhere as less likely to be appropriately diagnosed with CAS. This consistent finding (based on both the VMPAC subscores and the experts' opinions) that some of the children did not demonstrate strong symptoms of CAS could be the result of the very brief nature of the video clips used for judgment, of clinical progress rendering the signs of CAS more subtle in those children, of the overdiagnosis of CAS which is rampant in this country at this time (Davis et al., 1998), or some combina-

tion of these three. This issue is discussed in depth in Andrianopoulos, Velleman, Marilli, & Foreman (2005). For the purposes of this chapter, all of the children with a previous diagnosis of CAS will continue to be treated as one group, henceforth notated as "sCAS" ("suspected CAS"), given that they all had been given a diagnosis of CAS by their speech-language pathologists.

Instrumentation and Acoustic Analyses

Analysis and capture of acoustic signals followed guidelines set by the National Center for Voice and Speech (Titze, 1995). A miniature professional grade condenser microphone (AKG C-410) positioned 45 degrees off-axis with a one-inch mouth-to-microphone distance held constant to the right of each participant's mouth was head-mounted on each seated participant. Speech samples were recorded onto high-quality digital audio tapes using the Tascam, DA-P1 digital audio tape (DAT) recorder at a sampling rate of 48 kHz with an allowable headroom of 10 dB. The input level control was adjusted for each participant during three practice sessions to ensure signals did not overload. Once the necessary adjustments were made, the settings were held constant without adjustment throughout the remainder of each test session.

Spectrographic waveform, formant and voice analyses, and duration measurements of speech tokens were created or carried out using the Computerized Speech Lab (Kay Pentax, Model 4500). Speech tasks included prolongation of the vowel [a] and the fricative [f]; production of the vowels [a], [u], and [i]; and repetition of the sound sequences [o i] and [a m u], the short phrases "pea, tea, key," and "beet, boot, boat, bat," the sentences "Buy Bobby a puppy" and "Mommy bakes pot pies," Alternate Motion

Rates (AMRs) of the syllables [pʌ], [tʌ] and [kʌ], and Sequential Motor Rates (SMRs) of [pʌtʌkʌ]. Each stimulus was modeled by the examiner for each child and then the child was prompted to repeat the stimulus spontaneously three times on their own volition. Speech tokens were line-fed from the DAT recorder output to the line input of the CSL external module using an RCA output to a BNC plug connector. The CSL was set at a sampling rate of 50 kHz for vowel analyses. For each of the isolated [a], [i], [u] vowel prolongations, the middle 200 millisecond (msec) segment of each signal was trimmed, edited and saved digitally for acoustic analysis. Each 200-msec vowel token was downsampled to 12.5 kHz and analyzed using the LPC Formant History, Spectrogram, and Result Statistics functions. Mean fundamental frequency for the [a], [i], and [u] vowels in isolation and for the first formant (F1), second formant (F2), and third formant (F3) for each of the three tokens per vowel were calculated for all participants.

Total lengths of phrases, lengths of vowels and lengths of pauses between words, as well as maximum phonation time (in seconds) of [a] and [f] were also measured. The CSL software was utilized to make these temporal measurements directly from the acoustic signals and spectrograms on the monitor per participant. Table 7–2 enumerates the measurements obtained for each specific acoustic task and analyses calculated per token. In addition, gross lexical stress ratios were calculated for comparison to Shriberg, Campbell, et al. (2003). Unlike the Shriberg study, in the present research project, ratios of simple durations were used as a rough measure of lexical stress. Ratios of stressed to unstressed duration values (modified Lexical Stress Ratios, mLSR's) were calculated for three trochaic words with two target syllables each ("Mommy," "Bobby," "puppy").

Statistical Analyses

Mean scores were calculated for each vowel and speech token for each task for each participant. Standard deviations (SD) were also calculated on the three repetitions per task to determine the individual's variability across repetitions: "within task individual variability." Individual mean responses per task were subsequently averaged to calculate a group mean for each group (sCAS vs. TD). Standard deviations were also calculated for group means: "within task group variability." Standard error of measurement (SEM) was calculated for each group per task to determine the degree of variability among group means. F-tests were calculated using SPSS 13 software to identify differences between the two groups for each task and Tukey's "Honestly Significant Difference" procedure was used to correct for multiple comparisons. For statistical significance purposes, alpha was set at 0.05.

The primary differences between the children with a diagnosis of sCAS and those who were typically developing had to do with timing. The speech of the children with sCAS was consistently slower than that of the TD children. This difference reached statistical significance in comparisons of total phrase durations for "pea-tea-key" ($p = .004$) and "beet-boot-boat-bat" ($p = .036$) and of vowel duration for [i] in "key" ($p = .002$). Repetitions of [kʌ] and of [pʌtʌkʌ] by children with sCAS were also significantly slower ($p = .014$ and $p = .011$, respectively). Finally, the children with sCAS produced more extreme lexical stress ratios (as grossly measured via syllable durations only) than the children with typical speech patterns. Full results of this study are reported elsewhere (Andrianopoulos, et al., 2007). These results will be used here as points of contrast for the acoustic results from the children with ASD, below.

Table 7–2. Acoustic Measures

Stimulus	Measurements Performed
[f] prolongation	maximum phonation time (sec)
[ɑ] prolongation	maximum phonation time (sec), formant analysis (Hz), pitch extraction at midpoint (Hz), energy calculation at midpoint (dB), voicing analysis
[u]	formant analysis (Hz), pitch extraction at midpoint (Hz), energy calculation at midpoint (dB), voicing analysis
[i]	formant analysis (Hz), pitch extraction at midpoint (Hz), energy calculation at midpoint (dB), voicing analysis
[o i] & [ɑ m u]	formants (Hz), length of vowel, total duration (sec), pitch extraction at midpoint (Hz), energy calculation at midpoint (dB)
pea tea key	length of vowels (sec), length of pauses (sec), total duration (sec), vowels: formant analysis (Hz), pitch extraction at midpoint (Hz), energy calculation at midpoint (dB)
beet boot boat bat	length of vowels (sec), length of pauses (sec), total duration (sec), vowels: formant analysis (Hz), pitch extraction at midpoint (Hz), energy calculation at midpoint (dB)
Buy Bobby a puppy	length of vowels (sec), length of pauses (sec), total duration (sec), midpoints of vowels "Bobby" and "puppy" (dB): formant analysis (Hz), pitch extraction at midpoint (Hz), energy calculation at midpoint (dB)
Mommy bakes pot pies	length of vowels (sec), length of pauses (sec), total duration (sec), midpoints of vowels "Mommy" and "pies": formant analysis (Hz), pitch extraction at midpoint (Hz), energy calculation at midpoint (dB)
[pʌ]	alternate motion rate (syllables/second)
[tʌ]	alternate motion rate (syllables/second)
[kʌ]	alternate motion rate (syllables/second)
[pʌtʌkʌ]	sequential motor rate (syllables/second)

Acoustics of the Speech of Children with ASD

Having established the reliability and validity of our acoustic measures for the purposes of differentiating children who are TD versus those with a possible diagnosis of CAS, our next goal was to apply these measures to children with ASD in order to further explore the existence and nature of motor speech disorders in this population.

Participants

The ASD participants were 10 children between the ages of 4;0 and 6;5 (mean age 5;5) with a diagnosis of some type of ASD. To be included, potential participants had to have expressive vocabularies of at least

50 words (oral, signed, and/or picture communication), of which at least 10 had to be oral. As it turned out, all of the children had spoken vocabularies of at least 50 words and were producing many word combinations. Potential participants were excluded if they had any craniofacial or other structural differences, any uncorrected hearing or visual deficits, or any history within the previous six months of self-injury, injury to others, or damage to property. Hearing screenings were administered by supervised graduate students in Communication Disorders. The University of Massachusetts Psychological Services also screened all potential subjects to ensure that their verbal, nonverbal, or combined IQ's fell within the 70 to 90 range, unless there was previous documentation of an IQ within that range. Module 2 of The Autism Diagnostic Observation Schedule (ADOS; Lord, Rutter, DiLavore, & Risi, 2000) was administered to all participants to confirm their diagnosis. By chance

(and the nature of ASD), all but one of the participants were male. Table 7–3 presents individual participant profiles.

The Preschool Language Scale (PLS-4; Zimmerman, Steiner, & Pond, 2002) and the Hodson Assessment of Phonological Patterns–3 (HAPP-3; Hodson, 2004) were also administered to each participant; those results are summarized in Table 7–4. The VMPAC was additionally administered as one way to explore the oral motor and motor speech status of each participant. VMPAC results are given in Table 7–5.

Procedures

The acoustic recording and analysis procedures were the same as for the CAS study described above.

In addition, coefficients of variation for speech and pauses, and coefficient of variation ratios, were also calculated for the children as described in Shriberg, Green,

Table 7–3. ASD Participants

Participant Code	Age	Sex	Independent Diagnosis	ADOS Diagnosis (Score)
ASD1	4;5	Male	Autism	Autism (8+10)
ASD2	6;4	Male	Autism	Autism (10+11)
ASD3	6;3	Male	Autism	Mild Autism (5+9)
ASD4	6;3	Male	PDD-NOS	Autism (7+12)
ASD5	6;2	Male	Autism	Autism (11+16)
ASD6	6;3	Male	Autism	Autism (9+11)
ASD7	5;0	Male	Autism	Autism (9+12)
ASD8	4;2	Male	PDD-NOS	Autism (8+7)
ASD9	4;11	Female	PDD-NOS	Autism (10+13)
ASD10	4;4	Male	Autism	ASD (6+5)

ADOS Key:
1st number is Communication Score—cutoff for Autism: 5; cutoff for ASD: 3
2nd number is Social Interaction Score—cutoff for Autism: 6; cutoff for ASD: 4
Sum—cutoff for Autism: 12; cutoff for ASD: 8

Table 7–4. Language and Phonology Test Results

Participant Number	PLS			HAPP	
	AD	EC	TLS	Ability Score	%ile Rank
ASD1	92	81	85	74	7
ASD2	59	60	55	64	<1
ASD3	51	66	54	<55	<1
ASD4	93	73	83	68	2
ASD5	59	50	50	80	10
ASD6	83	90	85	77	7
ASD7	117	81	99	108	81
ASD8	75	56	62	<55	<1
ASD9	68	56	58	76	8
ASD10	104	95	100	92	24
Mean	**80.1**	**70.8**	**73.1**	**79.88**	**19.86**
St. dev.	**21.50**	**15.55**	**19.30**	**14.09**	**27.82**

Participant demographics in terms of tests administered as part of larger study.
PLS: AD (Auditory Comprehension), EC (Expressive Communication), TLS (Total Language Scale).
HAPP: Ability Score and Percentile Rank based upon Consonant Category Deficiencies Sum.

et al. (2003), except that instead of using spontaneous speech samples, the children's productions of the phrases "pea tea key" and "beet boot boat bat" (elicited using pictures from the VMPAC), and of the sentence "Buy Bobby a puppy" were used. Each of these phrases/sentences was produced one to three times by each participant; the first repetition of each was used to eliminate practice effects. The durations of syllables —rather than of uninterrupted stretches of speech, as in the Shriberg study—were measured. This eliminated the confounding variable of variable word lengths and variable lengths of speech events present in the Shriberg study. As in Shriberg, Green, et al. (2003) no pauses or speech durations less than 100 ms. were included. (*Note:* In almost all, but not quite all, cases there were pauses of more than 100 msec between syllables.)

Results

VMPAC Scores. VMPAC FOM and SEQ subscores for the children with ASD (presented in Table 7-5) indicated the likelihood that at least some of them exhibit several characteristics similar to some of the features of CAS. FOM scores ranged from 48% correct to 91% correct, with a mean of 75.7%. Using the age-based guidelines provided in the VMPAC manual, only three of these scores fell within normal limits for the child's age group; six of the remaining seven were at

Table 7–5. VMPAC Results for ASD Participants

Participant Number	Global Motor Contol		Focal Oromotor Control		Sequencing		Speech Characteristics	
	% Score	Severity Rating	% Score	Severity Rating	% Score	Severity Rating	% Score	Severity Rating
ASD1	90	Mod.	48	Severe	39	Severe	86	Mod.
ASD2	95	Mild	63	Severe	50	Mild	86	Mod.
ASD3	95	Mod.	76	Severe	59	Severe	100	W.N.L.
ASD4	100	W.N.L.	80	Severe	89	W.N.L.	71	Severe
ASD5	100	W.N.L.	67	Severe	67	Mod.	87	Severe
ASD6	100	W.N.L.	91	W.N.L.	98	W.N.L.	86	Mod.
ASD7	95	Mod.	90	W.N.L.	96	W.N.L.	86	Mod.
ASD8	100	W.N.L.	70	Severe	57	Mild	43	Severe
ASD9	95	Mod.	84	Mod.	87	W.N.L.	100	W.N.L.
ASD10	100	W.N.L.	88	W.N.L.	78	W.N.L.	43	Severe
Mean	97		75.7		72		78.8	

the "severe deficit" level, with the other one scoring within the "moderate deficit" range. Similarly, SEQ scores ranged from 39 to 98% correct, with a mean of 72%. Two scores fell at the "severe" level; one corresponded to a moderate deficit and two mild. The other five were within normal limits for the children's ages. Two children were within normal limits for both subscores; two were at the severe level for both. One child was within normal limits for sequencing but at the severe deficit level for focal oral motor skills.

Global Motor subscores which, according to Hayden and Square (1999), correspond more closely to symptoms of dysarthria (muscle tone differences, etc.), were also calculated. The ASD children's scores ranged from 90 to 100% correct, with a mean of 97%. These scores corresponded to moderate (4), mild (1), or no deficit (5) levels relative to VMPAC age norms. Perceptually based dichotic judgments of speech characteristics

(e.g., hoarseness judged to be present or not), such as pitch, resonance, and intensity, also ranged from 43% typical (severe deficit) to 100% typical (within normal limits). Thus, some children exhibited some features consistent with a diagnosis of dysarthria, especially with respect to perceptually-judged vocal quality.

Acoustic Results. With respect to the acoustic measures, a comparison group of children with speech sound disorders (of any type) matched to the participants with ASD for age and gender and who also have receptive language skills similar to those of the ASD participants (see Table 7–4), is currently being recruited. In the meantime, rough comparisons of these ASD participants to the two groups (sCAS, TD) described above will be made, keeping in mind that the ages of this ASD group do not quite match those of the other two groups. As the children with ASD are somewhat younger (mean age 5;5 versus 6;8), only very tentative hypotheses can be generated about tasks on which they perform more poorly than the other two groups.

Fundamental Frequency. Despite their younger ages, children with ASD demonstrated F_0 values below those of the children with sCAS and much below those of the TD children as well as below the norms reported in the literature for children in their age range. Age norms indicate that a male 5 to 8 year-old's pitch should fall between 250 and 265 hertz (Hz) (Roth & Worthington, 2005). As shown in Table 7–6, the TD children in our study produced F_0's between 212 Hz and 249 Hz during prolongation of the [i], [a], and [u] vowels; children with sCAS had F_0's between 212 and 238 Hz for the same vowel productions. According to Peterson and Barney (1952) and Thoonen, Maassen, Wit, Gabreels, and Schreuder (1999), average F_0 in children for the vowels [i], [a], and [u] range between 256 and 276 Hz; consequently, all three groups within this study produced F_0's well below those of their typical peers. Those of the children with ASD ranged from an average of 184 Hz while prolonging [u] to 212 Hz for [a], with [i] falling in between at 193 Hz. Pitch values for [u] and [i] were significantly different for the ASD versus the sCAS groups ([u] $p = .017$; [i] $p = .001$); the sCAS and TD groups did not differ significantly from each other. The group standard deviation for the ASD children was smaller than those for the sCAS and TD groups, possibly due at least in part to lower mean values. The children with ASD may also have performed similarly to each other on the tasks for a variety of other reasons, such as impairments in social emulation, imitation, comprehension, or motor execution and motor programming or planning. However, their individual standard deviations (for three repetitions) were as high or higher than those of the other groups.

Formant Values. Despite lower average fundamental frequencies per vowel prolongation, the children with ASD had generally higher formant values for the prolonged vowels [a], [u], and especially [i] (all produced in isolation) than the sCAS and TD children. For [a], the ASD children's F1 and F3 values were significantly above those of both other groups, as shown in Table 7–7; F2 was significantly above that of the TD group ($p = .005$) but barely missed significance ($p = .06$) in comparison to the sCAS group. In no case were the formants of the TDs versus the sCASs significantly different from each other.

However, these [a] formant values for the ASD children were within one standard deviation of those reported for American English-speaking five-year-olds producing the [a] in "pot" by Lee, Potamianos, and Narayanan (1999). In contrast, the sCAS and TD's F1 and F2 for [a] were more than 1 s.d. below the Lee et al. means for 7-year-olds.

As shown in Table 7–8, for the vowel [u], the mean F2 and F3 values of the ASD group were significantly above those of the other two groups. First formants did not differ for this vowel, nor did the sCAS and TD groups differ on any formants. Again, the ASDs' [u] F1 and F2 formants were within one standard deviation of those reported for American English-speaking five-year-olds producing the [u] in "boot" by Lee et al. (1999); their F3's were slightly more than one standard deviation above the Lee et al. mean. The TD's and sCAS's prolongations of the [u] vowel were at least 1 s.d below the Lee et al. means for 7-year-olds producing the [u] in "boot" for all three of the F1-F3 formants.

The formant differences for [i] were the most striking, as exhibited in Table 7–9.

Table 7-6. Pitch for [ɑ], [i], [u] Produced in Isolation

Task	Group	Mean Value (Hz)	Mean Individual Variability Within Task (SD)	Mean Group Variability Within Task (SD)	SEM	F-value	ANOVA	Significance	Tukey
[ɑ] pitch	ASD	212.36	15.73	24.57	15.76				
	CAS	231.97	30.40	39.42	13.938				
	TD	248.67	13.15	32.20	11.368				
	ASD & CAS					0.21			.075
	ASD & TD					0.46			.564
	CAS & TD					0.61			.438
	ANOVA						2.690	.09	
[u] pitch	ASD	184.43	68.59	18.93	13.03				
	CAS	237.93	39.65	31.90	11.279				
	TD	211.70	21.88	52.64	18.611				
	ASD & CAS					0.15			.017*
	ASD & TD					0.01			.292
	CAS & TD					0.21			.339
	ANOVA						4.572	.022*	
[i] pitch	ASD	192.96	11.65	17.83	11.99				
	CAS	212.15	26.15	31.76	11.227				
	TD	264.46	9.79	22.37	7.909				
	ASD & CAS					0.13			.001*
	ASD & TD					0.54			.000*
	CAS & TD					0.38			.259
	ANOVA						19.127	.000*	

*denotes statistically significant task ($p < 0.050$).

161

Table 7-7. Formants of [ɑ] Produced in Isolation

Task	Group	Mean Value (Hz)	Mean Individual Variability Within Task (SD)	Mean Group Variability Within Task (SD)	SEM	F-value	ANOVA	Significance	Tukey
[ɑ] F1	ASD	1078.94	463.67	165.47	112.18				
	CAS	681.00	85.90	165.49	58.511				
	TD	793.59	132.24	169.05	59.767				
	ASD & CAS					0.99			.005*
	ASD & TD					0.94			.000*
	CAS & TD					0.96			.383
	ANOVA						13.021	.000*	
[ɑ] F2	ASD	1896.36	372.50	611.42	419.35				
	CAS	1229.01	84.33	147.06	51.994				
	TD	1440.68	68.36	144.99	51.263				
	ASD & CAS					0.00			.060
	ASD & TD					0.00			0.005*
	CAS & TD					0.97			.527
	ANOVA						6.673	.005*	
[ɑ] F3	ASD	3091.61	1618.02	709.20	494.82				
	CAS	1941.64	85.90	268.43	94.903				
	TD	2348.49	132.24	391.61	138.455				
	ASD & CAS					0.02			.008*
	ASD & TD					0.14			.000*
	CAS & TD					0.34			.896
	ANOVA						12.885	.000*	

*denotes statistically significant task ($p < 0.050$).

Table 7–8. Formants of [u] Produced in Isolation

Task	Group	Mean Value (Hz)	Mean Individual Variability Within Task (SD)	Mean Group Variability Within Task (SD)	SEM	F-value	ANOVA	Significance	Tukey
[u] F1	ASD	436.43	54.2	59.55	38.07				
	CAS	398.03	38.65	51.83	18.324				
	TD	414.56	47.01	73.70	26.057				
	ASD & CAS					0.73			.752
	ASD & TD					0.56			.426
	CAS & TD					0.37			.857
	ANOVA						.817	.455	
[u] F2	ASD	1505.24	580.47	477.11	342.02				
	CAS	1007.96	122.34	170.10	60.139				
	TD	1051.38	106.12	145.86	51.570				
	ASD & CAS					0.01			.019*
	ASD & TD					0.01			.010*
	CAS & TD					0.70			.959
	ANOVA						6.634	.006*	
[u] F3	ASD	3457.37	233.63	456.85	225.31				
	CAS	2235.79	172.08	206.56	73.030				
	TD	2074.57	169.24	297.56	105.203				
	ASD & CAS					0.05			.000*
	ASD & TD					0.28			.000*
	CAS & TD					0.36			.621
	ANOVA						41.954	.000*	

*denotes statistically significant task ($p < 0.050$)

163

Table 7–9. Formants of [i] Produced in Isolation

Task	Group	Mean Value (Hz)	Mean Individual Variability Within Task (SD)	Mean Group Variability Within Task (SD)	SEM	F-value	ANOVA	Significance	Tukey
[i] F1	ASD	425.44	32.66	40.67	17.19				
	CAS	375.13	30.83	41.59	14.705				
	TD	348.13	21.24	23.82	8.423				
	ASD & CAS					0.94			.025*
	ASD & TD					0.18			.001*
	CAS & TD					0.16			.32
	ANOVA						9.895	.001*	
[i] F2	ASD	2648.59	260.38	610.45	150.92				
	CAS	1218.16	323.61	371.63	131.389				
	TD	1345.19	230.82	559.35	197.760				
	ASD & CAS					0.21			.000*
	ASD & TD					0.83			.000*
	CAS & TD					0.30			.881
	ANOVA						19.403	.000*	
[i] F3	ASD	3633.37	1486.92	521.47	123.89				
	CAS	2763.06	337.23	266.17	94.106				
	TD	2943.16	143.75	258.53	91.404				
	ASD & CAS					0.09			.000*
	ASD & TD					0.08			.003*
	CAS & TD					0.94			.613
	ANOVA						12.742	.000*	

*denotes statistically significant task ($p < 0.050$)

All three ASD mean formant frequencies were significantly higher than those of the other two groups ($p = .025$ and $p = .001$ for F1; $p < .0001$ in comparison to both groups for F2; $p < .0001$ and $p = .003$ for F3). Again the sCAS and TD groups did not differ on any formant values. Compared to Lee et al. (1999), the ASD participants' F1 and F3 frequencies are consistent with their published findings for 5-year-olds producing the [i] in "bead." However, our findings on ASD participants for F2 were more than 1 standard deviation below these authors' published findings for 5-year-olds. Moreover, the sCAS' and TDs' F2 and F3 frequencies are 1 to 2 standard deviations lower than the Lee et al. 7-year-olds.

The effect of the ASD group's somewhat younger mean age on these formant values cannot be determined, nor should it be ignored. However, it is important to note that formant values do not predictably nor linearly go either up or down between the ages of five and eight; changes in formants depend upon the vowel and the formant (Lee et al., 1999). These acoustic findings on our small sample of 10 participants with ASD should be interpreted with caution given the variability of results. The comparison to Lee et al. (1999) is also very tentative given the difference in sampling procedures (i.e., our analysis of prolonged vowels vs. their analysis of vowels embedded within b__t and b__d words).

Timing Measures

Maximum Phonation Time. Maximum phonation time for [a] could not be calculated for two of the children with ASD because they refused to produce prolongations of this sound. The remaining participants in this group produced significantly shorter prolongations of [a] than the sCAS group (group means 2.58 vs. 3.59; $p < .0001$), as shown in Tables 7–10 and 7–11. In turn, the

Table 7–10. Mean Length of [a] Prolongation (MPT)

ASD		CAS		TD	
Subject	Mean time (sec)	Subject	Mean time (sec)	Subject	Mean time (sec)
ASD1		M1	2.583	TDM1	14.442
ASD2	1.167	M2	6.775	TDM2	4.764
ASD3		M3	5.188	TDM3	6.716
ASD4	1.042	M4	1.808	TDM4	7.419
ASD5	3.16	M5	1.554	TDM5	11.887
ASD6	1.07	F1	4.579	TDF1	7.530
ASD7	1.55	F2	2.562	TDF2	9.921
ASD8	1.01	F3	3.562	TDF3	18.354
ASD9	1.50				
ASD10	2.91				

Table 7–11. [ɑ] Prolongation Statistics

Group	Mean Duration (sec)	Mean Individual Variability Within Task (SD)	Mean Group Variability Within Task (SD)	Standard Error of Measure-ment	F-value	ANOVA	Signifi-cance	Tukey
ASD	2.577	0.557	1.473	1.059				
CAS	3.588	1.020	1.808	0.639				
TD	10.129	2.358	4.534	1.603				
ASD & CAS					0.555			.000*
ASD & TD					0.003			.737
CAS & TD					0.010			.000*
ANOVA						16.086	.000*	

*denotes statistically significant task (p <0.050).

children with sCAS produced significantly shorter [a] prolongations that did the TD's (p <.0001). Both of these groups averaged prolongations well below age means of 8 to 11.5 seconds for children between the ages of four and seven years old (Robbins & Klee, 1987); the TD mean of 10 seconds was age-appropriate. Standard deviations for both disorder groups were very low (ASD 1.47; sCAS 1.81), most likely due to a floor effect. None of the ASD children prolonged [a] as long as the shortest TD [a] prolongation (4.76 sec.).

Prolongations of [f] showed a similar pattern: ASD [f]'s were significantly shorter than those of the sCAS group (p <.0001) which, in turn, were significantly shorter than those of the TD group (p = .002). Again, the disorder groups had smaller standard deviations than the TD group; however, in this instance there was overlap between durations of both ASD and sCAS children

and TD children. These results are displayed in Tables 7-12 and 7-13.

Speech Rate. There were some indications of slowed speech among the children with ASD. The durations of their productions of [i] in the word "key" (from the phrase "pea tea key") were significantly slower (p = .002) than those of the TD children. Other comparisons in which they appeared to be somewhat slower than the TD children (i.e., there was a statistical trend for a difference in that direction) included the [ɑɪ] in "pies" (p = .094) and repetitions of [pʌtʌkʌ] (p = .076). Cases in which the children with ASD appeared to be somewhat slower than the children with sCAS (i.e., there was a statistical trend for a difference in that direction) were the [i] in "key" (p = .086), the pause between "tea" and "key" in the phrase "pea-tea-key" (p = .110), the total duration of "pea-tea-key" (p = .101), and the duration of

Table 7–12. Mean Length of [f] Prolongation (MPT)

ASD		CAS		TD	
Subject	Mean time (sec)	Subject	Mean time (sec)	Subject	Mean time (sec)
ASD1	0.893	M1	2.660	TDM1	4.836
ASD2	1.630	M2	1.574	TDM2	3.315
ASD3	2.584	M3	3.725	TDM3	4.074
ASD4	3.729	M4	2.010	TDM4	3.536
ASD5	4.000	M5	2.469	TDM5	4.110
ASD6	5.371	F1	2.556	TDF1	4.525
ASD7	2.470	F2	2.167	TDF2	8.476
ASD8	0.722	F3	2.578	TDF3	7.308
ASD9	0.75				
ASD10	2.097				

Table 7–13. [f] Prolongation Statistics

Group	Mean Duration (sec)	Mean Individual Variability Within Task (SD)	Mean Group Variability Within Task (SD)	Standard Error of Measurement	F-value	ANOVA	Significance	Tukey
ASD	1.59	0.446	0.940	0.551				
CAS	2.467	0.760	0.625	0.221				
TD	5.023	0.902	1.863	0.659				
ASD & CAS					0.304			.000*
ASD & TD					0.092			.362
CAS & TD					0.027			.002*
ANOVA						17.526	.000*	

*denotes statistically significant task ($p < 0.050$).

[o] in "boat" (p = .122). The age differences among the groups could account, at least in part, for these differences and trends.

Lexical Stress Ratios. The children with ASD produced more extreme lexical stress ratios than the TD children, as measured by dividing the durations of the stressed vowels in "Bobby," "puppy," and "mommy" by the durations of the unstressed vowels in the same words. The mLSR's of the children with sCAS were also more extreme than those of the typically developing children. For both "Bobby" and "puppy," the eight most extreme values of each were produced by children with ASD or sCAS. These results are similar to those of Shriberg, Campbell, et al. (2003), who reported that five of the six most extreme LSR values (calculated using a more complex formula, based upon a larger sample of words) were attributable to children with sCAS ("sAOS") as opposed to children with speech delay (SD).

In the Shriberg study, the mean LSR's of all participants were very similar. The mean LSR of the SD group was 0.94 (median 0.94); the mean LSR of the sCAS group was 1.03 (median .96). (*Note:* These are means of means, as Shriberg, Campbell, et al. (2003) did not provide raw data in their article.)

In the present study, mean mLSR's for "Bobby" averaged somewhat above 1 among the sCAS children (1.23), indicating that stressed syllables were longer than unstressed ones. The "Bobby" mLSR's of the ASD children (1.08) were very similar to those of the TD children (1.1), with both very close to 1, indicating little difference between the stressed and unstressed syllables. For "puppy," the mLSR's of both the sCAS and the ASD children were quite close to one (sCAS 1.09; ASD 0.97), whereas the TD children had very low mLSR's (mean of 0.74), suggesting that the TD children's unstressed vowels

were longer than the stressed vowels, perhaps due to the sentence-final position of the unstressed syllable. One possible interpretation of this difference in the length of the final unstressed syllable in "puppy" is that the TD children, but not those from the other two groups, demonstrated phrase-final lengthening on this syllable, as would be expected in English.

The variability among the children with sCAS—and ASD—was much greater than among the children with TD/SD. For "Bobby," TD children's mLSR's ranged from 0.94 to 1.33, with a standard deviation of 0.13; those of children with sCAS ranged from 0.94 to 1.67 with a standard deviation of 0.31, and those of children with ASD ranged from .37 to 1.49, with a standard deviation of 0.40. For "puppy" TD mLSR's ranged from 0.48 to 1.07 (s.d. 0.23), sCAS mLSR's from 0.55 to 1.89 (s.d. 0.43), and ASD mLSR's from 0.36 to 2.52 (s.d. 0.67). The variability demonstrated by the children with sCAS and ASD in comparison to TD participants is exhibited in the boxplots provided in Figure 7–1. (Note that the boxplots are grouped by stimulus; the two leftmost boxplots represent the LSR's of the SD versus the sCAS children in the Shriberg study; the three other pairs of boxplots represent the modified LSR's calculated based on productions of "Bobby" and "puppy" by the TD, sCAS, and ASD groups, respectively, in the present study. Of course, this comparison is compromised by the fact that we did not use the same formula in our study as Shriberg et al. had used; we measured duration only. The point of including the Shriberg boxplots in this figure is to permit comparisons of the amounts of variability in the different groups.)

Coefficients of Variation. As seen in Table 7–14, coefficients of variation of speech (CVSpeech) for the individual TD children

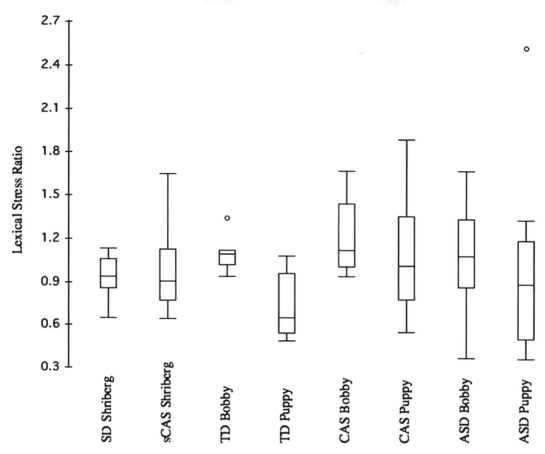

Figure 7–1. Lexical stress ratios for Shriberg, Campbell, et al. (2003) and the present study.

ranged from 0.05 (very little variation) to 0.76 (more variation). Average speech variation was greater for "Buy Bobby a puppy" than for "beet, boot, boat, bat," which was more variable than "pea tea key." The mean CVSpeech was 0.15 for "pea tea key," 0.25 for "beet boot boat bat," and 0.12 for "Buy Bobby a puppy." TD Pause CV's ranged from 0.04 to 0.55 (both from "beet, boot, boat, bat"), with means of 0.27 for "pea tea key" and 0.24 for "beet boot boat bat." CV's for pauses were not calculated for "Buy Bobby a puppy" for any group, as many partici-

pants omitted the word "a," and therefore there were many missing data points. Mean coefficient of variation ratios (CVR's) were 2.24 for "pea tea key," indicating that pauses were typically more than twice as long as syllables for this utterance, and 1.06 for "beet boot . . . " suggesting approximately equal durations.

Children with sCAS produced CV's for speech that ranged from 0.06 to 0.70, similar to the TD participants. However, the means were lower than for the TD children: 0.20 ("pea tea key"), 0.15 ("beet boot . . . "),

Table 7–14. Coefficient of Variation Results

Group	Utterance	Range of CVSpeech	Mean CVSpeech	Range of CVPause	Mean CVPause	CV Ratio (CVP/CVS)
Shriberg TD	conversation	0.46–0.52	0.50 (s.d. 0.26)	0.43–0.64	0.54 (s.d. 0.08)	1.08
Shriberg SD	conversation	0.43–0.50	0.46 (0.23)	0.43–0.57	0.49 (s.d. 0.05)	1.07
Shriberg sCAS	conversation	not available	0.43 (s.d. 0.22)	not available	0.54 (s.d. 0.32)	1.26
TD	pea tea key	0.05–0.44	0.21	0.05–0.51	0.27	2.24
	beet boot boat	0.12–0.76	0.33	0.04–0.55	0.24	1.06
	Buy Bobby a	0.42–0.72	0.56	N/A	N/A	N/A
sCAS	pea tea key	0.06–0.33	0.20	0.004–0.62	0.37	3.13
	beet boot boat	0.06–0.23	0.15	0.30–1.11	0.55	4.32
	Buy Bobby a	0.16–0.70	0.40	NA	NA	NA
ASD	pea tea key	0.02–0.74	0.17	0.0006–0.5	0.36	5.02
	beet boot boat	0.09–0.73	0.35	0.09–1.23	0.53	1.24
	Buy Bobby a . . .	0.18–0.58	0.40	1.02–1.06	1.04	0.49

and 0.4 ("Buy Bobby . . . "). sCAS Pause CV's ranged from 0.004 ("pea tea key") to 1.11 ("beet boot . . . "), a broader range than for the TD participants, with higher means as well, of 0.37 ("pea tea key") and 0.55 ("beet boot . . . "). Mean CVR's were 3.13 for "pea tea key" and 4.32 for "beet boot . . . "; thus pauses were generally much longer than syllables.

The speech CV's of the children with ASD ranged from 0.02 to 0.74 (both for productions of "pea tea key"), a range similar to that of the TD group, narrower than that of the sCAS group. CVSpeech means were slightly lower than the other two groups for "pea tea key" (0.17), slightly higher for "beet boot . . . " (0.35), and the same as the sCAS group for "Buy Bobby . . . " (0.40). ASD coefficients of variation of pauses ranged from 0.0006 (again for "pea tea key") to 1.23 (for "beet boot . . . "), a slightly wider range than the sCAS group. Mean pauses were even more similar to those of the participants with sCAS: 0.36 for "pea tea key" and 0.53 for "beet boot . . . " Mean CVR's were even higher than for the sCAS children for "pea tea key" at 5.02, but more similar to those of the TD participants for "beet boot . . . " at 1.24.

Thus, like the children with sCAS in Shriberg, Green, et al.'s (2003) study, our participants with sCAS and ASD had less average variation in their speech durations than TD children, although the range of variability across participants was higher for the sCAS group than for the other two groups (i.e., children with sCAS had both more variable and less variable speech durations than children in the other two groups). They also demonstrated more variable and longer pause durations than speech durations, as reported by Shriberg et al. As a result, their coefficient of variation ratios were higher overall than those of the TD participants (Figure 7–2).

Discussion and Conclusion

The results of this study strongly support the suggestions in previous literature and the finding of our initial parent survey that many children with ASD demonstrate some symptoms consistent with childhood motor speech disorders. Seven out of our 10 ASD participants exhibited deficits with respect to focal oral motor skills and five with respect to sequencing on the VMPAC. Half scored below age expectations on global motor skills, and 80% had voice characteristics that aroused concern. None of the children with ASD were within normal limits for their ages on all VMPAC scores. Due to the difficulty of relying on test scores alone for this population (given their potential lack of compliance or lack of comprehension; see below), acoustic analysis was used to explore these issues further.

These acoustic analyses revealed that, as a group, the children with ASD produced generally lower fundamental frequencies and higher vowel formants than TD children and those with a previous diagnosis of CAS, possibly accounting for the odd vocal quality often anecdotally associated with ASD. This finding is consistent with past findings of prosodic abnormalities in ASD, although no specific theory (such as deficits in imitation or procedural learning or lack of social emulation) can explain why these values might differ in these specific directions. Their maximum phonation times for both [a] and [f] were abnormally low, as were those of the children with sCAS. This confirms the report of Thoonen et al. (1999) that children with CAS have a decreased ability to prolong [f] compared to controls, although Thoonen and colleagues did not find a difference between CAS and TD groups on prolongation of [a]. Both the children with ASD and the children with sCAS produced

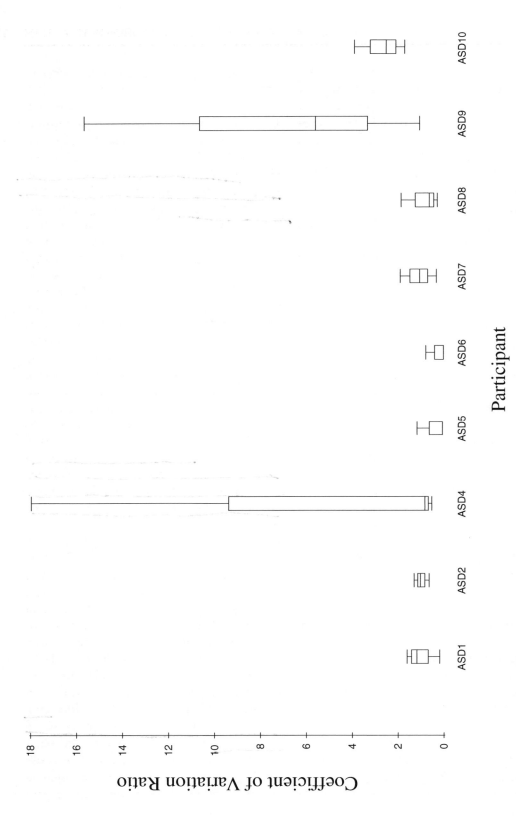

Figure 7–2. Coefficient of variation ratios by subject. (*Note*: ASD3 is omitted because his extremely high ratio, 90.89, for one production of "pea, tea, key," changes the scale to such an extent that the variability of the other participants is invisible.)

more extreme and more variable lexical stress ratios than the children who were TD. These results parallel those in the Shriberg, Campbell, et al. (2003) study despite the fact that duration alone was used as our measure of stress. As in the Shriberg et al. study, this result appears to contradict the many perceptual reports that the stress patterns of children with CAS are "excessive/equal" (i.e., closer to 1 than in typical children). Although our measure of lexical stress ratios differed from that of Shriberg et al., neither of the outcomes is consistent with syllables that do not differ with respect to the acoustic characteristics of stress, as one might expect from the description of apraxic child speech as having "excessive/equal" stress. These findings require further investigation and explanation.

In addition, the children with ASD and sCAS in this study did not appear to use phrase-final lengthening in the same way as the TD children. If it were only the children with ASD who demonstrated this lack of attunement to the native language (given that phrase-final lengthening is language-specific despite its physiologic basis), it would be reminiscent of a report by Baron-Cohen and Staunton (1994) that children with ASD do not adapt their speech patterns to those of their peers, although the participants in the latter study did attune their speech to that of their mothers. However, the fact that neither disordered group made this accommodation suggests that it may instead reflect a difficulty with planning adjustments to sentence context. Alternatively, there could be different explanations for the apparent lack of phrase-final lengthening in each of the two disorder groups.

Despite the differences in methodology, including participants' ages and the use of conversation versus imitation, our coefficient of variation ratio findings were similar

to those reported by Shriberg, Green, et al. (2003) for children with sCAS. Our participants with sCAS, as well as those with ASD, produced less variable syllable durations than pause durations, resulting in high coefficient of variation ratios. However, there was a great deal of variability across children, across repetitions, and across utterances. Shriberg et al. did not report individual data, so it is not possible to compare the two studies at this level. It appears, from the convergence of these two studies, that significant variability, with a lower range for speech duration and a higher range for pause duration, is a feature of the speech of children with CAS. Our participants with ASD demonstrated a similar pattern. The difference between speech and pause durations warrants further study and consideration, given that pause durations as well as speech durations—that is, overall speech rhythm—are language-specific and contextually determined. Thus, a timing deficit, as hypothesized by Shriberg, could be expected to affect both equally. It is not clear why the effects of a timing deficit on linguistic pauses (termed "juncture") would differ from its effects on speech.

Whether it is appropriate to categorize the speech difficulties of children with ASD as CAS or not remains an open question. As we have seen, there are both similarities and differences in the acoustics of speech production of the two disorder groups. In some respects, the speech of the children with ASD is more similar to that of the typically developing children, and in other ways it differs from that of both of the other two groups of children. Furthermore, the Shriberg et al. coefficient of variation ratio study suggests that this measure may not differentiate apraxia from dysarthria. Some hypotheses about CAS and ASD, specifically a possible impairment in direct-route encoding of speech, with resulting reliance on the far less efficient indirect encoding route, overlap. Yet, widespread reports of a more general impairment in imitation are unique to ASD. It is notable that imitation of oral-facial movements is reported to be more impaired than other types of imitation (Rogers et al., 2003); there is inconsistent evidence that this specific type of imitation deficit is associated with degree of speech delay (Stone, Ousley, & Littleford, 1997, as cited by Rogers et al., 2003). Thus, either an explanation for the increased severity of the oral motor imitation deficit must be devised, or some other oral motor deficit or disorder that interacts with the more general imitation deficit associated with ASD must be implicated. If such alternative models are developed, they may prove to be better able to account for the findings reported in the present study. These questions remain for future research.

There are many limitations to this preliminary study. The groups are small, especially the sCAS and TD groups, which only included eight children each. The sCAS and TD groups were not matched exactly to the ASD group by age or developmental level, which introduces an important extraneous variable. Furthermore, the group of children who had been previously diagnosed as having CAS was not homogeneous. In fact, their scores and also expert ratings of their apraxic symptoms were dichotomous; about half of this group either no longer demonstrated clear symptoms of apraxia or perhaps never did. In addition, quite a few of the tasks administered in the present study, especially those used for acoustic analysis, depended upon the children imitating speech stimuli (vowels, sequences of segments and phrases, and sentences). The role of the general deficit in imitation that has been proposed by many authors in the performance of children with ASD on these tasks cannot be specifically determined.

Comparisons to the Shriberg, Campbell, et al. (2003) and Shriberg, Green, et al. (2003) studies are tentative, as age ranges were much wider and procedures were somewhat different in those studies. However, the fact that our results largely concur with theirs for both measures provides some validation of our methods as well as further verification of their findings.

Finally, even though participants with ASD in this study were limited to children with IQ's between 70 and 90 (i.e., not lower), there are inherent difficulties with testing this group that probably impacted upon the results. Often, it is challenging to determine whether a child with ASD performed poorly on a task because he/she cannot perform it, does not understand it, or simply is not motivated enough to comply. Other researchers have reported children with ASD to be as cooperative as TD children and children with developmental delays (Rogers et al., 2003), but this factor was not measured here. Many measures, such as making available the child's usual rewards—(favorite foods, stickers, a favorite toy), providing breaks, using a "red timer," and cutting testing sessions short if needed, were taken to maximize compliance. In some cases, it was clear that the child was making every effort to perform the task, but was unable to do so. Other cases were ambiguous. Nonetheless, our research team was persistent in soliciting responses for every task so that the behaviors exhibited by our CAS and ASD participants could be empirically studied.

The PLS Auditory Comprehension standard scores of the ASD participants ranged from 46 to 117 (mean 69.9), so it is also important to consider whether some of the participants may not have understood all of the directions. Our future plans include testing children with phonological disorders, matched for age, sex, and receptive language level to the children with ASD reported here.

This will provide some measure of control for comprehension difficulties among the ASD participants, as well as a group of more closely age-matched peers without ASD.

Other future research goals include investigating the role of imitation deficits in the oral motor and motor speech performance of children with ASD, gathering similar expert judgments of the ASD group with respect to the apraxia versus dysarthria symptoms that they demonstrate, exploring the presence of motor speech symptoms in lower functioning groups of children with ASD, and assessing the effectiveness of motor speech intervention for young children with ASD.

The clinical implications of this research are critical, especially in conjunction with previous findings and suggestions in the literature. It cannot be assumed that the lack of speech output on the part of many children with autism is due solely to a lack of social motivation or of pragmatic understanding. Nor should it be assumed that oral communication is not possible for children with ASD. Thorough oral motor and motor speech assessments are vital for all children with disorders on the autism spectrum. As the prevalence of dysarthria and apraxia of speech in the pediatric ASD population is indeterminate to date, we need to rule in or out the presence of these motor speech disorders in individual children with ASD.

As previously stated, we speculate that dysarthria in children is not rare (van Mourik et al., 1997). We believe that the under-diagnosis of dysarthria in children is primarily due to these factors: (1) the application of the adult model and classification system for the differential diagnosis of dysarthria in children has not been validated; (2) few clinicians diagnose dysarthria or specific subtypes of dysarthria in the pediatric population in that children with congenital or developmental abnormalities are typically diagnosed by syndrome or disorder and not speech and/or language impairment; and (3) children with motor speech disorders may not always exhibit the same constellation of symptoms as adults with acquired motor speech disorders due to the beneficial effects of neurodevelopment and neuroplasticity in children.

The identification of symptoms of CAS in children with ASD is complicated by the fact that diagnostic markers to differentially diagnose childhood apraxia of speech are not universally agreed upon and that symptoms change over time within the same child due to the beneficial effects of neuroplasticity and neurodevelopment. It is plausible that a child may exhibit an apraxia of speech on initial evaluation and upon re-evaluation at a future date not appear to be apraxic or as apraxic as before (as may have been the case for some of our sCAS participants).

Given these challenges associated with diagnosing either dysarthria or CAS in any pediatric population, identification and treatment of specific motor speech symptoms in children with ASD is more important than deciding on the appropriate motor speech diagnostic label.

Techniques designed to improve speech production skills in children with motor speech disorders should be implemented in those children with ASD who do present with motor-speech-based deficits in oral communication; the current heavy reliance on augmentative communication strategies may be able to be reduced as a result. Admittedly, evidence-based treatment studies to explore the efficacy of various motor speech treatment approaches for this population are sorely needed. In the meantime, the selection of intervention strategies geared to children with CAS versus those with dysarthria, or both, should depend on the specific motor speech symptoms (if any) exhibited by the individual with ASD.

References

Allen, G. (2006). Cerebellar contributions to autism spectrum disorders. *Clinical Neuroscience Research*, 6, 195–207.

American Psychological Association. (2000). *Diagnostic and statistical manual of mental disorders: DSM-IV-TR* (4th ed., text revision). Washington, DC: Author.

American Speech-Language-Hearing Association. (2007a). *Childhood apraxia of speech* [Position statement]. Available from www.asha.org/policy

American Speech-Language-Hearing Association (ASHA). (2007b). Technical report on childhood apraxia of speech. Retrieved June 24, 2007, fromhttp://www.asha.org/NR/rdonlyres/1A85CA28-0B4D-4E56-B740-EF13C2F0D689/0/v3TRChildhoodApraxia.pdf2007

Amoroso, H. (1992). Disorders of vocal signaling in children. In H. Papousek, U. Jurgens, & M. Papousek (Eds.), *Nonverbal vocal communication: Comparative and developmental approaches* (pp. 192–204). Cambridge: Cambridge University Press.

Andrianopoulos, M. V., Velleman, S. L., Perkins, J. J., Boucher, M. J., & Van Emmerik, R. (June 3, 2007). *Acoustic speech characteristics of childhood apraxia of speech.* Paper presented at the Annual Voice Foundation Conference, Philadelphia.

Andrianopoulos, M. V., Velleman, S. L., Marilli, K., & Foreman, C. (November 20, 2005). *Communication and academic abilities of individuals with Autism and Asperger's.* Paper presented at the American Speech Language Hearing Association, San Diego, CA.

Ansel, B. M., & Kent, R. (1992). Acoustic-phonetic contrasts and intelligibility in the dysarthria associated with mixed cerebral palsy. *Journal of Speech and Hearing Research*, 35(2), 296–309.

Aram, D. (1984). Assessment and treatment of developmental apraxia. *Seminars in Speech and Language*, 5(2), 66–70.

Baltaxe, C. (1984). Use of contrastive stress in normal, aphasic, and autistic-children. *Journal of Speech and Hearing Research*, 27(1), 97–105.

Baron-Cohen, S., & Staunton, R. (1994). Do children with autism acquire the phonology of their peers? An examination of group identification through the window of bilingualism. *First Language*, 14(3), 317–352.

Bartolucci, G., Pierce, S., Streiner, D., & Eppel, P. T. (1976). Phonological investigation of verbal autistic and mentally retarded subjects. *Journal of Autism and Developmental Disorders*, 6(4), 303–316.

Bax, M., Goldstein, M., Rosenbaum, P., Paneth, N., Dan, B., Jacobsen, B., et al. (2005). Proposed definition and classification of cerebral palsy. *Developmental Medicine and Child Neurology*, 47(8), 571–576.

Berkeley, S., Zittel, L., Pitney, L., & Nichols, S. (2001). Locomotor and object control skills of children diagnosed with autism. *Adapted Physical Activity Quarterly*, 18, 405–416.

Boucher, J. (1976). Articulation in early childhood autism. *Journal of Autism and Developmental Disorders*, 6(4), 297–302.

Caruso, A., & Strand, E. (1999). *Clinical management of motor speech disorders in children.* New York: Thieme.

Chawarska, K., Klin, A., Paul, R., & Volkmar, F. (2007). Autism spectrum disorder in the second year: Stability and change in syndrome expression. *Journal of Child Psychology and Psychiatry*, 48(2), 128–138.

Chen, H., & Stevens, K. N. (2001). An acoustical study of the fricative /s/ in the speech of individuals with dysarthria. *Journal of Speech, Language, and Hearing Research*, 44, 1300–1314.

Darley, F. L., Aronson, A. E., & Brown, J. R. (1969a). Differential diagnostic patterns of dysarthria. *Journal of Speech and Hearing Research*, 12, 249–269.

Darley, F. L., Aronson, A. E., & Brown, J. R. (1969b). Cluster of deviant speech dimensions in dysarthria. *Journal of Speech and Hearing Research*, 12, 462–269.

Davis, B., Jakielski, K., & Marquardt, T. (1998). Developmental apraxia of speech: Determiners of differential diagnosis. *Clinical Linguistics and Phonetics*, 12, 25–45.

DeMyer, M. (1976). Motor, perceptual-motor and intellectual disabilities of autistic children. In L. Wing (Ed.), *Early childhood autism* (pp. 169–196). Oxford: Pergamon.

Diamond, L., Dobson, L., & Boucher, J. (1998). Is time a problem for children with autism as well as for children with SLI? *Child Language Teaching and Therapy, 14*(2), 181–198.

Eisenmajer, R., Prior, M., Leekam, S., Wing, L., Gould, J., Welham, M., et al. (1996). Comparison of clinical symptoms in autism and Asperger's disorder. *Journal of the American Academy of Child and Adolescent Psychiatry, 35*(11), 1523–1531.

Foreman, C. G. (2001). *The use of contrastive focus by high-functioning children with autism*. Unpublished doctoral dissertation, University of California, Los Angeles.

Ghaziuddin, M., Butler, E., Tsai, L., & Ghaziuddin, N. (1994). Is clumsiness a marker for Asperger syndrome? *Journal of Intellectual Disability Research, 38*(5), 519–527.

Gibbon, F. E., McCann, J., Peppe, S., O'Hare, A., & Rutherford, M. (submitted). *Articulation abilities in children with high functioning autism*. Journal of Communication Disorders.

Hamilton, A. F., de C., Brindley, R. M., & Frith, U. (2007). Imitation and action understanding in autistic spectrum disorders: How valid is the hypothesis of a deficit in the mirror neuron system? *Neuropsychologia, 45*, 1859–1868.

Hayden, D., & Square, P. (1999). *Verbal motor production assessment for children*. San Antonio, TX: Psychological Corporation.

Haynes, W. O., & Pindzola, R. H. (2004). *Diagnosis and evaluation in speech pathology* (6th ed.). Boston: Pearson Education.

Hodson, B. (2004). *Hodson assessment of phonological patterns* (3rd ed.). East Moline, IL: LinguiSystems.

Huber-Okraine, J., Dennis, M., Brettschneider, J., & Spiegler, B. J. (2002). Neuromotor speech deficits in children and adults with spina bifida and hydrocephalus. *Brain and Language, 80*(3), 592–602.

Johnson, M. H., Siddons, F., Frith, U., & Morton, J. (1992). Can autism be predicted on the basis of infant screening tests? *Developmental Medicine and Child Neurology, 34*(4), 316–320.

Kay Elemetrics. (1993). *Motor speech profile* (MSP) [Computer program]. Pine Brook, NJ: Author.

Kay Elemetrics. (1993). *Multi-dimensional voice program* (MDVP) [Computer program]. Pine Brook, NJ: Author.

Kay Elemetrics. (1993). *Multi-speech* [Computer program]. Pine Brook, NJ: Author.

Kay Elemetrics. (2004). *Computerized speech lab* (CSL) [Computer program]. Pine Brook, NJ: Author.

Kent, R. D., Kent, J. F., Duffy, J., Thomas, J. E., Weismer, G., & Stuntebeck, S. (2000). Ataxic dysarthria. *Journal of Speech, Language and Hearing Research, 43*, 1275–1289.

Kent, R. D., Vorperian, H. K., Kent, J. F., & Duffy, J. R. (2003). Voice dysfunction in dysarthria: Application of the multi-dimensional voice orogram. *Journal of Communication Disorders, 36*, 281–306.

Kent, R. D., Weismer, G., Kent, J. F., Vorperian, H. K., & Duffy, J. R. (1999). Acoustic studies of dysarthric speech: Methods, progress, and potential. *Journal of Communication Disorders, 32*, 141–186.

Kirkpatrick, E., & Ward, J. (1984). Prevalence of articulation errors in NSW school pupils. *Australian Journal of Human Communication Disorders, 12*, 55–62.

Kjelgaard, M. M., & Tager-Flushberg, H. (2001). An investigation of language impairment in autism: Implications for genetic subgroups. *Language and Cognitive Processes, 16*(2/3), 287–308.

Klin, A., Volkmar, F. R., Sparrow, S. S., Cichetti, D. V., & Rourke, B. P. (1995). Validity and neuropsychological characterization of Asperger syndrome: Convergence with nonverbal learning disabilities syndrome. *Journal of Child Psychology and Psychiatry and Allied Disciplines, 36*(7), 1127–1141.

Kreiman, J., Gerratt, B. R., & Precoda, K. (1990). Listener experience and perception of voice quality. *Journal of Speech and Hearing Research, 33*, 103–115.

Laures, J. S., & Weismer, G. (1999). The effects of a flattened fundamental frequency on intelligibility at the sentence level. *Journal of Speech, Language, and Hearing Research, 42*, 1148–1156.

Lee, S., Potamianos, A., & Narayanan, S. (1999). Acoustics of children's speech: Developmental changes of temporal and spectral parameters. *Journal of the Acoustical Society of America*, *105*(3), 1455–1468.

Lewis, B. A, Freebairn, L. A., Hansen, A. J., Iyengar, S. K., & Taylor, H. G. (2004). School-age follow-up of children with childhood apraxia of speech. *Language, Speech, and Hearing Services in Schools*, *35*, 122–140.

Lord, C., Rutter, M., DiLavore, P. C., & Risi, S. (2000). *Autism diagnostic observation schedule (ADOS)*. Los Angeles: Western Psychological Services.

Maasen, B., Nijland, L., & Van der Meulen, S. (2001). Coarticulation within and between syllables by children with developmental apraxia of speech. *Clinical Linguistics and Phonetics*, *15*(1&2), 145–150.

Manjiviona, J., & Prior, M. (1995). Comparison of Asperger syndrome and high-functioning autistic children on a test of motor impairment. *Journal of Autism and Developmental Disorders*, *25*(1), 23–39.

Marili, K. E., Andrianopoulos, M. V., Velleman, S. L., & Foreman, C. G. (November 18, 2004). *Incidence of motor speech impairment in autism and Aperger's disorders*. Paper presented at the American Speech-Language-Hearing Association Convention, Philadelphia.

McCabe, P., Rosenthal, J. B., & McLeod, S. (1998). Features of developmental dyspraxia in the general speech impaired population. *Clinical Linguistics and Phonetics*, *12*, 105–126.

Mostofsky, S. H., Goldberg, M. C., Landa, R. J., & Denckla, M. B. (2000). Evidence for a deficit in procedural learning in children and adolescents with autism: Implications for cerebellar contribution. *Journal of the International Neuropsychological Society*, *6*(7), 752–759.

Munson, B., Bjorum, E. M., & Windsor, J. (2003). Acoustic and perceptual correlates of stress in nonwords produced by children with suspected developmental apraxia of speech and children with phonological disorder. *Journal of Speech, Language, and Hearing Research*, *46*, 189–202.

Nijland, L., Maassen, B., & van der Meulen, S. (2003). Evidence of motor programming deficits in children diagnosed with DAS. *Journal of Speech, Language, and Hearing Research*, *46*, 437–450.

Nijland, L., Maassen, B., van der Meulen, S., Gabreels, F., Kraaimaat, F. W., & Schreuder, R. (2002). Coarticulation patterns in children with developmental apraxia of speech. *Clinical Linguistics and Phonetics*, *16*(6), 461–483.

Nishio, M. (2006). Comparison of speaking rate, articulation rate and alternating motion rate in dysarthric speakers. *Folia Phoniatrica et Logopaedica*, *58*(2), 114–131.

Noterdaeme, M., Mildenberger, K., Minow, F., & Amorosa, H. (2002). Evaluation of neuromotor deficits in children with autism and children with a specific speech and language disorder. *European Child and Adolescent Psychiatry*, *11*(5), 219–225.

Ornitz, E. M., Guthrie, D., & Farley, A. H. (1977). The early development of autistic children. *Journal of Autism and Developmental Disorders*, *7*(3), 207–229.

Page, J., & Boucher, J. (1998). Motor impairments in children with autistic disorder. *Child Language Teaching and Therapy*, *14*, 233–259.

Paul, R., Bianchi, N., Augustyn, A., & Volkmar, F. (2008). Production of syllable stress in speakers with autism spectrum disorders. *Research in autism spectrum disorders*, *2*(1), 110–124.

Peterson, G. E., & Barney, H. L. (1952). Control methods used in a study of vowels. *Journal of the Acoustical Society of America*, *24*(2), 175–184.

Portnoy, R. A. (1982). Diadochokinetic syllable rate and regularity in normal and in spastic and ataxic dysarthric subjects. *Journal of Speech and Hearing Disorders*, *47*(3), 324–328.

Prizant, B. M. (1996). Brief report: Communication, language, social, and emotional development. *Journal of Autism and Developmental Disorders*, *26*(2), 173–178.

Rabinov, C., Kreiman, J., Gerratt, B. R., & Bielamowicz, S. (1995). Comparing reliability of perceptual ratings of roughness and acoustic measures of jitter. *Journal of Speech and Hearing Research*, *38*, 26–32.

Reid, G., & Collier, D. (2002). Motor behavior and the autism spectrum disorders—introduction. *Palaestra*, *18*(4), 20–29.

Rinehart, N. J., Bradshaw, J. L., Brereton, A. V., & Tonge, B. J. (2001). Movement preparation in high-functioning autism and Asperger disorder: A serial choice reaction time task involving motor reprogramming. *Journal of Autism and Developmental Disorders*, *31*(1), 79–88.

Robbins, J., & Klee, T. (1987). Clinical assessment of oropharyngeal motor disorders in children. *Journal of Speech and Hearing Disorders*, *52*, 271–277.

Rodier, P. M. (2000). The early origins of autism. *Scientific American*, *282*(2), 56–63.

Rogers, S. J., Bennetto, L., McEvoy, R., & Pennington, B. F. (1996). Imitation and pantomime in high-functioning adolescents with autism spectrum disorders. *Child Development*, *67*(5), 2060–2073.

Rogers, S. J., Hepburn, S. L., Stackhouse, T., & Wehner, E. (2003). Imitation performance in toddlers with autism and those with developmental disorders. *Journal of Child Psychology and Psychiatry and Allied Disciplines*, *44*(5), 763–781.

Roth, F. P., & Worthington, C. K. (2005). *Treatment resource manual for speech-language pathology* (3rd ed.). Clifton Park, NY: Thomson Delmar Learning.

Seal, B. C., & Bonivillian, J. D. (1997). Sign language and motor functioning in students with autistic disorder. *Journal of Autism and Developmental Disorders*, *27*(4), 437–466.

Sheinkopf, S. J., Mundy, P., Oller, D. K., & Steffens, M. (2000). Vocal atypicalities of preverbal autistic children. *Journal of Autism and Developmental Disorders*, *30*(4), 345–354.

Shriberg, L. D., & Aram, D. M. (1997a). Developmental apraxia of speech: I. Descriptive and theoretical perspectives. *Journal of Speech, Language, and Hearing Research*, *40*(2), 273–285.

Shriberg, L. D., Aram, D. M., Kwiatkowski, J. (1997b). Developmental apraxia of speech: II. Toward a diagnostic marker. *Journal of Speech, Language, and Hearing Research*, *40*, 286–312.

Shriberg, L. D., Aram, D. M., Kwiatkowski, J. (1997c). Developmental apraxia of speech: III. A subtype marked by inappropriate stress. *Journal of Speech, Language, and Hearing Research*, *40*, 313–337.

Shriberg, L. D., Campbell, T. F., Karlsson, H. B., Brown, R. L., McSweeny, J. L., & Nadler, C. J. (2003). A diagnostic marker for childhood apraxia of speech: The lexical stress ratio. *Clinical Linguistics and Phonetics*, *17*(7), 549–574.

Shriberg, L. D., Green, J. R., Campbell, T. F., McSweeny, J. L., & Scheer, A. R. (2003). A diagnostic marker for childhood apraxia of speech: The coefficient of variation ratio. *Clinical Linguistics and Phonetics*, *17*(7), 575–595.

Shriberg, L. D., Paul, R., McSweeny, J. L., Klin, A., Cohen, D. J., & Volkmar, F. R. (2001). Speech and prosody characteristics of adolescents and adults with high functioning autism and Asperger syndrome. *Journal of Speech, Language, and Hearing Research*, *44*, 1097–1115.

Skinder, A., Connaghan, K., Strand, E., & Betz, S. (2000). Acoustic correlates of perceived lexical stress errors in children with developmental apraxia of speech. *Journal of Medical Speech Language Pathology*, *4*, 279–284.

Smith, I. M., & Bryson, S. E. (1994). Imitation and action in autism: A critical review. *Psychological Bulletin*, *116*(2), 259–273.

Shprintzen, R. J. (2000). *Syndrome identification for speech-language pathology: An illustrated pocket guide*. San Diego, CA: Singular.

Stark, S. (2006). *Neurodevelopmental disorders with genetic etiologies and speech and language disorders*. (Book in preparation).

Stone, W. L., Ousley, O. Y., & Littleford, C. D. (1997). Motor imitation in young children with autism: What's the object? *Journal of Abnormal Child Psychology*, *25*(6), 475–485.

Strand, E. A., & McNeil, M. R. (1996). Effects of length and linguistic complexity on temporal acoustic measures in apraxia of speech. *Journal of Speech and Hearing Research*, *39*(5), 1019–1033.

Szypulski, T. A. (2003). Interactive oral senso-rimotor therapy: One more weapon in the arsenal fight to combat the primary deficits of autism. *Advance for Speech-Language Pathologists and Audiologists*, 9–10.

Tager-Flusberg, H., Paul, R., & Lord, C. (2005). Language and communication in autism. In F. Volkmar, R. Paul, A. Klin, & D. Cohen (Eds.), *Handbook of autism and pervasive developmental disorders* (3rd ed., Vol. 1, pp. 335–364). New York: Wiley.

Thoonen, G., Maassen, B., Gabreels, F., & Schreuder, R. (1999). Validity of maximum performance tasks to diagnose motor speech disorders in children. *Clinical Linguistics and Phonetics*, *13*(1), 1–23.

Titze, I. (1995). *Workshop on acoustic voice analysis: Summary statement*. Iowa City, IA: National Center for Voice and Speech Report.

Tjaden, K., Rivera, D., Wilding, G., & Turner, G. S. (2005). Characteristic of the lax vowel space in dysarthria. *Journal of Speech, Language, and Hearing Research*, *48*, 554–566.

Tomik, B. (1999). Acoustic analysis of dysarthria profile in ALS patients. *Journal of Neurological Sciences*, *169*(1–2), 35–42.

Ullman, M. T. (2004). Contributions of memory circuits to language: The declarative/procedural model. *Cognition*, *92*(1–2), 231–270.

Van Mourik, M., Catsman-Berrevoets, C. E., Paquier, P. F., Yousef-Bak, E., & van Dongen, H. R. (1997) Acquired childhood dysarthria: Review of its clinical presentation. *Pediatric Neurology*, *17*, 299–307.

Velleman, S. L. (1996). The development of phonology and mental representations in a child with pervasive developmental disorder. In T. P. Powell (Ed.), *Pathologies of speech and language: Contributions of clinical phonetics and linguistics* (pp. 27–36). New Orleans, LA: International Clinical Phonetics and Linguistics Association.

Velleman, S. L., & Shriberg, L. D. (1999). Metrical analysis of speech of children with suspected developmental apraxia of speech. *Journal of Speech, Language, and Hearing Research*, *42*, 1444–1460.

Watson, L. R., Baranket, G. T., & DiLavore, P. C. (2003). Toddlers with autism-Developmental perspectives. *Infants and Young Children*, *16*(3), 201–214.

Wetherby, A. M., Yonclas, D. G., & Bryan, A. M. (1989). Communicative profiles of preschool children with handicaps. *Journal of Speech and Hearing Disorders*, *54*, 148–158.

Whiteside, S. P., & Varley, R. A. (1998). A reconceptualisation of apraxia of speech: A synthesis of evidence. *Cortex*, *34*, 221–231.

Williams, J. H. G., Whiten, A., & Singh, T. (2004). A systematic review of action imitation in autism spectrum disorder. *Journal of Autism and Developmental Disorders*, *34*(3), 285–299.

Williams, J. H. G., Whiten, A., Suddendorf, T., & Perrett, D. I. (2001). Imitation, mirror neurons, and autism. *Neuroscience and Biobehavioral Reviews*, *25*, 287–295.

Wing, L. (1981). Asperger's syndrome: A clinical account. *Psychological Medicine*, *11*(1), 115–130.

Wit, J., & Maassen, B. (1993). Maximum performance tests in children with developmental spastic dysarthria. *Journal of Speech and Hearing Research*, *36*(3), 452–459.

Wolk, L., & Edwards, M. L. (1993). The emerging phonological system of an autistic child. *Journal of Communication Disorders*, *26*(3), 161–177.

Wolk, L., & Giesen, J. (2000). A phonological investigation of four siblings with childhood autism. *Journal of Communication Disorders*, *33*(5), 371–389.

Ziegler, W. (2002). Task-related factors in oral motor control: Speech and oral diadochokinesis in dysarthria and apraxia of speech. *Brain and Language*, *80*, 556–575.

Zimmerman, I. L., Steiner, V. G., & Pond, R. E. (2002). *Preschool Language Scale* (4th ed.). San Antonio, TX: Harcourt.

CHAPTER 8

Vocal Production in Toddlers with Autism Spectrum Disorders

ELIZABETH SCHOEN, RHEA PAUL, AND KATARZYNA CHAWARSKA

Autism spectrum disorders (ASDs) are a group of severe neuropsychiatric conditions characterized by disturbances in social, cognitive, and communicative function that are not fully explained by developmental level. Communicative dysfunction is one of the core symptoms of autistic disorders, and delays in language development are highly prevalent in children with ASD (Chawarska et al., 2008; Tager-Flusberg et al., 2005; Wetherby et al., 2004). There has, however, been limited study of the course of acquisition of speech in this population.

There have, though, been hints in the literature about deviancies in vocal development in this population. Ricks and Wing (1976) studied parents' identification of the meaning of the prelinguistic vocalizations of preverbal preschoolers with ASD and found that their parents were unable to understand the intentions behind the vocalizations of other parents' children with ASD, even

though they could understand their own child's messages. In contrast, parents of typically developing children could understand vocalizations of typical children who were not their own, as well as those of their own child. These findings were not replicated, though, in a later study by Elliot (1993). Anecdotally, children with ASD have been described as babbling less frequently than other infants. However, Elliott (1993) found no difference in the average frequency with which preverbal, developmentally delayed two-year-olds, preverbal typically developing 10- to 12-month-olds, and two-year-olds with autism produced vocalizations in free play situations. It is noteworthy, however, that a greater number of children in the group with ASD produced no vocalizations. Moreover, the vocalizations of children with ASD were less likely than those of children in the other groups to be paired with nonverbal communication, such as shifts in gaze, gestures, or changes in facial expression. Sheinkopf and colleagues conducted a detailed examination of the vocal behavior of young preverbal children with ASD and a group of comparison children with developmental delays (Sheinkopf, Mundy, Oller, & Steffens, 2000). They showed that the children with ASD did not have difficulty with the expression of well-formed syllables (i.e., canonical babbling), but produced a greater proportion of syllables with atypical phonation than did comparison children. Wallace et al. (2008) performed acoustic analysis on the vocalizations of preschool children with ASD, comparing them to those of children with other developmental delays, and reported no differences in the vibratory quality (e.g., regular harmonic intervals, widely spaced harmonics, closely spaced harmonics) of the sound production. They did, however, see trends toward differences in the perceptual quality of phonation (e.g., breathy, tremors). Thus, acoustic analyses have not fully described the physical characteristics of these perceived differences in prelinguistic vocalization in ASD.

In terms of phonological development, articulation is often reported to be normal or even precocious in children with ASD who speak (Kjelgaard & Tager-Flusberg, 2001; Pierce & Bartolucci, 1977). However, Bartak and colleagues (Bartak, Rutter, & Cox, 1975) found articulation development to be somewhat slower than normal. These delays were more transient in a group of high-functioning boys with autism than in language-level matched nonautistic boys with severe receptive-expressive delays in middle childhood (Rutter et al., 1992) and were thought to be related to later onset of language milestones. Bartolucci, Pierce, Streiner, and Tolkin-Eppel, (1976) showed that phoneme frequency distribution and the distribution of phonological error types

in a small group of children with autism was similar to that of intellectually disabled and typical children matched for nonverbal mental age. The less frequent the phoneme's occurrence in their language, the greater was the number of errors. More recently, McCleery, Tully, Slevc, and Schreibman (2006) reported that minimally verbal 2 to 3-year old-children with ASD also showed a normal sequence of phonological acquisition in an elicited imitation task. On the other hand Wolk and Edwards (1993) and Wolk and Giesen (2000) report both delayed and atypical patterns of phonological production in a single case study and in a case series of four siblings with ASD. They observed some degree of chronologic mismatch in speech sound development, such that some early-developing sounds were absent whereas later developing sounds were present. Shriberg et al. (2001) reported that one-third of speakers with high functioning autism retained residual speech distortion errors on sounds such as /r/, /l/, and /s/ into adulthood, whereas the rate of these errors in the general population is 2 to 3% (Kirkpatrick & Ward, 1984). Gibbon, McCann, Peppe, O'Hare, and Rutherford (2004) reported similar findings. Thus, there remains some disagreement in the literature about the status of phonological development in children with ASD.

In this chapter, we compare the vocalizations of a group of toddlers with ASD to peers with typical development, both in terms of the acoustic properties of their sound production, and of its phonological characteristics. Our aim is to help to resolve some of the lingering questions about the nature of these productions in ASD, and to begin to think about their implications for the integration of vocal production into a meaningful speech system. Acoustic analysis was included because of its potential to highlight finer differences not readily available from perceptual analysis alone (see also Chapter 5 for more discussion of the advantages of such approaches).

Study 1: Acoustic Analysis of Nonlinguistic Vocalizations

Methods

Participants

Children aged 18–36 months suspected of ASD were seen for clinical evaluations at the Yale Child Study Center as part of a longitudinal study of toddlers presenting with autistic symptoms. Each toddler received a comprehensive evaluation including the Mullen Scales of Early Learning (MSEL; Mullen, 1995), the Vineland Adaptive Behavior Scales (VABS; Sparrow, Balla, & Cicchetti, 1984), the Autism Diagnostic Observation Schedule (ADOS; Lord et al., 2000), the Autism Diagnostic Interview, Revised (ADI-R; Rutter, LeCouteur, & Lord, 2002) and the Communication and Symbolic Behaviors Scales–Developmental Profile (CSBS-DP; Wetherby & Prizant, 1993).

Toddlers were given a diagnosis of ASD by a team of experienced clinicians using information derived from the ADOS and ADI in conjunction with other clinical observations. The ADOS examines the three major areas of impairment commonly seen in ASD, including communication, social interaction and imaginative play, in a semi-structured play interview. Twelve toddlers who met aforementioned criteria for an ASD and were included in Study 1.

Eleven typically developing (TD) toddlers were selected as a comparison group for this study. These participants were recruited from flyers distributed to local childcare centers and pediatric practices. The control group completed a single day evaluation that included a MSEL, VABS, and CSBS-DP to ensure global development was within normal limits. Control participants were selected to match the clinical group for chronologic age and sex ratio. Approximately 73% of the participants were males and 27% were females which is common of the gender distribution for ASD (Fombonne, 1999). Table 8–1 describes the participants in Study 1.

Recording Procedures

The CSBS-DP was administered to both groups during the comprehensive clinical evaluation. The CSBS-DP is a standardized tool used to evaluate speech and communication of typically developing children age 6 months to 24 months and can be used with children with delayed developed until 72 months of age. The CSBS-DP can be used as a screening tool for early social communication problems (Wetherby et al., 2004; Wetherby, Allen, Cleary, Kublin, & Goldstein, 2002). When administered to children with ASD and children with developmental language delay, the CSBS yields two distinctly different profiles, especially in the areas of gesture, social communication and symbolic behavior

During the CSBS-DP assessment, vocalizations produced by each participant were recorded. All vocalizations were captured using a Shure UT Series transmitter, receiver, and wireless microphone. A Marantz CDR300 compact disk (CD) recorder was used to record the vocalizations onto CD. The Marantz CD recorder captured the data as pulse-code modulation (PCM) format at 44,100 samples per second.

Table 8–1. Study 1 Participants

| Group | Age in Months (SD) | Visual Reception | | Receptive Language | | Expressive Language | |
| | | T–score (SD) | Age Equivalent in Months (SD) | T–score (SD) | Age Equivalent in Months (SD) | T–score (SD) | Age Equivalent in Months (SD) |
					MSEL* Scores		
ASD (*n* = 12)	27.87 (5.96)	33.42 (14.84)	20.58 (3.82)	26.67 (17.75)	13.33 (9.84)	26.58 (10.95)	13.08 (6.11)
TD (*n* = 11)	25.64 (6.03)	50.70 (8.82)	26.50 (8.26)	52.10 (12.02)	27.40 (8.68)	52.40 (12.21)	27.60 (10.47)

*Mullen Scales of Early Learning (Mullen, 1995).

Participants were fitted with a lavalier, cardioid microphone. The microphone was placed on the participant's shirt approximately three to five inches away from his or her mouth. If that was not tolerated, a parent or a research assistant held the microphone within three to five inches of the participant's mouth. The transmitter was secured to the participant's back via a small backpack. The receiver was connected to the CD recorder via an XLR cable.

Recording Editing

Each participant's CSBS-DP recording was edited using Adobe Audition 1.0 software by the first author. Extraneous noise (e.g., rustling of papers, banging of toys, adult speech) was removed from each recorded sample. All word or word approximations were also removed as the purpose of this study was to examine nonlinguistic vocalizations. Non-linguistic whining, crying and laughing were also removed. Two seconds of silence was placed between each of the remaining utterances to help facilitate analysis. Each sound file was saved in Waveform Audio Format (.WAV) to ensure high fidelity.

Acoustic Analysis

Waveforms, spectrograms and pitch contours were generated by PRAAT Software, Version 4.6.09 (Boersma, 2001). Figure 8–1 is a screenshot of PRAAT illustrating its waveform, spectrogram and pitch output capabilities.

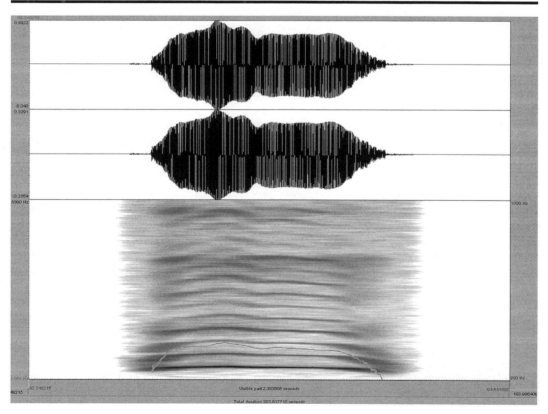

Figure 8–1. Screenshot of PRAAT analysis of vocalization used in study.

Waveforms and spectrograms were used for obtaining duration of vocalizations. Pitch points, the visual output of frequency range produced during a vocalization, assisted in perceptual coding of pitch contours. PRAAT also provided pitch analysis (e.g., high pitch, low pitch for each vocalization).

PRAAT generated wideband spectrograms using Fourier analysis with a viewing range of 0 Hz to 5000 Hz. Pitch range was set to capture the variation commonly observed in infant and toddler vocalizations. The pitch floor was set at 200 Hz and the pitch ceiling was set at 1000 Hz. Window length, for viewing spectrograms and pitch contours, was set at 250 milliseconds.

Acoustic Coding

A trained research assistant completed the acoustic coding. Using the edited recordings from the CSBS-DP assessments, each utterance was divided into smaller units, vocalizations, based on perceptual judgment. A vocalization was defined as any sound produced using vocal fold vibration containing a vowel (V) or consonant-vowel (CV) (e.g., CV, CVC, VC) combination. The first 50 vocalizations produced in each recording by each participant were acoustically analyzed and coded. If the participant did not produce 50 vocalizations, all vocalizations were analyzed and coded.

Each vocalization was analyzed and coded for the following information:

1. Duration of each vocalization (in seconds).
2. Highest pitch (Hz) and lowest pitch (Hz) produced for each vocalization.
3. Pitch range was manually computed by subtracting the lowest pitch from the highest pitch.

A perceptual measure for pitch contour was used for coding vocalization shape. Using the Kent and Murray (1982) classification system (Figure 8–2), each vocalization was assigned a shape based on perceptual judgment.

Any vocalization that contained pitch doubling was eliminated from analysis. Pitch doubling occurs when there is significant and rapid change during vocal fold vibration. These changes disrupt the acoustic software algorithm that computes pitch in computerized acoustic analysis programs. The algorithm output displays double the actual pitch produced (i.e., participant produced an F_0 of 350 Hz; however, the algorithm output displays 700 Hz). Pitch doubling is a common issue in acoustic signal processing (Wu, Wang, & Brown, 2003) as most algorithms require clean speech signals and minimal noise. Pitch doubled vocalizations were identified based on visual inspection of PRAAT pitch contours and pitch analysis.

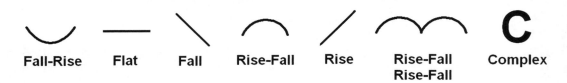

Figure 8–2. Pitch contours for vocalization coding. Adapted with permission from R. Kent and A. Murray (1982). Acoustic features of infant vocalic utterances at 3, 6, and 9 months. *Journal of the Acoustical Society of America, 72*, 353–365.

Reliability

Interrater agreement was established by having the first author independently code a 10% sample of recordings using the aforementioned methods. A point-to-point reliability method was utilized. Interrater reliability was 94.1% agreement on vocalization duration, 95.3% agreement on low pitch point production, 96.0% agreement on high pitch point production and 78.2% agreement on pitch contours.

Data Analysis

Descriptive statistics were computed for the following behaviors: number of vocalizations produced, vocalization duration (in seconds), pitch range and number of different pitch contours produced. Inferential statistics (i.e., ANOVAs, chi-square, independent t-tests) were utilized to measure differences between diagnostic groups on quantity of vocalization production, duration and pitch information.

Results: Study 1

Vocalization Production

The ASD group produced a mean of 38 non-linguistic vocalizations ($SD = 16.00$) whereas the TD group produced a mean of 25 ($SD = 9.74$). Independent t-tests indicated that the ASD group produced significantly more non-linguistic vocalizations than the TD group ($t = 2.47$, $p = .02$). It should be noted that since the meaningful words and approximations were excluded from this analysis, the higher level of nonmeaningful productions by the ASD group reflects not greater total amount of vocal production, but higher levels of nonmeaningful production.

Vocalization Duration

The mean length of vocalization was .44 seconds ($SD = .16$) and .36 seconds ($SD = .16$) for the ASD and TD groups, respectively. Independent t-tests indicated that these differences were not statistically significant ($t = 1.67$, $p = .13$). Further examination of vocalization duration, through additional independent t-tests, indicated the ASD group produced a significantly higher number of vocalizations greater than 0.5 seconds long when compared to the TD group ($t = 3.13$, $p = .016$). The ASD group also showed a trend toward more frequent productions with a duration of 1.0 second or greater but this difference did not reach significance. ($t = 2.00$, $p = .117$). Figure 8–3 represents the percentage of vocalizations produced with duration of greater than .5 and 1.0 seconds.

Pitch Information

Acoustic Analysis. Independent t-tests revealed no significant differences between groups for high pitch, low pitch, and pitch range. Table 8–2 presents pitch information.

A chi-square analysis was performed to compare the distributions of low and high pitched productions in the ASD and TD groups. Results of the χ^2 suggest the ASD group produced a higher proportion of vocalizations with high pitch above the median high pitch for all subjects, with a significance level at $p < .059$ (Table 8–3).

Perceptual Judgment of Pitch Contour. The most frequently produced pitch contour (per Kent & Murray, 1982) used by the ASD group was Complex, comprising 29.84% of vocalizations produced. The second most frequently utilized pitch contour

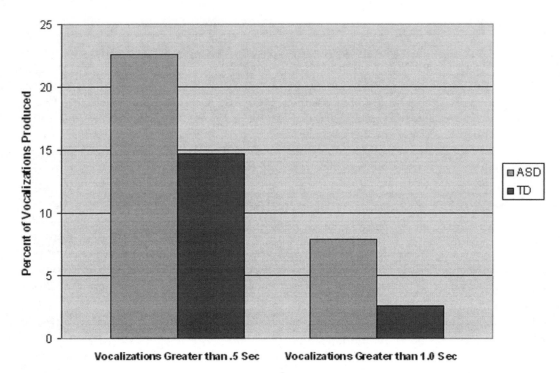

Figure 8–3. Frequency of longer vocalization durations in two diagnostic groups.

Table 8–2. Acoustic Pitch Information in Hz

Group	Mean Low Pitch (SD)	Mean High Pitch (SD)	Mean Pitch Range (SD)
ASD (n = 12)	301.53 (41.90)	425.79 (58.26)	113.49 (44.00)
TD (n = 11)	288.12 (40.34)	391.81 (48.53)	100.98 (30.16)

Table 8–3. Participants Producing Pitch Above the Median Pitch

	ASD n (%)	TD n (%)	χ^2	p
Participants producing pitch >400 Hz	8 (66.7)	3 (27.3)	3.57	.059

was Rise-Fall, comprising 25.28% of vocalizations produced. The TD group used the Flat pitch contour most frequently comprising 33.08% of their vocalization productions. The second most frequently produced pitch contour for the TD group was Rise-

Fall. A total of 26.31% of their vocalization productions utilized this contour. The least used pitch contour by both groups was Rise-Fall-Rise-Fall comprising only 4.55% and 3.00% of vocalizations produced by ASD and TD groups respectively. Figure 8–4 displays the frequency of each contour by diagnostic group.

A chi-square was computed to examine pitch contour distributions within the TD and ASD groups. The χ^2 showed no significant difference in distribution among pitch contours for either the ASD and TD group (Table 8–4). However, further analysis through independent *t*-tests indicated that the ASD group produced a significantly greater proportion of Complex Pitch ($M = 29.84\%$) contours compared to their TD ($M = 10.07\%$) counterparts ($t = 500.50$, $p = .0001$).

Study 2: Perceptual Analysis of Speech and Nonspeech Vocalizations

Methods

Participants

Toddlers were evaluated as part of the same longitudinal study examining ASD as Study 1. Identical diagnostic criteria were utilized for inclusion into the ASD group. Thirty (30) toddlers who were not included in Study 1 comprised the ASD group for Study 2.

Fifteen (15) typically developing toddlers were selected as a comparison group for this study. These 15 TD toddlers were also not included in Study 1. These participants

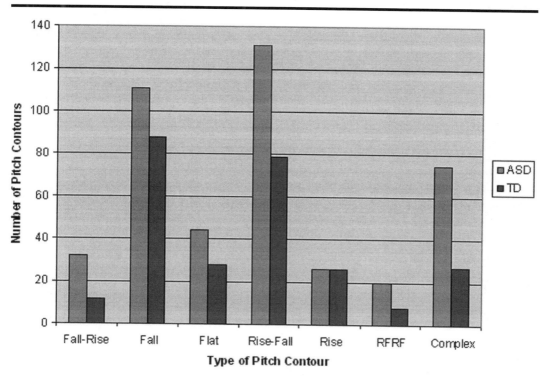

Figure 8–4. Frequency of occurrence of pitch contours in two diagnostic groups.

Table 8–4. χ^2 of Pitch Contours Produced by ASD and TD Groups

| | Group | | | |
| | ASD (n = 12) | | TD (n = 11) | |
Pitch Contour Type	χ^2	df	χ^2	df
Fall-Rise	2.17	4	2.36	2
Flat	3.00	9	2.36	6
Fall	2.00	6	1.55	5
Rise-Fall	1.33	9	1.36	7
Rise	1.33	4	1.55	5
Rise-Fall-Rise-Fall	2.17	4	2.36	4
Complex	2.67	7	1.27	4

Note: No statistical differences.

were recruited from flyers distributed to local child care centers and pediatric practices. The control group completed a single day evaluation that included a MSEL, VABS, and CSBS-DP to ensure global development were within normal limits. All control participants received a standard score of 70 or greater on each of the aforementioned measures. The control group was matched for chronologic age and sex ratio to the group with ASD. The mean age for the control group was 24 months ($SD = 7$ months). The group was 80% males and 20% females. Table 8–5 provides a detailed description of participants.

Procedures

A certified speech-language pathologist administered the CSBS-DP to the ASD group; a research assistant with a B.S. in communication disorders administered the CSBS-DP to the control group. The research assistant was provided with training and supervision by a certified speech-language pathologist to ensure correct administration. The CSBS-DP assessments were videotaped by trained research assistants onto digital media. A timed, 15-minute segment from the CSBS-DP interaction from each participant provided the data for Study 2.

All transcription and coding was completed by the first author. The second author completed reliability coding.

Transcription

Categorization of Vocal Productions. Vocalizations were first, separated into two categories:

1. Speechlike vocalizations, characterized by the production of consonants and/or vowels that could be represented by phonetic symbols and contained speech-like resonance, and
2. Nonspeech vocalizations, including sounds produced without speech resonance and no recognizable consonants.

Table 8–5. Study 2 Participants

Group	Age in Months (SD)	Visual Reception T-score (SD)	Visual Reception Age Equivalent in Months (SD)	Receptive Language T-score (SD)	Receptive Language Age Equivalent in Months (SD)	Expressive Language T-score (SD)	Expressive Language Age Equivalent in Months (SD)
				M and SD MSEL* Scores			
ASD (n = 30)	28.33 (5.08)	31.93 (12.03)	20.13 (4.08)	23.43 (9.24)	11.87 (5.53)	27.60 (9.57)	15.00 (6.63)
ASD PS (n = 21)	27.05 (5.05)	33.76 (12.23)	19.90 (3.65)	23.24 (10.07)	10.66 (4.76)	25.19 (7.17)	12.23 (5.10)
ASD MS (n = 9)	31.33 (3.91)	27.67 (11.03)	20.67 (5.17)	23.89 (7.46)	14.67 (6.46)	33.22 (12.34)	21.44 (5.27)
TD (n = 15)	24.40 (7.37)	52.11 (11.86)	26.00 (10.16)	48.80 (9.57)	25.11 (9.31)	51.00 (11.22)	25.06 (9.46)
TD PS (n = 4)	15.25 (0.96)	51.25 (10.59)	21.50 (12.44)	43.75 (12.45)	19.75 (12.84)	53.75 (13.20)	22.5 (15.15)
TD MS (n = 11)	27.73 (5.50)	54.45 (12.76)	27.63 (9.33)	50.63 (8.23)	27.09 (7.49)	50.00 (10.95)	26.00 (8.12)

*Mullen Scales of Early Learning (Mullen, 1995).

Any vocalization that occurred simultaneously with any other sound on the videotape, such as a cough, adult speech, toy noises or rustling of supplies, was not transcribed in order to avoid errors and reductions in transcription reliability.

Transcription of Speechlike Vocalizations. Rules for transcription of speechlike vocalizations were adapted from Olswang, Stoel-Gammon, Coggins, and Carpenter (1987). The first 50 speechlike vocalizations produced during the 15 minute sample were transcribed utilizing phonemic transcription. If the toddler produced more than 50 utterances during this time period, these were tallied, but not transcribed. Some toddlers did not produce 50 vocalizations in the 15-minute videotaped segment; in these instances all utterances produced by the toddler were transcribed. Any cries, screams, and other nonspeech vocalizations produced by the toddler were analyzed separately. Vegetative sounds including coughing, burping or sneezing were discarded from all analyses.

Transcription of Nonspeech Vocalizations. The same 15-minute segments transcribed for speechlike vocalizations were also coded for nonspeech productions. All nonspeech vocalizations occurring within the same 15-minute time period as the speechlike vocalizations were tallied and coded using rules adapted from Sheinkopf et al. (2000). Nonspeech vocalizations were segmented into utterances based on breath groups (all productions within one breath), or into separate utterances when a pause of greater than one second occurred between productions. Breath groups were determined through visual and auditory inspection of the video recordings. Only the first 50 nonspeech vocalizations were coded. If the participant produced more than 50 nonspeech

vocalizations, the excess were tallied but not coded. If a participant produced fewer than 50 nonspeech vocalizations, all vocalizations were coded.

Coding

Coding was completed on the transcribed speech and recorded nonspeech vocalizations produced by each toddler.

Speechlike Vocalization Coding. Phonemic transcription with International Phonetic Alphabet (IPA) symbols was utilized to transcribe the speechlike vocalizations in the 15-minute sample of each participant. Any utterance that could not be transcribed after four playbacks was eliminated. These transcriptions formed the basis for the construction of consonant and consonant blend inventories. Counts of consonant blend tokens for each participant were also tallied.

In addition to transcribing the speechlike vocalizations phonemically, each utterance was assigned to a syllable structure level (SSL), in order to assess overall level of syllable complexity. SSL values were computed in a manner adapted from Olswang and colleagues (1987), as follows:

> Level 1 utterances: vowels or continuant single consonants (i.e., /mmm/).
>
> Level 2 utterances: syllables comprised of a single consonant-vowel combination, which could include reduplicated syllables. Voicing differences (e.g., /paba/) were disregarded, as per Olswang et al. (1987).
>
> Level 3 utterances: syllables containing two or more different consonants (disregarding voicing

differences) plus vowels (e.g., /pati/).

The number of meaningful words produced by each participant was also tallied and percent consonants correct (PCC) was tabulated (relative to adult targets) for participants who produced at least 10 different recognizable words. Procedures for computing PCC followed those outlined by Shriberg and Kwiatkowski (1982).

Nonspeech Vocalization Coding. Five categories of nonspeech vocalizations were identified, following Sheinkopf et al. (2000):

1. *Distress* was coded when the participant produced crying, whining, or fussing.
2. *Hum* was coded when the participant produced continuous phonation with a closed mouth and no consonants, which contained pitch variation.
3. *Delight* was coded when the participant produced laughter, giggles, or other pleasure sounds.
4. *Atypical vocalization* was coded when the participant produced an example of one of the following categories:
   a. *Squeal*: An utterance containing a perceptually high-pitched vocalization with no consonants,
   b. *Growl*: An utterance containing a perceptually low-pitched vocalization with no consonants,
   c. *Yell*: An utterance containing a loud, neutrally pitched vocalization with no consonants
5. *Other* was coded when the vocalization could not be placed into any of the aforementioned categories.

Each utterance, whether speechlike or nonspeech was also coded based on function. An utterance was coded as communica-

tive if it was directed to the communication partner (i.e., through gaze or gesture) and appeared to convey a message. An utterance was coded as noncommunicative if not directed to the communication partner and did not appear to convey any intentional meaning.

Reliability

Interrater reliability was computed by having a second trained individual independently transcribe and code a 10% sample of videotapes using the aforementioned methods. Point-to-point reliability method was utilized for both speechlike and nonspeech coding. Transcription and coding for speechlike vocalizations, using a point-to-point method, yielded 87.7% reliability for consonants produced in meaningful utterances, 71.9% reliability for consonants produced in nonmeaningful utterances, 87.8% agreement on SSL and 89.6% agreement on PCC, for an average reliability of 84.3% on coding. Coding for nonspeech vocalizations, using a point-to-point method, yielded 96.3% agreement on Distress category, 86.6% on Hum category, 97.7% on Delight category, 91.8% on Atypical category, and 78.6% on Other category, for an average reliability of 90.2%.

Analysis

The following indexes were used to examine the speechlike and nonspeech vocalizations of the participants.

Consonant Inventories. Consonant and consonant blend inventories were assembled for each participant. In addition to compiling a consonant inventory, consonants produced were divided into three categories as outlined by Shriberg (1993) (Table 8–6).

Table 8–6. Sounds Based on Developmental Acquisition

Early-8	/m/	/b/	/j/	/n/	/w/	/d/	/p/	/h/
Middle-8	/t/	/ŋ/	/k/	/g/	/f/	/v/	/tʃ/	/dʒ/
Late-8	/s/	/θ/	/s/	/z/	/ð/	/l/	/r/	/ʒ/

Source: Adapted with permission from "Four new speech and prosody-voice measures for genetics research and other studies in developmental phonological disorders," by L. D. Shriberg. *Journal of Speech and Hearing Research, 36*(1), 105–140. Copyright 1993 by American Speech-Language-Hearing Association. All rights reserved.

These categories reflect relative order of acquisition of consonants in young children with typical development (Shriberg, Kwiakowski, & Gruber, 1994).

Syllable Structure Complexity. A mean SSL was computed for each participant by assigning each speechlike vocalization to the highest SSL level appropriate, then summing these scores and dividing by the number of speechlike vocalizations coded (see Paul & Jennings, 1992). Number and percentage of closed syllables (i.e., VC, CVC) produced by each participant was also calculated (Olswang et al., 1987).

Percent Consonants Correct. Toddlers who produced 10 or more different words or word approximations were classified as meaningful speech stage (MS) participants, following Thal, Oroz, and McCaw (1995). Toddlers who produced fewer than 10 different words or word approximations were classified as premeaningful speech stage (PS) participants. Percent consonants correct (PCC) was tabulated for each participant in the MS group.

Type and Frequency of Nonspeech Vocalizations. The type and frequency of nonspeech vocalizations were tallied for each participant, and group means were computed, following Sheinkopf et al. (2000)

Results: Study 2

The data were first analyzed descriptively; means and standard deviations for each variable are reported. Inferential statistics were used to compare ASD and TD groups.

Descriptive Data

Speech Sound Inventories. Speech sound inventories were tallied and mean number of different consonants produced by each participant in each group is presented in Table 8-7. Specific consonant types produced and the frequencies of use for each appear in Table 8-8. In both diagnostic groups, the subjects with MS produced more consonant types than subjects with PS. No participants in the ASD group produced the /ŋ/, /ʒ/, or /r/ phonemes. The TD MS participants generally appeared to produce more later developing phonemes than the ASD PS and MS groups.

Consonant blend inventories were also tallied. In the ASD group, 29% of subjects

Table 8–7. Number of Different Consonant Types Produced

Number of Different Consonants	Group			
	ASD		TD	
	PS (n = 21)	MS (n = 9)	PS (n = 4)	MS (n = 11)
M	5.33	10.00	6.50	13.82
SD	2.52	1.80	2.08	2.93

Table 8–8. Consonant Inventories of ASD and TD Groups

Sound Stage	Phoneme	Percentage of Participants Producing	
		ASD	TD
Early-8	/m/	83	100
	/b, p/	77	100
	/j/	57	73
	/n/	67	80
	/w/	70	73
	/d/	80	93
	/h/	36	53
Middle-8	/t/	80	73
	/ŋ/	0	20
	/k,g/	80	80
	/f,v/	27	47
	/tʃ/	3	20
	/dʒ/	3	7
Late-8	/ʃ/	7	20
	/θ, ð/	3	27
	/s, z/	40	80
	/l/	13	47
	/r/	0	27
	/ʒ/	0	0

with PS and 67% of participants with MS produced consonant blends compared to 0% and 63% in the PS TD and MS TD, respectively. Table 8–9 outlines the type and frequency of consonant blends produced by all participants. All participants in the MS ASD group produced idiosyncratic consonant blends including /vw/, /tj/, and /θs/, whereas none of those in the TD group did.

Syllable structure complexity. Syllable structure complexity was examined for shape of syllables and use of closed syllables. Means and standard deviations were computed for syllable structure level and percentage of closed syllables for each group and displayed in Table 8–10. Subjects with MS in both the ASD and TD groups produced a mean syllable structure level greater than 2, indicating the majority of their utterances contained some consonant-vowel combinations and at least one CVC.

Speech Stage. Seventy percent of the children with ASD scored in the PS group; 27% of those with TD were PS. The mean and standard deviations for age of participants in each of these four groups (ASD MS, ASD PS, TD MS, TD PS) were shown in Table 8–5. It is noteworthy that the mean age for the TD PS group was significantly younger than the ASD PS group ($t = 4.58$, $df = 23$, $p = .0001$).

Table 8–9. Number of Participants Producing Each Consonant Blend

	Group			
	ASD		TD	
Blends	PS (n = 21)	MS (n = 9)	PS (n = 4)	MS (n = 11)
/w/ blends	3	6	–	2
/j/ blends	1	1	–	1
/s/ blends	–	1	–	5
/l/ blends	–	1	–	4
/r/ blends	–	–	–	1
Other	1	6	–	4

Note: Dash denotes no production.

Table 8–10. Syllable Structure Complexity Level*

	Group			
	ASD		TD	
Syllable Structure Complexity	PS (n = 21)	MS (n = 9)	PS (n = 4)	MS (n = 11)
Syllable Structure Level				
M	1.52	2.08	1.89	2.28
SD	0.35	0.26	0.47	0.26
Percentage of Closed Syllables				
M	4.96	30.84	19.46	44.53
SD	8.21	18.14	28.97	22.38

*Based on Olswang et al (1987).

Word Productions. Table 8–11 outlines the mean number of different words and PCC produced by each group.

Nonspeech Vocalizations. Nonspeech vocalizations were tallied for all four participant groups. Means and standard deviations are displayed in Table 8–12. All but three participants produced at least one nonspeech vocalization. The mean number of nonspeech vocalizations produced by the ASD PS and MS groups were 18 and 14 respectively. The mean number of nonspeech vocalizations produced by the TD

Table 8–11. Word Productions and PCC

	Group			
	ASD		TD	
	PS (n = 21)	MS (n = 9)	PS (n = 4)	MS (n = 11)
Mean Number of Different Words Produced (*SD*)	3.52 (2.73)	15.89 (6.47)	1.27 (1.50)	30.36 (16.13)
Range	0–8	10–30	0–3	10–62
Mean PCC (SD)	–	58.72 (9.34)	–	65.84 (10.99)

Note: Dash denotes too few words for analysis.

Table 8–12. M Number of Nonspeech Vocalizations Produced by ASD and TD groups

	Group							
	ASD				TD			
Number of Nonspeech Vocalizations	PS (n = 21)		MS (n = 9)		PS (n = 4)		MS (n = 11)	
	M	SD	M	SD	M	SD	M	SD
Atypical	4.8	6.1	4.4	4.1	0.5	1.0	1.1	1.9
Squeal	2.9	3.8	3.8	3.6	–	–	0.2	0.6
Growl	1.7	3.0	0.3	0.5	–	–	0.9	1.8
Yell	0.3	0.6	0.4	1.1	0.5	1.0	–	–
Distress	4.8	10.0	1.3	2.8	5.3	9.8	0.4	0.7
Delight	5.1	10.3	6.9	8.6	1.8	2.4	1.7	2.1
Hum	0.4	0.8	0.4	0.7	–	–	0.2	0.6
Other	0.3	0.5	0.6	1.1	0.3	0.5	0.1	0.3

Note: Dashes indicate absence of production.

PS and MS groups were 8 and 4, respectively. *Delight* was the most commonly produced nonspeech vocalization in all four groups. High-pitched squeal was the most commonly produced atypical vocalization produced by both the ASD PS and MS groups.

Communicativeness. Each nonspeech vocalization was coded as either communicative (i.e., conveying a message) or noncommunicative (i.e., not conveying a message). The mean number of communicative nonspeech vocalizations produced by the four groups is illustrated in Table 8–13.

Table 8–13. Communicativeness of Nonspeech Vocalizations

Number of Communicative Nonspeech Vocalizations Produced	Group			
	ASD		TD	
	PS (n = 21)	MS (n = 9)	PS (n = 4)	MS (n = 11)
M (SD)	2.8 (4.1)	3.3 (6.6)	3.3 (4.7)	1.6 (2.6)

Statistical Comparisons

Speechlike Vocalizations. Statistical tests were used to investigate group differences in the use of speechlike data among the three larger subject groups (ASD MS, ASD PS, TD MS). The TD PS group was eliminated from analyses due to its small size ($n = 4$). One-way ANOVAs were performed to examine differences on mean number of different consonants and consonant blends produced. ANOVA results revealed significant differences on both variables (Table 8–14). Posthoc comparisons indicated participants in the TD MS group produced significantly more different consonants than participants in the ASD PS and MS groups (Table 8–15). Moreover, participants in the ASD MS produced a significantly greater number of different consonants than their ASD PS counterparts (see Table 8–14). Additionally, the TD group produced each consonant more frequently with the exception of /t/, where there was no difference between the groups.

Posthoc analysis also revealed that TD MS participants produced significantly more consonants blends overall than ASD PS participants (see Table 8–15), although both groups had a similar chronologic age. In general, TD groups produced more typical consonant blends (i.e., /s/ blends, /l/ blends) whereas the ASD groups produced idiosyncratic consonant blends (i.e., /wp/, /tj/, /hm/).

A one-way ANOVA revealed statistically significant differences in SSL between ASD

MS and PS groups, but no differences between the ASD MS and TD MS groups (see Tables 8–14 and 8–15). The same findings pertained for percentage of closed syllables. There was a correlation between the number of different words produced and percentage of closed syllables for both the TD group ($r = .64$, $p = .009$) and ASD groups ($r = .87$, $p < .0001$).

Analysis of Shriberg's (1993) classification of developmental acquisition of sounds revealed no difference among diagnostic groups for Middle-8 sound production ($t = .79$, $df = 43$, $p = .43$) through an independent t-test. Significant differences were noted within Early-8 and Late-8 sound production. The ASD group produced fewer Early ($t = 2.78$, $p = .008$) and Late ($t = 3.64$, $p = .0007$) developing sounds compared to the TD group.

No significant group differences were observed relative to PCC ($t = 1.53$, $df = 18$, $p = .14$) indicating ASD MS and TD MS participants are producing a similar number of correct consonants per word.

Nonspeech Vocalizations. An independent t-test was used to compare the total number of nonspeech vocalizations used by the ASD and TD groups. The ASD group produced a significantly greater total number of nonspeech vocalizations ($t = 2.10$, $df = 43$, $p = .04$). Further statistical analyses of nonspeech data were also completed to examine the frequency of nonspeech vocalization categories (e.g., atypical vocaliza-

Table 8–14. ANOVA Comparison of ASD PS, ASD MS, and TD MS Groups on Speechlike Variables

Speech Variables	df	F	p
Different Consonants	2, 38	43.15	.00001
Different Consonant Blends	2, 38	5.63	.007
SSL	2, 38	24.16	.001

Table 8–15. Post Hoc Results from One-Way ANOVAs of Speechlike Variables

Speech Variables	Difference (M)	Significance
Number of Different Consonants		
ASD PS vs. ASD MS	−4.67	.0001*
ASD PS vs. TD MS	−8.48	.0001*
ASD MS vs. TD MS	−3.82	.005
Number of Different Consonant Blends		
ASD PS vs. ASD MS	−1.79	.111
ASD PS vs. TD MS	−2.57	.008*
ASD MS vs. TD MS	−0.77	.709
Closed Syllables		
ASD PS vs. ASD MS	−25.88	.002*
ASD PS vs. TD MS	−39.57	.001*
ASD MS vs. TD MS	−13.68	.280
SSL		
ASD PS vs. ASD MS	−0.55	.001*
ASD PS vs. TD MS	−0.75	.001*
ASD MS vs. TD MS	−0.20	.340

*Statistically significant.

tions, delight, and distress) within the diagnostic subgroups (e.g., TD PS, TD MS, ASD PS, ASD MS). One-way ANOVAs on each variable indicated no significant differences between groups for nonspeech vocalizations classified in the major categories (Table 8–16). However, an unpaired *t*-test revealed the ASD group produced

Table 8–16. Comparison of ASD PS, ASD MS, TD PS, and TD MS Groups on Nonspeech Variables

Nonspeech Variables	df	F	p
Atypical	3, 41	2.09	.119
Distress	3, 41	1.07	.373
Delight	3, 41	.860	.471

significantly more vocalizations in the "squeal" subcategory, compared to the TD group ($t = 3.18$, $df = 43$, $p = .003$).

Another independent *t*-test was computed to determine differences for communicative use of nonspeech vocalizations between diagnostic groups. No significant differences were noted relative to communicative function of nonspeech vocalizations between ASD ($M = 2.72$, $SD = 4.65$) and TD groups ($M = 2.00$, $SD = 3.20$), $t = .05$, $p = .59$.

Discussion: Studies 1 and 2

The participants in Study 2 with ASD in this study produced more atypical vocalizations than their typically developing peers. Similar results were found in studies by Sheinkopf et al. (2000) and Wetherby et al. (1989); however, control groups in the previous studies were composed of children with developmental delays, Down syndrome and specific language impairment, rather than the children with TD in this report. These findings suggest that even when they begin speaking, children with ASD continue to include noncanonical forms in their production repertoire. Although these nonspeech forms were not used with great frequency, their co-occurrence with more typical babble and word use represents a qualitative

difference from the observations of children with TD. Children with ASD appear less able or willing to transition fully from sound-making to speech and retain their use of primitive forms, even when more mature forms become available.

Most vocalizations produced by both groups of children were less than 0.5 seconds in duration. The syllable durations observed in both groups are consistent with earlier-reported data on syllable production in this age group, in which average syllable duration ranged from 0.1 to 0.5 seconds with the median between 0.2 and 0.3 seconds (Oller, 2000). Although the majority of the ASD group's vocalizations were similar in duration to these values, the ASD group produced a significantly greater number of long vocalizations, over 0.5 seconds in duration. There could be a number of reasons for this lengthening, including motoric slowness or a failure to tune vocalizations toward the parameters of the speech community. Since the children with ASD did produce many vocalizations of appropriate duration, it seems unlikely that a purely motor explanation can account for this difference. Again, it may be the case that children with ASD are less able to, or more delayed in the transition from earlier developing vocal behavior to sound production that conforms to the general rules of speech.

Pitch information was examined both acoustically and perceptually in Study 1. The acoustic analysis suggested an elevation of pitch on the part of children with ASD. More participants in the ASD group produced pitch points above the median pitch of 400 Hz, when compared to participants in the TD group. This acoustic measure of high-pitch vocalizations supports perceptual reports of high-pitched vocal behaviors in young children with ASD (e.g., Sheinkopf et al., 2000). Failure to move pitch into the more typical speech register may reflect excessive tension in the vocal folds which could be related to poor motor control, or may be another example of a failure to tune in to the characteristics of speech produced by others.

Information on prelinguistic intonation was collected through perceptual analysis of pitch contour, following Kent and Murray (1982). The Complex pitch contour was the most commonly utilized for the group with ASD. The most frequently used for the TD group was the Flat contour. Although the contours produced by children with ASD are generally similar to those seen in previous research on typical children (Flax, 1986; Kent & Murray, 1982; Robb et al., 1989) as well as to the children in the present TD sample, the ASD group did produce a significantly greater number of Complex pitch contours compared to the TD group. These Complex contours, in which pitch fluctuated irregularly within a breath group could, again, have several explanations. Lack of precise motor control and coordination in the larynx could lead to pitch fluctuations, as laryngeal tension is managed imperfectly. An alternative explanation is that these vocalizations may have less communicative intent and more perceptual-motor play, or self-stimulatory, function so that the variation in sound is an end in itself. The degree to which motor deficits contribute to the observed differences is a hotly debated issue (see Chapter 7) that cannot be settled by the present data. What does seem clear is that roots of the well-documented deficits in prosodic production that are common in speakers with ASD (Shriberg et al., 2001) can be observed in the pitch and timing parameters of their early, prelinguistic productions.

Turning to the phonological findings of the current study, our data tend to support the observation that phonological production in this population generally follows a typical developmental sequence. As McCleery et al. (2006) found in an elicited imitation task, we observed that toddlers with ASD who were just emerging into spoken language produced a range of consonant sounds in free speech similar to that seen in the normal course of development. Early developing consonants were produced more frequently than those seen later in typical acquisition; syllable structure levels and PCC in children with ASD who produced some meaningful speech were similar to those seen in age-mates with TD.

Nonetheless, children with ASD appear from these data to be delayed in their speech acquisition, just as they are delayed in their development of language, as many studies have shown (e.g., Chawarska et al., 2008 LeCouteur et al., 1989; Tager-Flusberg, 1994; Wetherby et al., 2004). Toddlers with ASD had significantly smaller consonant inventories than TD children at a similar developmental level, and produced fewer closed syllables and typical consonant blends. Although the participants with ASD produced classes of sounds similar to those of typically developing participants, they did not acquire the range of consonants within each class at the same rate as peers, nor did they use each phoneme in their repertoire as often as did typical peers. Not surprisingly, then, the children with ASD scored lower on our measures of language as well as on speech measures. Besides scoring lower on standardized language measures, they produced approximately half of the number of different word types as their same-age peers, and used fewer word tokens overall than typical age peers. A smaller proportion of two year olds in the group with ASD met criteria for using Meaningful Speech; that is, production of at least 10 different spontaneous words; than did peers with TD, and as we might expect in delayed—rather than deviant—development, toddlers with ASD, like their

TD counterparts (Stoel-Gammon, 1998), showed a correlation between number of words produced and phonological complexity of vocalization, indexed in this study by the number of closed syllables produced. In this way, toddlers with ASD resemble late talkers who also produce smaller than normal sound inventories and syllable structure levels, in conjunction with reduced expressive vocabulary size (Paul & Jennings, 1992; Rescorla & Ratner, 1996).

Despite the fact that toddlers with ASD in this study appear to demonstrate a sloweddown version of normal phonological development that aligns with their language delays, they did produce more atypical consonant blends. The typically developing participants produced common, adultlike consonant blends, whereas only speakers in the ASD group produced idiosyncratic blends. This suggests that the speakers with ASD were not acquiring the phonotactic rules of their language at the same rate as their peers. Research suggests that children with TD limit phonological production to the sounds and acceptable sound combinations of their native language by 12 months of age (Vihman, Macken, Miller, Simmons, & Miller, 1985). The participants with ASD in this study continued to produce atypical blends in their speechlike vocalizations well into their third year. This may indicate that young children with ASD fail to tune in to the particular properties of the language of their environment.

The findings of this study suggest a generally slowed down version of normal development in the phonological acquisition patterns of children with ASD, with little evidence of significant deviances, and many similarities to the development of children with more specific language delays. However, there were findings that could suggest that vocalizations are not being aligned to the duration, pitch, and phonotactic properties of the ambient language. Whether these findings are related to motoric delays, lack of social attunement, some combination of these, or some other factor entirely cannot be determined by these data. However, it is noteworthy that the majority of differences found tend to be those more closely related to suprasegmental, rather than segmental production. In spite of the generally typical sequence of phonological development seen in these toddlers with ASD, the retention of aberrant pitch and timing patterns in their nonlinguistic vocalizations suggests a connection to the prevalent prosodic deficits in ASD and may point toward a link between the vocal characteristics of lower functioning individuals and the speech characteristics of high functioning speakers. It will be important to follow this development from prelinguistic vocal production through the language learning process in order to elucidate speech and language learning, as well as prosodic development, in this population. Further investigation is needed to determine the etiology and the consequence of these observations in children with ASD who do and do not develop spoken language. Better understanding of these early segmental and suprasegmental characteristics may lead to more focused methods of improving spoken language outcomes and thus provide greater opportunities for education and independence for individuals with ASD.

References

Bartak, L., Rutter, M., & Cox, A. (1975). A comparative study of infantile autism and specific developmental receptive language disorder: I. The children. *British Journal of Psychiatry, 126,* 127–145.

Bartolucci, G., Pierce, S., Streiner, D., & Tolkin-Eppel, P. (1976). Phonological investigation of verbal autistic and mentally retarded subjects. *Journal of Autism and Childhood Schizophrenia, 6,* 303–315.

Bauman-Waengler, J. (2004). *Articulatory and phonological impairments: A clinical focus* (2nd ed.). New York: Pearson Education.

Boersma, P. (2001). PRAAT: Doing phonetics by computer (Version 4.6.09) [Computer software]. Retrieved from http://www.praat.org/

Chawarska, K., Klin, A., & Volkmar, F. (Eds.). (2008). *Autism spectrum disorders in infants and toddlers.* New York: Guilford Press.

Elliott, M. J. (1993). *Prelinguistic vocalizations in autistic, developmentally delayed, and normally developing children.* Unpublished master's thesis, University of North Carolina, Greensboro.

Flax, J. (1986). *Functional intonation in the prelinguistic and early linguistic child.* Unpublished doctoral dissertation. City University of New York.

Gibbon, F., McCann, J., Peppe, S., O'Hare, A., & Rutherford, M. (2004, September). *Articulation disorders in children with high functioning autism.* Paper presented at the World Congress of the International Association of Logopedics and Phoniatrics. Brisbane, Australia.

Fombonne, E. (1999). The epidemiology of autism: A review. *Psychological Medicine, 29,* 769–786.

Kent, R., & Murray, A. (1982). Acoustic features of infant vocalic utterances at 3, 6, and 9 months. *Journal of the Acoustical Society of America, 72,* 353–365.

Kirkpatrick, E., & Ward, J. (1984). Prevalence of articulation errors in NSW school pupils. *Australian Journal of Human Communication Disorders, 12,* 55–62.

Kjelgaard, M., & Tager-Flusberg, H. (2001). An investigation of language impairment in autism: Implications for genetic subgroups. *Language and Cognitive Processes, 16,* 287–308.

Le Couteur, A., Bailey, A., Rutter, M., & Gottesman, I. (1989, August). *Epidemiologically based twin study of autism.* Paper presented at the First World Congress on Psychiatric Genetics, Churchill College, Cambridge.

Lord, C., Risi, S., Lambrecht, L., Cook E. H., Leventhal, B. L., DiLavore, P. C., et al. (2000). The autism diagnostic observation schedule-generic: A standard measure of social and communication deficits associated the spectrum of autism. *Journal of Autism and Developmental Disorders, 30,* 205–223.

McCleery, J., Tully, L., Slevc, L., & Schreibman, L. (2006). Consonant production patterns of young severely language-delayed children with autism. *Journal of Communication Disorders, 39,* 217–231.

Mullen, E. M. (1995). *Mullen Scales of Early Learning–AGS Edition.* Circle Pines, MN: American Guidance Services.

Oller, D. K. (2000). *The emergence of the speech capacity.* Mawah, NJ: Lawrence Erlbaum Associates.

Olswang, L., Stoel-Gammon, C., Coggins, T., & Carpenter, R. (1987). *Assessing prelinguistic and early linguistic behaviors in developmentally young children.* Seattle, WA: University of Washington Press.

Paul, R., & Jennings, P. (1992). Phonological behavior in normal and late talking toddlers. *Journal of Speech and Hearing Research, 35,* 99–107.

Pierce, S., & Bartolucci, G. (1977). A syntactic investigation of verbal autistic, mentally retarded and normal children. *Journal of Autism and Childhood Schizophrenia, 7,* 121–143.

Rescorla, L., & Ratner, N. B. (1996). Phonetic profiles of toddlers with severe expressive language impairments (SLI-E). *Journal of Speech and Hearing Research, 39,* 153–165.

Ricks, D. M., & Wing, L. (1976). Language, communication and use of symbols. In L. Wing (Ed.), *Early childhood autism* (pp. 93–134). Oxford: Pergamon.

Robb, M., Saxman, J., & Grant, A. (1989). Vocal fundamental frequency characteristics during the first two years of life. *Journal of the Acoustical Society of America, 85,* 1708–1717.

Rutter, M., LeCouteur, A., & Lord, K. (2002). *The autism diagnostic interview–revised.* Los Angeles: Western Psychological Services.

Rutter, M., Mawhood, L., & Howlin, P. (1992). Language delay and social development. In P. Fletcher & D. Hall (Eds.), *Specific speech and language disorders in children: Correlates, characteristics and outcomes* (pp. 63–78). London: Whurr.

Sheinkopf, S., Mundy, P., Oller, D. K., & Steffens, M. (2000). Vocal atypicalities of preverbal autistic children. *Journal of Autism and Developmental Disorders, 30,* 345–354.

Shriberg, L. (1993). Four new speech and prosody-voice measures for genetics research and other studies in developmental phonological disorders. *Journal of Speech and Hearing Research, 36,* 105–140.

Shriberg, L., & Kwiatkowski, J. (1982). Phonological disorders, III: A procedure for assessing severity of involvement. *Journal of Speech and Hearing Disorders, 47,* 256–270.

Shriberg, L., Kwiatkowski, J., & Gruber, F. (1994). Developmental phonological disorders: II. Short-term speech-sound normalization. *Journal of Speech and Hearing Research, 37,* 1127–1150.

Shriberg, L., Paul, R., McSweeney, J., Klin, A., Cohen, D., & Volkmar, F. (2001). Speech and prosody characteristics of adolescents and adults with high functioning autism and Asperger syndrome. *Journal of Speech, Language, and Hearing Research, 44,* 1097–1115.

Sparrow, S. S., Balla, D. A., & Cicchetti, D. V. (1984). *Vineland Adaptive Behavior Scales–Interview Edition.* Circle Pines, MN: American Guidance Services.

Stoel-Gammon, C. (1998). Sounds and words in early language acquisition: The relationship between lexical and phonological development. In R. Paul (Ed.), *Exploring the speech-language connection* (pp. 25–52). Baltimore: Paul H. Brookes.

Tager-Flusberg, H. (1994). Dissociations in form and function in the acquisition of language by autistic children. In H. Tager-Flusberg (Ed.), *Constraints on language acquisition: Studies of atypical children* (pp. 175–194). Hillsdale, NJ: Erlbaum.

Tager-Flusberg, H., Paul, R., & Lord, K. (2005). Language and communication in autism. In D. Cohen & F. Volkmar (Eds.), *Handbook of autism and pervasive developmental disorders* (3rd ed., pp. 335–364). New York: John Wiley & Sons.

Thal, D. J., Oroz, M., & McCaw, V. (1995). Phonological and lexical development in normal and late-talking toddlers. *Applied Psycholinguistics, 16,* 407–424.

Vihman, M., Macken, R., Simmons, H., & Miller, J. (1985). From babbling to speech: A reassessment of the continuity issue. *Language, 61,* 397–445.

Wallace, M., Cleary, J., Buder, E., Oller, D., Sheinkopf, S., Mundy, P., et al. (May, 2008). *An acoustic inspection of vocalizations in young children with ASD.* Poster presented at the International Meeting for Autism Research, London.

Wetherby, A., Allen, L., Cleary, J., Kublin, K., & Goldstein, H. (2002). Validity and reliability of the Communication and Symbolic Behavior Scales Developmental Profile with very young children. *Journal of Speech, Language, and Hearing Research, 45,* 1202–1218.

Wetherby, A., & Prizant, B. (1993). *Communication and Symbolic Behaviors Scales Developmental Profile.* Baltimore: Brookes.

Wetherby, A., Woods, J., Allen, L., Cleary, J., Dickinson, H., & Lord, C. (2004). Early indicators of autism spectrum disorders in the second year of life. *Journal of Autism and Developmental Disorders, 34,* 473–493.

Wetherby, A., Yonclas, D., & Bryan, A. (1989). Communicative profiles of preschool children with handicaps: Implications for early identification. *Journal of Speech and Hearing Disorders, 54,* 148–158.

Wolk, L., & Edwards, M. (1993). The emerging phonological system of an autistic child. *Journal of Communication Disorders, 26,* 161–177.

Wolk, L., & Giesen, J. (2000). A phonological investigation of four siblings with childhood autism. *Journal of Communication Disorders, 33,* 371–389.

Wu, M., Wang, D., & Brown, G. (2003). A multi-pitch tracking algorithm for noisy speech. *IEEE Transactions on Speech and Audio Processing, 11,* 229–241.

CHAPTER 9

Understanding Speech-Sound Change in Young Children Following Severe Traumatic Brain Injury

THOMAS F. CAMPBELL, CHRISTINE A. DOLLAGHAN, AND JANINE E. JANOSKY

Introduction

Many of the tasks we perform as speech-language pathologists involve forecasting and facilitating changes in communication behavior. Such tasks are particularly challenging for clinicians who work with children who have experienced severe traumatic brain injury (TBI). Because such children's speech production skills can change dramatically over short periods of time, especially in the acute stages of recovery (Campbell & Dollaghan, 1994), interpreting the significance of these changes would ideally be done by comparing them to the variations seen in typical children sampled at comparable points in time. However, the paucity of fine-grained longitudinal data concerning speech development even in uninjured children represents a serious obstacle to the objective of understanding, and ultimately predicting, the course of individual children's speech recovery after TBI.

For a number of years we have studied the rate and extent of recovery of speech skills following pediatric TBI, both in children injured during the earliest and most dynamic stages of speech development and in children injured at later ages. Much of our work has been longitudinal; our interest in children at the early stages of speech development, and in the early stages of recovery from TBI, presented us with a number of methodological roadblocks concerning the measurement, analysis, and interpretation of speech sound change in this heterogeneous population. In this chapter we consider the issues associated with measuring and interpreting fine-grained changes in children's speech-sound production skills after TBI. We summarize an early attempt to evaluate speech-sound change in these children and describe how our dissatisfaction with that approach led us to explore a new procedure for deriving normal performance curves using data from typically developing children (Campbell, Dollaghan, Janosky, & Adelson, 2007). We demonstrate how to generate such a performance curve for another speech metric, and conclude by illustrating the potential of the performance curve approach to inform our efforts to document and understand changes in the speech production skills of children recovering from severe TBI.

Challenges in Studying Children with TBI

The conceptual and practical problems of measuring cognitive-linguistic recovery after acquired pediatric brain injury have been discussed for more than 20 years (Brooks et al., 1984; Dicker, 1989). Cognitive, motoric and linguistic impairments may persist long after the acute stages of recovery in these children (e.g., Anderson, Morse, Catroppa, Haritou, & Rosenfeld, 2004; Barlow, Thomson, Johnson, & Minns, 2005), but until recently (e.g., Cahill, Murdoch, & Theodoros, 2005) few empirical data concerning these children's speech production skills were available. Early reports of speech skills following pediatric TBI focused on school-aged children and adolescents and generally concluded that these children's speech skills did not differ significantly from those of age-matched controls, although there was noted variability in performance across subjects (Jordan, Ozanne, & Murdoch, 1988; Thompson, 1988). However, speech production in these studies was generally measured at only one or two points during the recovery process, usually by means of single-word articulation tests or subtests from language and cognitive scales. In addition, the ages of participants in these studies placed them well beyond the period of intensive speech production development. Accordingly, fine-grained analyses of the course of speech recovery as compared to the course of speech development were impossible.

In fact, fine-grained longitudinal data concerning the rate and extent of speech development in typical children are also surprisingly scarce. Many of the "normative" expectations concerning speech development have been derived from cross-sectional studies in which single-word articulation tests were administered at lengthy (e.g., yearly) intervals. Shriberg and colleagues (e.g., Shriberg & Kwiatkowski, 1982) were among the first to emphasize the value of assessing children's speech skills in connected speech contexts; measures derived from more typical speaking events have greater face validity and are less vulnerable to the effects of repeated administrations than formal measures that are not designed for such uses. Accordingly, in our studies of speech change after TBI we have relied heavily on these investigators' rigorous development and validation of two measures derived from connected speech samples, the Percentage of Consonants Correct (PCC; Shriberg & Kwiatkowski, 1982) and the Percentage of Consonants Correct–Revised (PCC-R; Shriberg, Austin, Lewis, McSweeny, & Wilson, 1997a). The information made available concerning these metrics in large samples of typically developing and speech-disordered children at yearly intervals (Austin & Shriberg, 1997) has been instrumental in our efforts to understand speech changes in children recovering from TBI.

An Initial Study of Changes in PCC After Pediatric TBI

We first attempted to address the methodological limitations of the early studies of speech recovery in a longitudinal study of nine English-speaking children and adolescents with TBI, ranging in age from 5:8 to 16:2 (years:months) at the time of injury (Campbell & Dollaghan, 1990). Employing conversational sampling techniques, we obtained continuous speech samples from these children seven times during a one-year period. The first sample was collected during the week in which the child was discharged to a rehabilitation hospital and demonstrated some attempt at intentional communication; speech was sampled again on each of the next three successive weeks, and at 3, 6, and 12 months after the fourth weekly sample. The challenge was to establish some standard of "typical" performance against which to evaluate each speech sample, given the differing ages at which participants had been injured and sampled and the lack of normative information on age-matched uninjured children undergoing similar sampling and analyses. In our first effort to solve this problem, we matched each child with TBI with an uninjured same-age, same-sex peer allowing us to sample both children's continuous speech on the same schedule and with the same sampling procedures. We analyzed seven global measures of expressive speech and language production; the measure of speech production was percentage of consonants correct (PCC; Shriberg & Kwiatkowski, 1982), in which each consonant produced is scored as correct or incorrect (i.e., omitted, substituted, or distorted) with reference to the adult target.

Results of this study showed that, as a group, children with TBI had significantly lower PCCs than controls at the first sampling session but that group mean PCCs did not differ at the final sampling session, approximately 13 months later. PCCs of the group with TBI, but not the control group, increased significantly over this interval. However, scatterplots showed that although the brain-injured group as a whole showed substantial improvements in speech production skills, group averages were poor reflections of the speech changes observed in some of the individual children with TBI, whose PCCs were never commensurate with those of their matched controls. In an effort to better represent the variations among individual children's speech production skills across the 13 months of sampling, we calculated a simple "normal performance quotient" (Bagnato & Mayes, 1986) for each subject pair at each sampling session by dividing the PCC from the child with TBI by the PCC from his or her control; a quotient of 1.0 would indicate that their PCCs were equivalent. Figure 9–1 illustrates changes in the normal performance quotient for PCC from one child with TBI over the seven sampling sessions. This child's normal performance quotient was approximately 0.8 by sampling session 4, approximately 1 month after sampling began, but his PCC had not reached the level of his uninjured control at the end of the 12-month sampling period.

The normal performance quotient was a preliminary attempt to gauge the amount of speech recovery by individual brain injured children in relation to typical peers. However, the normal performance quotient approach can be criticized on several grounds. First, the reliability of using a measure from a single child to estimate "normal" performance is unknown and certainly suspect; without large-sample estimates of PCC from typical children at each sampling

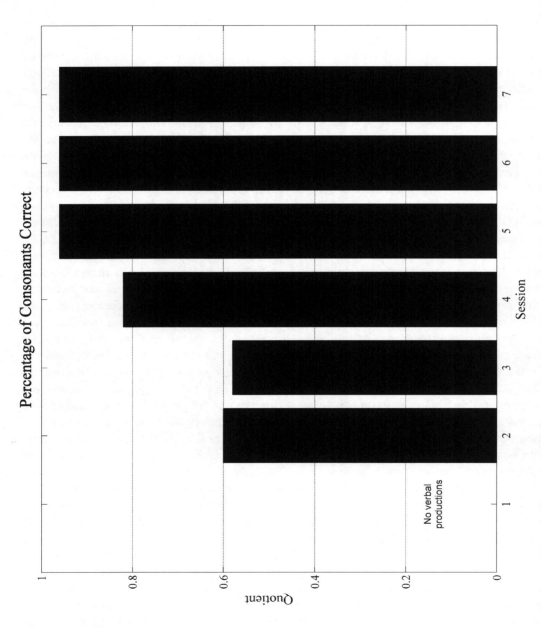

Figure 9–1. The "Normal Performance Quotient" for the PCC for one child with traumatic brain injury at each sampling session.

session the significance of the variations in PCC observed after TBI cannot be determined. Second, and relatedly, the normal performance quotient approach depends on the unsupportable assumption (Plante, Swisher, Kiernan, & Restrepo, 1993) that children in each pair were well matched on variables other than the presence or absence of TBI that could influence PCC in these sampling sessions (e.g., Campbell et al., 2003). Differences in volubility, vocabulary size, and fluency are just a few of many potential confounds that might contribute to differences in PCC, and it is impossible to anticipate all or even most of the relevant variables that would need to be controlled for an ideal match. Our dissatisfaction with the normal performance quotient motivated us to develop a new approach for analyzing longitudinal changes in speech production in a larger cohort of children with severe TBI.

A Performance Curve Approach to Speech Change after Severe TBI

In 2000 we began a longitudinal investigation of speech development in children following severe pediatric TBI sustained between the ages of 18 and 134 months (Campbell et al., 2001). The primary objective of the study was to examine the rate and level of speech-sound change in 60 children who were severely injured at various points in the speech development process. Twelve monthly conversational speech samples, starting at the point postinjury at which the child began speaking, were transcribed phonetically by a team of research assistants according to procedures outlined in Shriberg, Allen, McSweeny, and Wilson (2000).

As mentioned previously, one of the most problematic aspects of studying the speech recovery process in brain-injured children longitudinally is determining what constitutes an appropriate comparison group. One approach would be to assemble a matched comparison group of typically developing children at each monthly age of interest in the investigation. Due to the fact that the 60 children with TBI in the study were injured at different and unpredictable ages, this approach would be both costly and impractical. An alternative approach would be to simply use previously published mean and standard deviation values of a speech metric from typically developing children as a yardstick against which to compare the performance of the children with TBI.

For this analysis, the metric we chose was the Percentage of Consonants Correct-Revised (PCC-R; Shriberg et al., 1997a), a measure of consonantal accuracy that like PCC can be applied to multiple samples from an individual child without concern about practice effects. By contrast with PCC, however, PCC-R consonant distortions or allophonic errors are not scored as errors; only consonant omissions and substitutions are counted as errors. As noted by Shriberg et al. (1997a) PCC-R is preferred over PCC for comparisons in samples of children having diverse ages and diverse speech characteristics.

Importantly, some PCC-R values from children at varying ages were available in the literature, although they were available only at yearly intervals for children from three to eight years and at longer intervals thereafter (Austin & Shriberg, 1997; Shriberg et al., 1997b). That meant that PCC-R values were lacking for the large majority of monthly ages between 18 and 172 months. Accordingly, it would be difficult to interpret the PCC-Rs from children with TBI obtained at the monthly ages for which no normative data were available.

To address this problem we employed a curve-fitting technique to generate a PCC-R performance curve against which the monthly PCC-R values of each child with TBI could be compared. As described in Campbell et al. (2007), we first compiled 16 PCC-R means from samples of typically developing children between 18 to 172 months of age that had been published previously (Austin & Shriberg, 1997; Paradise et al., 2001; Paradise et al., 2003; Shriberg et al., 1997b; Stoel-Gammon, Kelly, Tinsley, & Kellogg, 1987) and used curve fitting to test more than 11,000 statistical models of monthly growth in PCC-R. A parsimonious and developmentally plausible model was selected with a R^2 = .9829 (p <.0005), sug-

gesting that more than 98% of the variance in PCC-R was accounted for by age in months. From this model, the PCC-R, standard deviation, and standard error expected at each monthly age were generated.

This procedure represented a new approach to the problem of interpreting rapid changes in the speech-sound production skills of children recovering from TBI or other neurological injuries. Using the generated PCC-R performance curve shown in Figure 9–2, the child's speech production skills can be charted month by month to ascertain the point at which PCC-R enters the normal range, which can be defined according to either confidence intervals or standard deviation (z) scores. This approach could also be applied to other conversational measures of speech-sound production, as long as the empirical data are sufficient to fit a develop-

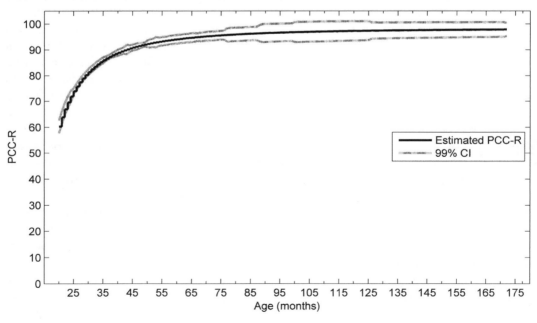

Figure 9–2. Performance curve generated from the model $\left[PCC - R = \dfrac{98.39 - 15256.53}{age\ (months)^2} \right]$ with upper and lower limits of the 99% confidence interval for each month of age from 20 to 172 months.

mentally plausible curve that accounts for a significant amount of the variance.

In the next section, we briefly illustrate how to generate a performance curve for a second measure of speech-sound production, Percentage Consonants Correct (PCC; Shriberg et al., 1997a). As mentioned earlier, PCC is a metric that expresses the percentage of intended consonant sounds in a conversational sample that are articulated correctly, giving equal weight to speech-sound omissions, substitutions and distortions. Recall that PCC-R gives equal weight to omissions and substitutions, while counting distortions as correct. This fundamental difference in the scoring of the two measures enables the prediction that the performance curves for PCC-R and PCC will differ, especially during the early period of speech-sound development when a child may have achieved correct phonemic production but still lack the phonetic precision required for adult-like articulation. The differences in the normal performance curves generated for these two measures will be discussed after we describe the process of calculating a normal performance curve for the PCC speech metric.

Steps in Calculating a PCC Performance Curve

The initial step in generating a performance curve for any measure of speech and language production is to search the literature for representative data. In the context of our longitudinal investigation of speech recovery after severe TBI, we first reviewed relevant databases to identify studies of typically developing children in which the PCC metric had been reported. Special attention was given to identifying those studies that used methods similar to those suggested

by Shriberg et al. (1997a, 1997b) with respect to continuous speech sampling, phonemic transcription, and calculation of PCC. Selected studies had to include PCC means and standard deviations, preferably with comparable numbers of boys and girls, at a specific age.

PCC data at 14 different ages were available (Austin & Shriberg, 1997; Paradise et al., 2001; Paradise et al., 2003; Shriberg et al., 1997b; Stoel-Gammon, Kelly, Tinsley, & Kellogg, 1987). Means, standard deviations and *N*s for the PCC data at each of these 14 ages are shown in Table 9–1. We used the 14 empirical data points to calculate a statistical model that could be used to generate predicted PCCs at each month over the age span from 20 months to 172 months.

The second step in the process was to generate and select a growth curve model. Statistical models were generated from the 14 empirical PCC values using curve fitting (Table Curve 3D, 1997). Over 11,000 possible PCC models were generated, ranging from simple linear models with slope and intercept to nonlinear fourth order polynomial models. Our criteria for selecting a model from among the various alternatives included: (1) amount of variance accounted for; (2) parsimony in estimation terms; and (3) developmental plausibility given other known information regarding growth in PCC. These criteria allowed us to maximize the percentage of variance accounted for, minimize the number of parameters contained within the model and select a performance curve that was developmentally plausible. Based on these criteria a model was selected that had an $R^2 = 0.96$ ($p < 0.0005$), representing 96% of the variance accounted for with the following equation: PCC = [103.46 − (887.9/age in months)]. The standard error of measurement (SEM) for the model was 1.52, which represents a statistically significant fit.

Table 9–1. Information on the 14 Empirical Data Points Used to Calculate the PCC Performance Curve

Age (mos)	N	% male	PCC M	SD	Source
21	32	50	62.1	15.3	Stoel-Gammon et al. (1987)[a]
24	34	50	70.1	14.3	Stoel-Gammon et al. (1987)[a]
36	245	49	79.5	7.0	Paradise et al. (2001)[b]
37	291	50	80.3	6.5	Paradise et al. (2001)[b]
38	186	49	80.1	7.7	Paradise et al. (2001)[b]
43	52	42	80.3	6.9	Austin & Shriberg (1997)[c]
48	215	49	86.0	6.2	Paradise et al. (2003)[b]
49	378	49	86.0	6.4	Paradise et al. (2003)[b]
50	107	48	86.0	5.9	Paradise et al. (2003)[b]
67	109	54	87.1	7.7	Austin & Shriberg (1997)[c]
76	76	59	91.2	4.4	Austin & Shriberg (1997)[c]
88	23	39	95.7	2.3	Austin & Shriberg (1997)[c]
125	14	64	97.2	3.0	Austin & Shriberg (1997)[c]
172	25	60	98.1	2.2	Austin & Shriberg (1997)[c]

[a]Data from a sample of 40 children developing normally (20 males) who were followed longitudinally from 9 to 24 months of age. Not all children were assessed at every age and the exact percentage of males at ages 18, 21, and 24 months was not reported. Percentage Consonants Correct (PCC) was determined from broad phonemic transcription of a corpus of approximately 50 different words audio-recorded during a 30-minute spontaneous language sample and during efforts to elicit approximately 10 to 15 object labels by the examiner. Because distortion errors are not captured by broad phonetic transcription, the resulting PCC corresponds to PCC-R as described by Shriberg et al. (1997a).

[b]Data from a sample of healthy children being followed in the course of another investigation who were tested within two months of their third birthday (at ages 36, 37, or 38 months) and/or within two months of their fourth birthday (at ages 48, 49, or 50 months). PCC was determined from an audio-recorded 15-minute spontaneous language sample according to procedures described by Shriberg, Allen, McSweeney, and Wilson (2000); data reported reflect all children whose PCC results classified them as having Normal Speech Acquisition (Shriberg et al., 1997b).

[c]Data from conversational samples audio-recorded from healthy Wisconsin children who were followed in several studies. PCC values are those for children whose speech met criteria for Normal Speech Acquisition at their current age according to the Speech Disorders Classification System (Shriberg et al., 1997b).

The next step was to use the parameters of the fitted model to calculate PCC means and standard deviation values at each monthly age. Each of these predicted monthly PCC values was generated by the formula PCC = [103.46 − (887.9/age in months)]. We will illustrate how the predicted PCC value at 25 months of age was generated using two simple steps: (1) divide the term 887.93 by the months of age (887.93/25 = 35.52); and (2) subtract this value from the term 103.46 (103.46 − 35.52 = predicted PCC value of 67.94). The monthly PCC values derived from the fitted curve appear in the Appendix of this chapter. For those interested in the derived monthly values for PCC-R, please refer to the appendix in Campbell, Dollaghan, Janosky, and Adelson (2007).

The final step in the process was to derive confidence intervals for each monthly PCC value. This was done by first calculating the *SEM* for each monthly age using the formula *SEM = SD*/square root of sample size. For those ages lacking empirical PCC data from the literature, we calculated SEM based on the average sample size of the two adjacent observed data points. We then generated the 99% confidence interval (CI) surrounding the expected PCC at each monthly age using the formula PCC + 2.58 *SEM*, providing a definition of normal range PCC values at each monthly age. Figure 9–3A shows the resulting curve of PCC values at each monthly age surrounded by the upper and lower bounds of the 99% CI.

Comparison of the PCC and PCC-R Performance Curves

Before we turn to the validity and potential applications of the normal performance curve approach, it should be emphasized that such curves can only be used to interpret children's performances on the same measures that were used to generate the curves. For example, it would not be appropriate to compare a PCC derived from a single-word articulation test to the PCC values from the normal performance curve,

which were derived from conversational speech samples and transcribed according to the specific procedures (Shriberg et al., 1997b). Of course, if developmental data on PCC from other conditions were available, it would be possible to generate a normal performance curve for them. Similarly, PCC and PCC-R values must be interpreted with reference to their respective performance curves.

To illustrate this point, consider the differences and similarities in the developmental trajectories of the 99% confidence intervals for the PCC and PCC-R performance curves shown in Figure 9–3B. There are obvious differences at the earlier ages, particularly between 24 to 48 months of age, but the two curves gradually approximate each other at the older ages and overlap completely at approximately 145 months (12 years). These differences in the developmental trajectories of the two performance curves are quite predictable. As noted above, PCC-R treats consonant distortions as correct, while PCC treats them as errors. Accordingly, the developmental trajectory of PCC necessarily lags behind that of PCC-R until the phonetic precision that enables adultlike articulation, free of distorted sound productions, has been achieved. Again, specific speech production measures must be interpreted with respect to their corresponding performance curves. Interpreting PCC by comparing it to the performance curve generated for PCC-R would lead to incorrect inferences about the speech status of children at ages for which the curves differ.

Validity of the PCC Performance Curve

As a prelude to using the PCC performance curve to identify clinically important changes in the course of recovery from severe TBI,

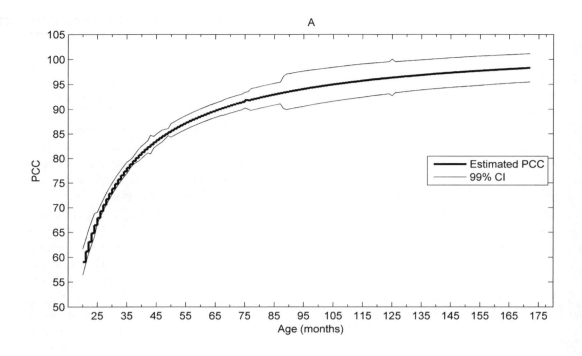

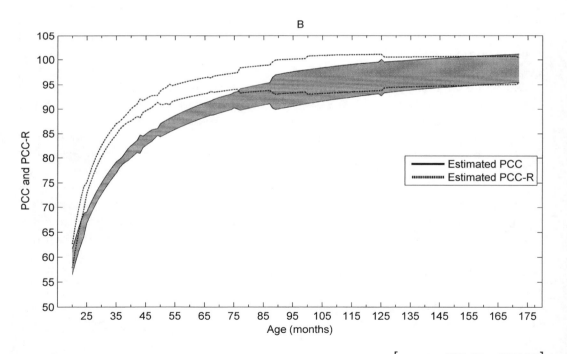

Figure 9–3. A. Performance curve generated from the model $\left[PCC = \dfrac{103.46 - 887.93}{\text{age (months)}} \right]$ with upper and lower limits of the 99% confidence interval for each month of age from 20 to 172 months. **B**. Comparison of upper and lower limits of the 99% confidence interval for PCC-R (*dashed*) and PCC (*shaded*) for each month of age from 20 to 172 months.

we examined PCC scores obtained from 105 children from 37 to 57 months of age who were participating in a separate investigation of normal and disordered speech development (Moore et al., 2006). None of the PCC data from these 105 children had been used to develop the fitted model and all had been evaluated and diagnosed independently of the present investigation. Forty-nine of the children had been recruited to the study as normal speakers based on a lack of parental concern about their speech and met criteria for Normal Speech Acquisition (NSA); 56 had been recruited as having an

articulation disorder based on a clinical evaluation by a speech-language pathologist and met criteria for Speech Delay of unknown origin (SD; Shriberg et al., 1997b).

If the curve provides a valid reflection of typical development, we would expect children with normal speech acquisition to have PCCs greater than the PCC at the lower boundary of the 99% CI for their age in months, and children with speech delay of unknown origin to have PCCs below this threshold value. As illustrated in Figure 9–4, 42 of 49 (86%) children classified as having normal speech acquisition had PCCs above

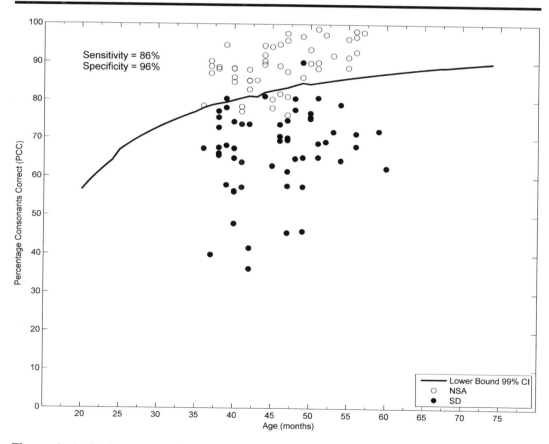

Figure 9–4. Performance of children with normal speech acquisition (NSA; *open circles*) and speech delay (SD; *filled circles*) compared to the lower bound of the 99% confidence interval of the PCC performance curve.

the threshold value for their age, and 54 of 56 (96%) children classified as having speech delay of unknown origin had PCCs below the threshold value for their age. These data suggest that the PCC performance curve may be clinically useful in interpreting speech performance at discrete monthly ages.

Some Potential Applications of Performance Curves

The most obvious application for the PCC performance curve in evaluating recovery after TBI would be to compare a child's PCC to the normal performance curve at a single monthly age. In addition, if multiple data points are available for a child the slope of change in his or her PCC can also be compared to that of the slope of the performance curve by calculating the z slope of the child's PCC growth curve and statistically comparing it to the corresponding portion of the performance curve (e.g., Campbell et al., 2007).

For example, Figure 9–5 shows data from five children recovering from severe traumatic brain injury whose percentage of consonants correct (PCC) values were calculated at 12 successive monthly sampling sessions, plotted against the lower bound of

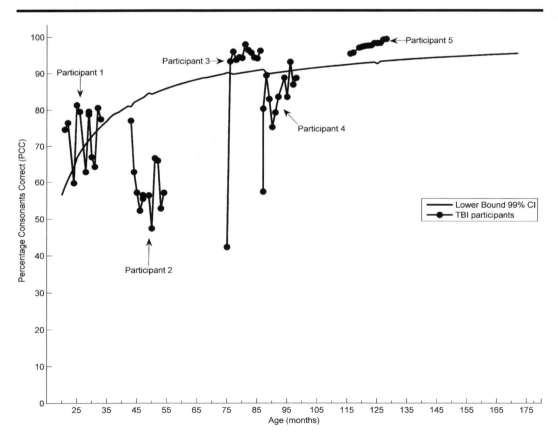

Figure 9–5. Individual growth curves for 12 PCC values (sampled monthly) for five children recovering from severe traumatic brain injury, plotted against the lower bound of the 99% confidence interval.

the 99% confidence interval from the PCC performance curve for the child's age in months at each session. As discussed above, this lower bound can be used as a threshold value for normal-range PCC, so data points that fall above it indicate PCCs that are within this broadly defined range of normal performance for children at that monthly age. These five children's performance curves nicely illustrate the heterogeneity that has been said to characterize the course of recovery in other developmental domains following severe TBI during childhood. The differences among the individual curves from these five children are striking, as are the differences within the curves from the first four individual children. However, in addition to validating the observation of heterogeneity after TBI, depicting individual children's PCC performance curves in this fashion also motivates additional hypotheses and suggests future studies that might ultimately enable predictions about the course of recovery in an individual child. For example, for all but one child (Participant 2) performance curves trend upward, although for most it is a bumpy ride. Are there physiologic, psychologic, or sampling issues that might explain why consonant production accuracy consistently declines over the first four months of recovery for Participant 2, and is it coincidental that this is the only child whose PCC values remain substantially below the normal range a full year postinjury? Similarly, for the remaining children it appears that once PCC crosses into the normal range, its variability in subsequent months rarely takes it substantially below this threshold. Might the point at which a child achieves a normal-range PCC serve as an indication that additional major decrements in consonant accuracy are not expected (and conversely, that if such decrements occur there might be physiologic bases for them)? Does a child's distance from the PCC threshold have meaningful

implications for clinical efforts aimed at improving either intelligibility or normalcy of the child's speech production?

At this point such questions are nothing more than speculations, but the performance curve approach seems to offer a means of both generating and testing hypotheses that may take us closer to the ultimate goal of understanding and predicting an individual child's course of recovery from severe TBI. With additional performance curves from larger numbers of children injured at various ages it will be possible to determine whether we can identify reliably different types of performance curves (e.g., von Eye, Young Mun, & Indurkhya, 2004) that are predicted by pre- or postinjury variables and that are predictive of a child's subsequent clinical course.

Conclusion

We believe that the performance curve approach holds promise for addressing questions about fine-grained longitudinal changes in children's communication performance. The fact that it is already possible to generate and test performance curves for measures of children's speech is largely a result of Larry Shriberg's work to discover psychometrically adequate measures of speech production and to make normative data for these measures freely accessible. For this and his many other contributions, those of us who are interested in children's speech development and disorders owe him a great debt of gratitude.

References

Anderson, V. A., Morse, S. A., Catroppa, C., Haritou, F., & Rosenfeld, J. V. (2004). Thirty-month outcome from early childhood head injury:

A prospective analysis of neurobehavioural recovery. *Brain, 127,* 2608–2620.

Austin, D., & Shriberg, L. D. (1997, Revised). *Lifespan reference data for ten measures of articulation competence using the Speech Disorders Classification System (SDCS)* (Phonology Project Tech. Rep. No. 3). Madison: University of Wisconsin, Waisman Center on Mental Retardation and Human Development.

Bagnato, S. J., & Mayes, D. D. (1986). Patterns of developmental and behavioral progress for young children during interdisciplinary intervention. *Developmental Neuropsychology, 2,* 213–240.

Barlow, K. M., Thomson, E., Johnson, D., & Minns, R. A. (2005). Late neurologic and cognitive sequelae of inflicted traumatic brain injury in infancy. *Pediatrics, 116,* 174–185.

Brooks, D. N., Deelman, B. G., van Zomeren, A. H., van Dongen, H., van Harskamp, F., & Aughton, M. E. (1984). Problems in measuring cognitive recovery after acute brain injury. *Journal of Clinical Neuropsychology, 6,* 71–85.

Cahill, L., Murdoch, B. E., & Theodoros, D. G. (2005). Articulatory function following traumatic brain injury in childhood: A perceptual and instrumental analysis. *Brain Injury, 19,* 55–79.

Campbell, T. F., & Dollaghan, C. A. (1990). Expressive language recovery in severely brain-injured children and adolescents. *Journal of Speech and Hearing Disorders, 55,* 567–581.

Campbell, T., & Dollaghan, C. (1994). Phonological and speech production characteristics of children following traumatic brain injury: Principles underlying assessment and treatment. In J. Bernthal & N. Bankson (Eds.), *Child phonology: Characteristics, assessment, and intervention with special populations* (pp. 140–160). New York: Thieme.

Campbell, T. F., Dollaghan, C. A, Adelson, P. D., Janosky, J., Balason, D., Nash, T., et al. (2001). Speech change in young children after severe traumatic brain injury. In B. Maassen, W. Hulstijn, R. Kent, H. F. M. Peters, & P. H. M. M. van Lieshout (Eds.), *Proceedings of the 4th International Speech Motor Conference* (pp. 106–109). Netherlands: University of Nijmegen.

Campbell, T. F., Dollaghan, C. A., Janosky, J. E., & Adelson, P. D. (2007). A performance curve for assessing change in Percentage Consonants Correct-Revised (PCC-R). *Journal of Speech, Language, and Hearing Research, 50,* 1110–1119.

Campbell, T. F., Dollaghan, C. A., Rockette, H. E., Paradise, J. L., Feldman, H. M., Shriberg, L.D., et al. (2003). Risk factors for speech delay in three-year-old children. *Child Development, 74,* 346–357.

Dicker, G. D. (1989). Preinjury behavior and recovery after minor head injury: A review of the literature. *Journal of Head Trauma Rehabilitation, 4,* 73–81.

Jordan, F. M., Ozanne, A. E., & Murdoch, B. E. (1988). Long-term speech and language disorders subsequent to closed head injury in children. *Head Injury, 2,* 179–185.

Moore, C. A., Campbell, T. F., Shriberg, L. D., Green, J. R., Venkatesh, L., Vick, J., et al. (2006). Physiologic and behavioral classification of delayed speech. In B. Maassen (Ed.), *Proceedings of the 5th International Speech Motor Conference* (p. 109). Netherlands: Nijmegen University.

Paradise, J. L., Dollaghan, C. A., Campbell, T. F., Feldman, H. M., Bernard, B. S., Colborn, D. K., et al. (2003). Otitis media and tympanostomy tube insertion during the first three years of life: Developmental outcomes at the age of four years. *Pediatrics, 112,* 265–277.

Paradise, J. L., Feldman, H. M. Campbell, T. F., Dollaghan, C. A., Colborn, D. K, Bernard, B. S., et al. (2001). Effect of early or delayed insertion of tympanostomy tubes for persistent otitis media on developmental outcomes at the age of three years. *New England Journal of Medicine, 344,* 1179–1187.

Plante, E., Swisher, L., Kiernan, B., & Restrepo, M. A. (1993). Language matches: Illuminating or confounding? *Journal of Speech and Hearing Research, 36,* 772–776.

Shriberg, L. D., Allen, C. T., McSweeny, J. L., & Wilson, D. L. (2000). *PEPPER: Programs to examine phonetic and phonologic evaluation records* [Computer software and manual]. Madison: University of Wisconsin, Waisman Center on Mental Retardation and Human Development.

Shriberg, L. D., Austin, D., Lewis, B. A., McSweeny, J. L., & Wilson, D. L. (1997a). The Percentage of Consonants Correct (PCC) metric: Extensions and reliability data. *Journal of Speech, Language, and Hearing Research, 40,* 708–722.

Shriberg, L. D., Austin, D., Lewis, B. A., McSweeny, J. L., & Wilson, D. L. (1997b). The Speech Disorders Classification System (SDCS): Extensions and lifespan reference data. *Journal of Speech, Language, and Hearing Research, 40,* 723–740.

Shriberg, L. D., & Kwiatkowski, J. (1982). Phonological disorders III: A procedure for assessing severity of involvement. *Journal of Speech and Hearing Disorders, 47,* 256–270.

Stoel-Gammon, C., Kelly, C., Tinsley, S., & Kellogg, S. (1987). Language production scale. In L. B. Olswang, C. Stoel-Gammon, T. E. Coggins, & R. L. Carpenter (Eds.), *Assessing pre-linguistic and early linguistic behaviors in developmentally young children* (pp. 120–150). Seattle, WA: University of Washington Press.

Table Curve 3D. (1997). Chicago: AISN Software.

Thompson, C. K. (1988). Articulation disorders in the child with neurogenic pathology. In N. J. Lass, L. V. McReynolds, J. L. Northern, & D. E. Yoder (Eds.), *Handbook of speech-language pathology* (pp. 548–491). Philadelphia: DC Becker.

von Eye, A., Young Mun, E., & Indurkhya, A. (2004). Typifying developmental trajectories—A decision making perspective. *Psychology Science, 46,* 65–98.

APPENDIX

PCC Values Derived From the Performance Curve, by Age in Months

Age	M	SD	SE	99% CI	
				Lower	Upper
20	59.06	5.39	1.02	56.43	61.69
21	61.18	5.36	0.95	58.73	63.63
22	63.10	5.34	0.93	60.70	65.50
23	64.85	5.32	0.93	62.46	67.24
24	66.46	5.30	0.91	64.12	68.80
25	67.94	5.28	0.45	66.79	69.09
26	69.31	5.26	0.45	68.16	70.46
27	70.57	5.25	0.44	69.42	71.72
28	71.75	5.23	0.44	70.61	72.89
29	72.84	5.22	0.44	71.70	73.98
30	73.86	5.21	0.44	72.72	75.00
31	74.82	5.20	0.44	73.68	75.96
32	75.71	5.19	0.44	74.58	76.84
33	76.55	5.18	0.44	75.42	77.68
34	77.34	5.17	0.44	76.21	78.47
35	78.09	5.17	0.44	76.96	79.22
36	78.80	5.16	0.33	77.95	79.65
37	79.46	5.16	0.30	78.68	80.24
38	80.09	5.17	0.38	79.11	81.07
39	80.69	5.20	0.48	79.46	81.92
40	81.26	5.22	0.48	80.03	82.49
41	81.80	5.25	0.48	80.56	83.04
42	82.32	5.27	0.48	81.07	83.57
43	82.81	5.31	0.74	80.91	84.71
44	83.28	5.34	0.46	82.09	84.47
45	83.73	5.37	0.47	82.53	84.93
46	84.16	5.40	0.47	82.95	85.37
47	84.57	5.43	0.47	83.36	85.78
48	84.96	5.46	0.37	84.00	85.92

Age	M	SD	SE	99% CI	
				Lower	Upper
49	85.34	5.49	0.28	84.61	86.07
50	85.70	5.52	0.53	84.32	87.08
51	86.05	5.56	0.53	84.67	87.43
52	86.38	5.59	0.54	84.99	87.77
53	86.71	5.62	0.54	85.31	88.11
54	87.02	5.65	0.54	85.62	88.42
55	87.32	5.67	0.55	85.91	88.73
56	87.60	5.69	0.55	86.19	89.01
57	87.88	5.71	0.55	86.46	89.30
58	88.15	5.73	0.55	86.73	89.57
59	88.41	5.74	0.55	86.98	89.84
60	88.66	5.76	0.55	87.23	90.09
61	88.90	5.77	0.56	87.47	90.33
62	89.14	5.78	0.56	87.71	90.57
63	89.37	5.79	0.56	87.93	90.81
64	89.59	5.80	0.56	88.15	91.03
65	89.80	5.81	0.56	88.36	91.24
66	90.01	5.81	0.56	88.57	91.45
67	90.21	5.82	0.56	88.77	91.65
68	90.40	5.83	0.61	88.84	91.96
69	90.59	5.83	0.61	89.03	92.15
70	90.78	5.84	0.61	89.21	92.35
71	90.95	5.84	0.61	89.38	92.52
72	91.13	5.84	0.61	89.56	92.70
73	91.30	5.85	0.61	89.73	92.87
74	91.46	5.87	0.61	89.89	93.03
75	91.82	5.89	0.61	90.24	93.40
76	91.78	5.91	0.68	90.03	93.53
77	91.93	5.92	0.84	89.76	94.10
78	92.08	5.94	0.84	89.90	94.26
79	92.22	5.95	0.85	90.04	94.40

continues

Age	M	SD	SE	99% CI Lower	99% CI Upper
80	92.36	5.96	0.85	90.17	94.55
81	92.50	5.97	0.85	90.31	94.69
82	92.63	5.98	0.85	90.44	94.82
83	92.76	5.97	0.85	90.57	94.95
84	92.89	5.96	0.85	90.70	95.08
85	93.01	5.96	0.85	90.83	95.19
86	93.14	5.95	0.85	90.96	95.32
87	93.25	5.95	0.85	91.07	95.43
88	93.37	5.94	1.24	90.17	96.57
89	93.48	5.94	1.38	89.92	97.04
90	93.59	5.93	1.38	90.03	97.15
91	93.70	5.93	1.38	90.14	97.26
92	93.81	5.93	1.38	90.25	97.37
93	93.91	5.92	1.38	90.36	97.46
94	94.01	5.92	1.38	90.46	97.56
95	94.11	5.92	1.38	90.56	97.66
96	94.21	5.88	1.37	90.68	97.74
97	94.31	5.85	1.36	90.80	97.82
98	94.40	5.82	1.35	90.91	97.89
99	94.49	5.79	1.35	91.02	97.96
100	94.58	5.76	1.34	91.12	98.04
101	94.67	5.74	1.33	91.23	98.11
102	94.75	5.72	1.33	91.32	98.18
103	94.84	5.70	1.33	91.42	98.26
104	94.92	5.69	1.32	91.51	98.33
105	95.00	5.67	1.32	91.60	98.40
106	95.08	5.66	1.32	91.69	98.47
107	95.16	5.65	1.31	91.77	98.55
108	95.24	5.64	1.31	91.86	98.62
109	95.31	5.63	1.31	91.93	98.69
110	95.39	5.62	1.31	92.02	98.76

Age	M	SD	SE	99% CI	
				Lower	Upper
111	95.46	5.61	1.30	92.09	98.83
112	95.53	5.60	1.30	92.17	98.89
113	95.60	5.60	1.30	92.24	98.96
114	95.67	5.59	1.30	92.32	99.02
115	95.74	5.56	1.29	92.41	99.07
116	95.81	5.53	1.28	92.50	99.12
117	95.87	5.50	1.28	92.57	99.17
118	95.94	5.47	1.27	92.66	99.22
119	96.00	5.45	1.27	92.73	99.27
120	96.06	5.43	1.26	92.80	99.32
121	96.12	5.41	1.26	92.87	99.37
122	96.18	5.40	1.25	92.94	99.42
123	96.24	5.38	1.25	93.01	99.47
124	96.30	5.37	1.25	93.08	99.52
125	96.36	5.36	1.43	92.67	100.05
126	96.41	5.35	1.21	93.29	99.53
127	96.47	5.31	1.20	93.36	99.58
128	96.52	5.29	1.20	93.43	99.61
129	96.58	5.26	1.19	93.51	99.65
130	96.63	5.24	1.19	93.57	99.69
131	96.68	5.22	1.18	93.63	99.73
132	96.73	5.20	1.18	93.69	99.77
133	96.78	5.18	1.17	93.75	99.81
134	96.83	5.17	1.17	93.81	99.85
135	96.88	5.15	1.17	93.87	99.89
136	96.93	5.14	1.16	93.93	99.93
137	96.98	5.13	1.16	93.98	99.98
138	97.03	5.12	1.16	94.04	100.02
139	97.07	5.11	1.16	94.08	100.06
140	97.12	5.10	1.16	94.14	100.10
141	97.16	5.10	1.15	94.18	100.14

continues

Age	M	SD	SE	99% CI Lower	99% CI Upper
				Lower	Upper
142	97.21	5.09	1.15	94.24	100.18
143	97.25	5.08	1.15	94.28	100.22
144	97.29	5.08	1.15	94.32	100.26
145	97.34	5.07	1.15	94.38	100.30
146	97.38	5.07	1.15	94.42	100.34
147	97.42	5.06	1.15	94.46	100.38
148	97.46	5.06	1.15	94.50	100.42
149	97.50	5.06	1.15	94.54	100.46
150	97.54	5.06	1.14	94.59	100.49
151	97.58	5.05	1.14	94.63	100.53
152	97.62	5.05	1.14	94.67	100.57
153	97.66	5.05	1.14	94.71	100.61
154	97.69	5.05	1.14	94.74	100.64
155	97.73	5.02	1.14	94.79	100.67
156	97.77	5.00	1.13	94.85	100.69
157	97.80	4.99	1.13	94.89	100.71
158	97.84	4.97	1.13	94.94	100.74
159	97.88	4.95	1.12	94.99	100.77
160	97.91	4.94	1.12	95.02	100.80
161	97.94	4.93	1.12	95.06	100.82
162	97.98	4.92	1.11	95.11	100.85
163	98.01	4.91	1.11	95.14	100.88
164	98.05	4.90	1.11	95.19	100.91
165	98.08	4.89	1.11	95.22	100.94
166	98.11	4.88	1.11	95.26	100.96
167	98.14	4.88	1.10	95.29	100.99
168	98.17	4.87	1.10	95.32	101.02
169	98.21	4.87	1.10	95.37	101.05
170	98.24	4.86	1.10	95.40	101.08
171	98.27	4.86	1.10	95.43	101.11
172	98.30	4.85	1.10	95.46	101.14

CHAPTER 10

Factors Associated with the Intelligibility of Conversational Speech Produced by Children with Cochlear Implants

PETER FLIPSEN, JR.

Introduction

Intelligibility has been described as " . . . the functional common denominator of verbal behavior" (Kent, Miolo, & Bloedel, 1994, p. 81). It should not therefore come as a surprise that intelligibility of speech has been the focus of investigations into speech problems associated with a number of different populations (this issue is also discussed in Chapter 5). Studies in this area have included adults with acquired dysarthria (e.g., Dykstra, Hakel, & Adams, 2007; Yorkston & Beukelman, 1978), individuals with dysarthria secondary to cerebral palsy (e.g., Hustad, 2007), those born with palatal clefts (e.g., Whitehill, 2002), individuals with congeni-

tal syndromes (e.g., Iosub, Fuchs, Bingol, & Gromisch, 1981; Kumin, 1994; Von Berg, McColl, & Brancamp, 2007), as well as individuals with hearing impairments (e.g., Osberger, 1992). They also have included the population at the center of Dr. Shriberg's work, children with speech sound disorders. It was in large part my work with Dr. Shriberg on his SD-OME category and the intelligibility findings we obtained that motivated me to begin the work discussed in this chapter.

Beyond merely documenting intelligibility deficits, studies in this area have attempted to isolate particular speaker-related factors such as severity of involvement, prosodic skill, speech sound accuracy, or specific error patterns that might be contributing to those deficits. These studies have been motivated by several goals. For example, given that so many different disorders include intelligibility deficits, studies of the specific factors contributing to such deficits for particular populations have attempted to expand our theoretical understanding of the nature of the disorders being studied. As well, such studies have sought to help refine our diagnostic schemes by helping differentiate among potential subgroups of particular populations. That was, for example, Dr. Shriberg's initial goal. More clearly defined subgroups may then offer insight into both distal causes and proximal mechanisms that may be operating for particular populations. As noted by Flipsen (2002a), insight into causal mechanisms combined with the identification of specific intervention targets, may then allow clinicians to fine tune their intervention efforts Indeed many of the studies in this area (including the work documented in the current chapter) have had the improvement of intervention efforts as their primary goal.

The goal of this chapter is to attempt to isolate the aspects of speech-output that contribute to intelligibility deficits in children with severe and profound hearing impairments who have been fitted with cochlear implants (CIs). These devices represent a significant technologic advance, in part, because they bypass the external and middle ear systems and more directly stimulate the auditory nerve. As a result, they effectively negate the usual transmission loss of those systems and individuals fitted with these devices have hearing sensitivity that improves from a severe or profound level of impairment to that of a mild or mild-moderate impairment. For example, Nicholas and Geers (2007) presented data from 76 children implanted on average at 23 months of age (range 12–38 months) whose pre-implant unaided pure tone averages had a

mean value of 107 dB HL (range 77–120 dB). After surgery, cochlear implant thresholds averaged 30 dB HL (range 20–43 dB). Severity gains aside, the new technology raises other questions. Unlike hearing aids which simply amplify the incoming sound and stimulate the auditory nerve using the typical mechanical-chemical process provided by the bending of hair cells in the inner ear (Vollrath, Kwan, & Corey, 2007), CIs electrically stimulate the nerve (Wilson, 2000). Thus, the nature of the input provided (whether from the speech of others or during self-monitoring) and perhaps even the way in which the auditory system processes that input may be qualitatively different. It would therefore seem appropriate to ask whether the resulting speech output from these individuals also differs. The focus of the present chapter is, first, to document the degree to which intelligibility is impacted in children with CIs, and, second, to investigate the relationship between speech production abilities in children with CIs and any reduction in the intelligibility of their speech.

Factors Affecting Intelligibility

According to Kent (1993), intelligibility is part of the larger notion of communicative competence. Although intelligibility could be generally defined as " . . . the capability of the speaker to produce an intelligible spoken message," (Kent, 1993, p. 224), a more precise perspective would be that intelligibility reflects the ability to produce an intelligible message with a particular speaker, under particular listening conditions, given a particular social context and a particular linguistic context. Thus, making oneself understood really involves a complex interaction of the vocal behaviors of the speaker with the nature of the listener, the social context, and the listening conditions (Kent, 1993). For current purposes however, it is assumed that the contribution of factors beyond the speaker is controlled. Even with such controls in place, however, making oneself intelligible goes beyond simply being able to produce the sounds of speech accurately (although clearly that is a major factor). A variety of directly related factors such as prosodic variables (e.g., speaking rate, lexical and contrastive stress, intonation, loudness), appropriate use of resonance and voice quality are also part of the process. Indeed, although not considered here, expressive language skill might also contribute. The speaker whose utterances are filled with interjections, vague vocabulary, or mazes may be very difficult for a listener to follow even if the particular words being produced are phonetically accurate.

Two measurement factors potentially complicate any discussion of intelligibility. The first is the nature of the material being produced. Individuals with various types of speech impairments have been shown to differ in the degree to which their message is understood depending on linguistic complexity. Iosub et al. (1981), for example, tested 63 individuals with Fetal Alcohol Syndrome and noted that "[I]n many patients, single words were more intelligible than connected speech" (p. 477). Similarly, Wagner, Nettelbladt, Sahlen, and Nilholm (2000) reported that 28 preschool children with language impairments were more intelligible in conversation than in narratives. The second measurement factor is the nature of the judgment task. Put another way, how does one go about deciding what is being understood? Flipsen, Khwaileh, and Erickson (2007), for example, demonstrated that intelligibility scores for single words produced by children with CIs were significantly different depending on whether the judgments are made by blind transcription

(i.e., "What word do you think you heard?") or a multiple choice task (i.e., "Which one of these particular words was said?"). Similar findings were reported by Yorkston and Beukelman (1978) who evaluated a group of adults with dysarthria. Considering just these two factors, it may be that no single measure is sufficient to adequately capture intelligibility (Kent, 1992, p. 9). In an effort to make the current discussion more manageable, however, this report focuses on factors affecting the intelligibility of conversational speech as measured by transcription. Conversational speech was chosen because it is the most ecologically valid output mode (i.e., it represents the most common speaking situation). It also represents the context in which speakers likely have to demonstrate their greatest communicative competence because of the continuous tradeoffs involved (i.e., the shared information from the context may improve intelligibility, while at the same time the rapid generation of full utterances makes messages more difficult to follow). Transcription (also called a "write-down" approach) was chosen because it was thought to represent the harshest test of intelligibility as every word that was produced needed to be evaluated. The alternative for scoring at the conversational level would have been the use of some sort of intelligibility rating scale. Such scales are frequently used because of their convenience for busy practitioners. Schiavetti (1992) reviewed the research on such scales and concluded that they are problematic on at least three counts. First, listeners are often unable to treat all parts of such scales equally. Second, the confidence intervals around points on such scales (particularly in the middle of the range) are often very large. Third, and most relevant to the current analysis, such scales do not allow for specific examination of factors contributing to intelligibility deficits.

Intelligibility and the Speech of the Deaf

Individuals born with severe and/or profound hearing impairments (i.e., those fitting the historical sense of the term "deaf") represent a population where reduced intelligibility has long been noted. Gold (1980), for example, reviewed several studies of spontaneous speech in this population and noted " . . . that only about 20% of the speech output of the deaf is understood by inexperienced listeners" (p. 397). However, studies have shown that even experienced listeners may not fare that much better. For example, Markides (1970) noted that a group of teachers of the deaf only understood 31% on average compared to 19% for a group of "laymen" listeners. A similar conclusion might be reached from the results of a survey of classroom teachers reported by Jensema, Karchmer, and Trybus (1978). Findings indicated that of 741 children with hearing losses of at least 71 dB, only 56 (7.6%) were reported to be as intelligible as a normal hearing person of the same age. Another 199 (26.9%) were reported to be "somewhat difficult to understand." The remaining 486 (65.6%) were rated as "barely intelligible" or worse. Together these reports suggest that spoken language would appear to be seriously impacted as a communication option for the majority of the members of this population, at least prior to the introduction of the cochlear implant.

There has been a long-standing interest in understanding the speech output of those with severe and profound hearing impairments. Levitt and Stromberg (1983) noted that production errors may occur on all phoneme types including consonants, vowels and diphthongs. Parker (2005) reviewed the literature on error patterns (defined using phonological process descriptors) in this population and found many reports of developmental patterns commonly seen in younger, typically developing children with normal hearing (e.g., stopping, fronting, final consonant deletion). At the same time Parker also noted reports of nondevelopmental error patterns not usually associated with typical development (e.g., backing, initial consonant deletion). Problems with the suprasegmental aspects of speech have also been noted. For example, inappropriate voice pitch is frequently reported (e.g., Angelocci, Kopp, & Holbrook, 1964; Boone, 1966) as are problems with word duration and pausing (e.g., Parkhurst & Levitt, 1978), and difficulty with intonation (e.g., Allen & Arndorfer, 2000). Studies such as these have motivated a number of reports (e.g., Gold, 1980; Hudgins & Numbers, 1942; Markides, 1970; Smith, 1975) which have attempted to identify specific speech deficits associated with reduced intelligibility. Statistical correlations have been shown with both segmental and suprasegmental aspects of speech. Smith (1975) noted that although both types of errors may be involved, segmental errors appeared to account for a greater portion of the problem. Given the limitations inherent in the use of correlations, a more direct analysis of the impact of various types of errors on intelligibility was carried out by Maassen and Povel (1985). Using digital signal processing, Maassen and Povel modified the acoustic characteristics (both segmental and suprasegmental) of sentences produced by 10 Dutch-speaking deaf children, and then asked normal-hearing listeners to write down what they heard. Findings indicated that, consistent with the general conclusions by Smith, correction of segmental errors improved intelligibility from 24% to as much as 72%, while correction of segmental/word durations and intonation improved intelligibility to no more than 34%. Interestingly, Maassen and Povel noted that the greatest improvements were generated by correcting errors on the production of vowels.

Intelligibility and Children with CIs

Cochlear implants were introduced in the 1960s; however, the first multichannel implants were not approved for use in adults in the United States until 1984. They were subsequently approved for use in children as young as 2 years of age in 1990 and in children as young as 1 year in 2002. Although much of the research attention to date with this population has focused on speech perception, at least 21 studies have included findings on the intelligibility of speech produced by these children (Allen, Nikolopoulos, & O'Donoghue, 1998; Bakhshaee et al.,

2007; Beadle et al., 2005; Calmels et al., 2004; Chin, Finnegan, & Chung, 2001; Chin, Tsai, & Gao, 2003; Dawson et al., 1995; Flipsen & Colvard, 2006; Geers, 2004; Inscoe, 1999; Löhle et al., 1999; Loundon, Busquet, Roger, Moatti, & Garabedian, 2000; Miyamoto, Iler Kirk, Robbins, Todd, & Riley, 1996; Miyamoto, Iler Kirk, Svirsky, & Sehgal, 1999; Mondain et al., 1997; Osberger, Robbins, Todd, Riley, & Miyamoto, 1994; Peng, Spencer, & Tomblin, 2004; Ramirez Inscoe & Nikolopoulos, 2004; Tye-Murray, Spencer, & Woodsworth, 1995; Uziel et al., 2007; Vieu et al., 1998). These studies have tended to focus at either the sentence or the conversational speech level. Seven of these studies reported sentence-level data and their findings are summarized in Table 10–1 with the studies ordered by the mean age at which the children received their implants. Although findings vary somewhat across the studies (likely as a result of

Table 10–1. Findings from Studies of Sentence-Level Intelligibility for Children Fitted With Cochlear Implants[a]

Study	Mean Age of Implantation	Amount of Implant Experience				
		1 year	2 years	3 years	4 years	7 years
Chin et al. (2003)	3.2 years		~35%			
Chin et al. (2001)	3.42 years			~61%		
Tye-Murray (1995)[b]	4 years			~30%		
Miyamoto et al. (1996)	5.0 years	~10%	~15%	~25%	~40%	
Peng et al. (2004)	5.0 years					~72%
Osberger et al. (1994)	5.7 years		~20%	~35%	~40%	
Tye-Murray (1995)[b]	5.9 years			~25%		
Tye-Murray (1995)[b]	11.5 years			~20%		
Dawson (1995)	14.4 years		~45%			

[a]Cell entries = percentage words understood; NB: most values estimated by the current author from graphs in the publications.
[b]Tye-Murray (1995) reported findings for three groups who differed by age of implantation.

variations in the tasks and judgment formats used), two trends are evident. First, if one scans Table 10–1 vertically, there is a trend for sentence-level intelligibility outcomes to increase as age of implantation gets younger. Second, if one scans Table 10–1 horizontally, intelligibility appears to increase as children gain more experience with their implants. Flipsen (2008) conducted a similar analysis of 10 studies that reported findings for spontaneous conversational speech and reached similar conclusions. More relevant to the current report, Flipsen concluded that intelligibility outcomes in these children appear to be significantly better than we have historically seen when these children would have been provided with hearing aids. This conclusion is supported by findings from studies such as that of Horga and Liker (2006) who directly compared children with CIs to similar children who used hearing aids on several voice and articulation variables. Flipsen also concluded that, unlike the conclusions reached in the older studies of children with hearing aids (Gold, 1980; Jensema et al., 1978; Markides, 1970), fully intelligible conversational speech may be an attainable goal for many children who receive their CIs early.

Despite the improved outcomes, there are several reasons why it remains important to understand intelligibility deficits in this population. First, universal newborn hearing screening is not yet truly universal, and thus not all of these children are identified at birth. Second, even for those who are so identified, implantation may be delayed for a variety of reasons (e.g., medical considerations, funding issues, or concerns about surgical risks). Findings reported for children receiving implants at somewhat older ages suggest that intelligibility deficits remain for significant numbers of children. For example, several such studies (Allen et al., 1998; Bakhshaee et al., 2007; Beadle et al., 2006;

Calmels et al., 2004; Inscoe, 1999) reported 5-year follow-up outcomes using the Speech Intelligibility Rating (SIR) scale. Keeping in mind the previously cited concerns with the use of rating scales (Schiavetti, 1992), the SIR is a 5-point scale in which the highest rating of 5 corresponds to "connected speech is intelligible to all listeners." Across these studies the mean age of implantation ranged from 3;6 to 5;3, and findings indicated that anywhere from 27% to 78% of the children received an SIR rating of 5. Put another way, anywhere from 22% to 73% of these children did not achieve fully intelligible speech even after using their implants for at least 5 years. Recall that typically developing children are usually completely intelligible (in spite of some remaining speech sound errors) by age 4 years (Coplan & Gleason, 1988). A third reason for continuing the search for factors related to reduced intelligibility is that even for those children who are both identified at birth and implanted early, it is still not certain that fully intelligible speech will be the outcome for all of these children; few studies to date have specifically reported intelligibility outcomes for children implanted before age 2 years. Some findings in related domains are emerging however. For example, normal or near-normal outcomes have been reported for such children on language measures such as the Peabody Picture Vocabulary Test (Manrique, Cervera-Paz, Huarte, & Molina, 2004) or the Preschool Language Scale (Nicholas & Geers, 2007). As well, a study by Connor, Craig, Raudenbush, Heavner, and Zwolen (2006) reported superior outcomes on the Percentage Consonants Correct (PCC; from single word productions) metric for children implanted before age 2.5 years compared to those implanted later. However, statistical projections by Connor et al. suggested an average PCC score of only 75 for such children by age 6 years (none of the children in the youngest group had used their implants for more than 4 years). It is not clear how such PCC values might translate into intelligibility of conversational speech, although Shriberg and Kwiatkowski (1982) used a cut-off of 80% for "fair" intelligibility. Until intelligibility findings from these earliest of implantees are reported, it may be prudent to be prepared for less than optimal outcomes for at least some of these children.

A review of the literature to date suggests that there have not yet been any comprehensive attempts to identify the specific factors that impact speech intelligibility in this population. This was, in part, the motivation for the current report.

The Current Analysis

To begin to understand the nature of the intelligibility deficits in children fitted with CIs, a longitudinal study was undertaken. Potential participants were recruited from Child Hearing Services (CHS), a clinical service program for children with hearing impairments which is part of the University of Tennessee Speech and Hearing Center. Initially, children were only recruited if they had received their implants by their third birthday. Given an initial minimum implant age of 24 months, this meant a relatively narrow window for implantation age. However, during the course of the study the minimum age for implantation was lowered to 12 months and children implanted earlier than 24 months were subsequently permitted to enroll. A second inclusionary criterion was that participants had to have at least 18 months of implant experience at the start of the study in order to avoid reliance on samples that might consist mostly of single word productions. Data from a range

of speech outcome variables were obtained from recordings of these children and a series of studies was subsequently carried out (Flipsen, 2006; Flipsen & Colvard, 2006; Flipsen & Parker, 2008; Lenden & Flipsen, 2007). The current analysis is an attempt to tie together findings from these studies along with some additional analyses.

Study Participants

Details on the six children who ultimately participated are shown in Table 10-2. Note that the mean age of implantation was 2;4. Given that only one participant (6) was implanted under the lowered age guidelines, as a group these participants would not be classed as "early implantees" by current standards. The cause of hearing loss was unknown for all but participant 6 who was diagnosed with partial agenesis of the cochlea. At the beginning of the study all of the participants had between 23 and 42 months of experience with their implants (indicated in Table 10-2 in the column labeled PIA or post-implantation age).

Test Protocol

The children were tested every 3 months for periods ranging from 12 to 21 months with variations due largely to participant attrition over the course of the study. Each participant contributed between 5 and 8 samples (see Table 10-2) to the total of 40 samples that were available.

All testing was carried out inside a single-wall sound-treated booth by one of two trained graduate student clinicians. For many of the samples, a parent or the clinician who was providing treatment to the child was also present in the booth and participated in the interaction. The samples

Table 10–2. Participant Information

Partic-ipant	Gender	Age of ID[a]	Implan-tation Age[a]	Initial CA[a, b]	Initial PIA[a, c]	Implant Type	Number of Samples	PPVT-III[d]
1	F	0;8	2;4	5;2	2;11	Clarion	8	89
2	F	0;0	2;6	4;5	1;11	Nucleus-24	5	99
3	F	1;0	3;0	6;2	3;2	Clarion	8	72
4	F	0;3	2;0	5;5	3;6	Nucleus-22	7	77
5	F	1;3	2;7	4;10	2;3	Clarion	6	81
6	M	0;11	1;8	3;9	2;1	Nucleus-24	6	76
Mean (SD)		0;8 (0;6)	2;4 (0;6)	5;0 (0;10)	2;8 (0;8)			82.3 (10.0)

[a]Expressed in years; months.
[b]Chronologic age at start of current study.
[c]Postimplantation age (amount of cochlear implant use) at start of current study.
[d]Standard Score on the Peabody Picture Vocabulary Test-Third Edition (Dunn & Dunn, 1997).
Source: Adapted from Flipsen & Parker (2008).

were recorded on digital audiotape using a tabletop mounted microphone.

Several tasks were administered at each test time, but only two are relevant to the current report. The Peabody Picture Vocabulary Test (PPVT-III; Dunn & Dunn, 1997) was administered at the initial session as a measure of receptive vocabulary; findings are reported in Table 10-2 and as indicated all 6 participants scored within 2 standard deviations of their normal-hearing age peers. Conversational speech samples were evoked at each test time using a variety of topics (e.g., favorite movies or cartoons, current activities in therapy) and materials such as activity pictures from the Bracken Concept Development Program (Bracken, 1998). Narratives were avoided because of concerns about the use of nontypical prosody in the narrative register (Shriberg, Kwiatkowski, & Rasmussen, 1990). Examiners were instructed not to gloss the child's utterances (a common practice in collecting speech samples), because the intent was to look at intelligibility and such glossing might have artificially inflated intelligibility values. Samples lasted at least 10 minutes. A target sample size of at least 90 different words was selected because samples of this size have been shown to provide a representative sample of English phonemes and canonical forms (Shriberg, 1986). The current author monitored each test session via headphones from outside the booth and kept a running tally of unique intelligible words. One sample contained only 67 different words because the sample was terminated after 25 minutes in order to avoid fatigue effects. All other samples included at least 92 different words. Sample length varied from 67 to 199 different intelligible words (mean = 139.0; SD = 26.1) and included between 65 and 216 utterances (mean = 134.3, SD = 35.5).

Sample Transcription and Data Analysis

The conversational speech samples were transcribed by a trained graduate student clinician who had not been present for the sample collection. She had recently completed an undergraduate course in phonetics. The transcripts included three lines for each utterance (X: an orthographic gloss of the adult target; Y: a phonetic transcription of the adult target; Z: a phonetic transcription of the child's productions). For the Y and Z lines of the transcript, narrow phonetic transcription conventions were based on the system of Shriberg and Kent (1995). In order to avoid possible familiarity effects of listening to the same speaker multiple times in a row, the 40 samples were transcribed in random order. Transcription reliability procedures and results are reported in Flipsen and Colvard (2006). Transcripts were entered into the Programs to Examine Phonetic and Phonologic Evaluation Records (PEPPER) software tool (Shriberg, Allen, McSweeny, & Wilson, 2001).

Intelligibility Index (II; termed II-original in Flipsen & Colvard, 2006) served as the outcome variable for the current study. During transcription of unintelligible portions of the sample, the transcriber would (by definition) not know what the words were but would count unintelligible syllables (heard as peaks of sonority or relative loudness). Each unintelligible syllable would be indicated by a ∗, and syllables would be grouped into words (with boundaries indicated by spaces) using any available prosodic and/or contextual cues. Where such cues were unavailable or not definitive, unintelligible syllables were grouped into words using a rule of 3 monosyllabic words for every 1 disyllabic word. For example, if the transcriber heard a stretch of unintelligible speech that included 10 syllables where

prosodic and contextual cues were not helpful, the syllables would be grouped into 8 words as follows ∗ ∗ ∗ ∗∗ ∗ ∗ ∗ ∗∗. For purposes of the current analysis intelligibility was defined as the percentage of words understood by a transcriber who was not present for sample collection and who did not have the benefit of examiner glossing. II values were obtained from PEPPER (Shriberg et al., 2001).

Relative to variables potentially influencing intelligibility, both segmental and suprasegmental variables were included. PEPPER was used to calculate the segmental metrics which included those presented by Shriberg, Austin, Lewis, McSweeny, and Wilson (1997); many of these measures represent extensions to the PCC (Percentage Consonants Correct; Shriberg & Kwiatkowski, 1982). To provide an index of vowel production, Shriberg et al. suggested calculating Percentage Vowels Correct (PVC) and Percentage Phonemes Correct (PPC; a metric also proposed by Dollaghan, Biber, & Campbell, 1993) which includes both consonants and vowels. To address the broad (phonemic) level of transcription and to address concerns about the reliability of narrow phonetic transcription, Shriberg et al. proposed "revised" versions of these three metrics (PCCR, PVCR, & PPCR) that score distortion-level errors (as indicated by diacritics) as correct. To address the question of differentiating between common distortion errors and uncommon or idiosyncratic distortion errors, Shriberg et al. proposed Percentage Consonants Correct-Adjusted (PCCA). In this case, common distortion errors (e.g., dentalized or lateralized fricatives, derhotacized /r/, velarized /l/) are assumed to be correct; only uncommon distortions are counted as errors. The question of the breadth of the speech sound inventory is addressed with Percentage Consonants in the Inventory (PCI). To address concerns that measures such as PCC may mask important differences in terms of specific sounds or groups of sounds, analysis for the three consonant accuracy metrics (PCC, PCCA, & PCCR) was also conducted separately for three Development Sound Classes termed the Early 8 (/m,b,j,n,w,d,p,h/), Middle 8 (/t,ŋ,k,g,f,v,tʃ,dʒ/), and Late 8 (/s,z,ð,θ,r,l,ʃ,ʒ/), as well as totals for the 24 consonants.

Error patterns on speech sounds were examined as part of a master's thesis project (Parker, 2005). Analyses of 15 developmental phonological patterns (i.e., processes) were carried out using the Natural Process Analysis (NPA; Shriberg & Kwiatkowski, 1980) routine of PEPPER. Analyses of 9 nondevelopmental phonological patterns were carried out manually using procedures described in Flipsen and Parker (2008). The particular set of nondevelopmental patterns (shown later in the bottom half of Table 10–4) was chosen to reflect patterns regularly attested in the prior literature on speech production by the hearing impaired. Reliability procedures for the analysis of non-developmental patterns are reported in Flipsen and Parker.

Data on the suprasegmental variables were obtained separately as part of an undergraduate honors thesis project (Lenden, 2005). Following initial transcription, the 40 samples were analyzed manually for 7 prosody and voice characteristics using the conventions of the Prosody Voice Screening Profile (PVSP; Shriberg et al., 1990). Reliability procedures and results for the PVSP analyses are reported in Lenden and Flipsen (2007).

Instrumental analysis of articulation rate (beyond the perceptual impressions obtained with the PVSP) was carried out using Computerized Speech Lab (CSL 4400). Articulation rate was measured from broadband spectrograms in both syllables per second and phones per second. Findings for the syllables per second analysis were reported by Flipsen (2006). The phonetic phrase, a stretch of speech bounded by pauses, was used as the unit of analysis. Pauses were defined as periods of silence in the acoustic record of at least 250 msec except when potential pauses were bounded by contiguous stop consonants. For such exceptions, the silent period needed to be at least 400 msec in duration to avoid confusing two contiguous stop closures with a pause (see Flipsen, 1999, p. 163). As part of the articulation rate measurement process, data on length of phonetic phrase (in both syllables and phones) were gathered and were also considered in the current analysis.

A total of 52 variables were thus examined as potentially influencing intelligibility (II). Each of the variables was separately correlated with II. The significant correlations ($p <.05$) were then rank-ordered and fit into a stepwise regression model. Note that given the exploratory nature of the current analysis, Bonferroni-correction was not applied in any of the analyses as it was considered overly conservative. The risk of Type II errors was judged to be as much of a concern as the risk of Type I errors.

Findings

Individual Variables

Values for II (as reported in Flipsen & Colvard, 2006) ranged from 65.6 to 96.5% words understood (mean = 85.7; SD = 7.9). Of the 40 samples, 12 (30%) had II values of at least 90%.

Findings for the segmental analyses are shown in Table 10–3. Vowel accuracy (PVC, PVCR) was higher than consonant accuracy

Table 10–3. Values Obtained for the Segmental Analyses Across the 40 Samples

	Mean	SD	Range
Percentage Consonants Correct-Early 8 (PCC-E)	92.8	5.4	73.7–100.0
Percentage Consonants Correct-Middle 8 (PCC-M)	81.6	17.1	16.2–98.2
Percentage Consonants Correct-Late 8 (PCC-L)	67.1	13.6	29.5–91.0
Percentage Consonants Correct-Total (PCC)	81.8	10.1	47.0–94.4
Percentage Consonants Correct-Revised-Early 8 (PCCR-E)	93.1	5.4	73.7–100.0
Percentage Consonants Correct-Revised-Middle 8 (PCCR-M)	82.2	16.7	18.9–98.8
Percentage Consonants Correct-Revised-Late 8 (PCCR-L)	71.5	13.6	32.1–93.1
Percentage Consonants Correct-Revised (PCCR)	83.4	9.9	49.0–96.4
Percentage Consonants Correct-Adjusted-Early 8 (PCCA-E)	92.8	5.4	73.7–100.0
Percentage Consonants Correct-Adjusted-Middle 8 (PCCA-M)	81.6	17.1	16.2–98.2
Percentage Consonants Correct-Adjusted-Late 8 (PCCA-L)	71.0	13.8	29.5–93.1
Percentage Consonants Correct-Adjusted (PCCA)	83.0	10.1	47.8–95.5
Percentage Vowels Correct (PVC)	94.5	3.3	85.1–99.8
Percentage Vowels Correct-Revised (PVCR)	96.6	2.8	87.6–100.0
Percentage Phonemes Correct (PPC)	86.9	7.1	61.9–95.7
Percentage Phonemes Correct-Revised (PPCR)	88.7	6.9	64.1–97.3
Percentage Consonants in Inventory (PCI)	96.5	5.5	70.0–100.0

(PCC, PCCR, PCCA). Regardless of which version of PCC was used, accuracy on the Early 8 consonants was higher than accuracy on the Middle 8 consonants which was higher than accuracy on the Late 8 consonants. An examination of the findings for individual speakers revealed 2 samples (both from Participant 6) in which accuracy on the Late 8 consonants was higher than accuracy on the Middle 8 consonants. Values for PCC, PCCR, and PCCA were all relatively similar suggesting that relatively few of the remaining errors were distortions (whether common or uncommon).

Findings for the developmental and non-developmental phonological pattern analyses (Flipsen & Parker, 2008) are presented in Table 10-4. Both types of patterns were in evidence, although non-developmental patterns were far less common overall.

Table 10–4. Percentage Occurrence of Developmental and Non-Developmental Phonological Patterns Across the 40 Samples

Developmental Pattern[a]	Mean	SD	Range
Regressive Assimilation	0.1	0.2	0.0–0.8
Progressive Assimilation	0.1	0.3	0.0–1.1
Cluster Reduction-Initial	36.3	25.8	0.0–88.2
Cluster Reduction-Final	32.1	23.5	0.0–85.7
Final Consonant Deletion	14.1	9.8	0.0–34.2
Liquid Simplification-Initial	17.8	24.8	0.0–100.0
Liquid Simplification-Final	12.7	17.2	0.0–60.0
Palatal Fronting-Initial	0.4	1.7	0.0–10.0
Palatal Fronting-Final	0.3	2.0	0.0–12.5
Stopping-Initial	36.8	20.3	0.0–75.0
Stopping-Final	1.8	3.8	0.0–21.1
Unstressed Syllable Deletion-2 Syllables	2.8	3.0	0.0–13.4
Unstressed Syllable Deletion-3+ Syllables	16.0	17.7	0.0–66.7
Velar Fronting-Initial	5.5	18.4	0.0–92.3
Velar Fronting-Final	0.5	2.1	0.0–11.1
Nondevelopmental Pattern[b]			
Initial Consonant Deletion	2.0	3.0	0.0–18.5
Glottal Stop Substitution-Initial	0.0	0.0	0.0–0.0
Glottal Stop Substitution-Medial	1.6	4.8	0.0–26.7
Glottal Stop Substitution-Final	0.1	0.4	0.0–2.2
Backing-Initial	0.8	1.3	0.0–5.0
Backing-Final	0.6	1.4	0.0–7.1
Vowel Substitution	2.4	2.0	0.0–8.6
Vowel Neutralization	1.6	1.7	0.0–6.0
Diphthong Simplification	1.2	1.7	0.0–8.9

[a]Values derived using NPA output from PEPPER software (Shriberg et al., 2001).
[b]Values derived manually.
Source: Adapted from Flipsen & Parker, (2008).

One nondevelopmental pattern (Glottal Stop Substitution–Initial) never occurred in any of the samples.

Findings from the prosody and voice analysis, as reported in Lenden and Flipsen (2007), are shown in Table 10-5. Resonance Quality and Stress were the most problematic issues in this set of samples. Although mean values for Laryngeal Quality and Loudness were relatively high, considerable variability on both variables was present with samples containing as few as 36% and 56% appropriate utterances, respectively. Articulation rate and phonetic phrase length findings are presented in Table 10-6.

Zero-Order Correlations

Of the 52 variables examined, 32 were significantly correlated with II (p <.05), and these are listed in rank order in Table 10-7. Note that the directions of the correlations for the phonological pattern variables were all negative (i.e., as II increased, frequency of the pattern occurrence decreased). This is as expected given that the pattern variables reflect the proportion of errors. All of the other variables, which reflect proportion correct, were positively correlated with II.

The significant variables in Table 10-7 include segmental errors (related to both consonants and vowels), phonological patterns (both developmental and nondevelopmental), and prosody and voice variables. Relative to consonants, all three of the developmental sound classes (early, middle, and late) were included. The only instrumentally measured variable that was significantly correlated with II was Phonetic Phrase Length in phones.

Table 10–5. Prosody and Voice Screening Profile (PVSP) Findings Across the 40 Samples[a]

	Mean	*SD*	*Range*
Phrasing	97.1	4.3	86–100
Rate	88.4	10.0	60–100
Stress	48.2	26.9	0–96
Loudness	92.4	10.8	56–100
Pitch	97.6	4.3	80–100
Laryngeal Quality	87.3	15.0	36–100
Resonance Quality	10.4	20.8	0–84

[a]Cell entries = percentage of utterances rated as "appropriate" across the 40 samples.
Source: Adapted from Lenden & Flipsen, (2007).

Table 10–6. Articulation Rate and Phonetic Phrase Length Findings Across the 40 Samples

	Mean	*SD*	*Range*
Articulation Rate (syllables per second)[a]	3.15	0.45	2.15–3.92
Articulation Rate (phones per second)	7.26	1.24	4.92–10.21
Phonetic Phrase Length (syllables)	4.10	0.72	2.68–5.58
Phonetic Phrase Length (phones)	9.00	1.76	5.17–12.09

[a]As reported in Flipsen (2006).

Table 10–7. Variables Significantly Correlated with II

	r	p		r	p
PCC	.696	.000	Initial Consonant Deletion	−.493	.001
PCCR	.693	.000	Liquid Simplification-Final	−.467	.002
PPCR	.691	.000			
PCCA	.690	.000	Cluster Reduction-Initial	−.449	.004
PCC-M	.684	.000	Stress	.446	.004
PCCA-M	.684	.000	PVC	.428	.006
PCCR-M	.679	.000	Cluster Reduction-Final	−.427	.006
PPC	.677	.000	Laryngeal Quality	.423	.007
PCC-L	.578	.000	Glottal Stop Substitution-Medial	−.419	.007
PCCR-L	.568	.000	Pitch	.415	.008
PVCR	.559	.000	Vowel Neutralization	−.409	.009
PCCA-L	.558	.000	Final Consonant Deletion	−.397	.011
PCC-E	.546	.000			
PCCA-E	.546	.000	Phonetic Phrase Length-Phones	.364	.021
PCCR-E	.543	.000			
Vowel Substitution	−.539	.000	Resonance Quality	.334	.035
PCI	.517	.001	Backing-Initial	−.323	.045
Diphthong Simplification	−.495	.001			

$p < .05$

Regression Model

The 32 variables in Table 10–7 were then entered into a forward selection stepwise regression analysis with alpha to enter set at .25 using the software program MINITAB (Version 13.3). The analysis generated a model suggesting that a combination of six variables could account for 60% of the adjusted variance in II. The largest contributor to the model was PCC (48.4%), followed by Pitch (3.1%), Backing-Initial (2.8%), PCC-E (2.8%), Laryngeal Quality (2.0%), and Glottal Stop Substitution–Medial (0.9%). The model thus included overall consonant accuracy, accuracy on early developing consonants, two voice variables, and two nondevelopmental phonological patterns.

Discussion

Overall Performance

Intelligibility of conversational speech for the children in the current study was relatively high (mean = 85.7%). Segmental analyses indicated an average of 80% or more correct on consonant production and 94% or better on vowel production. Error patterns still in evidence indicated that the vast majority of errors were those usually seen in normal-hearing, typically developing children although a small proportion on non-developmental error patterns were observed. Prosody and voice analysis (Lenden & Flipsen, 2007) indicated some remaining problems with Resonance Quality and use of Stress. Articulation rate and phonetic phrase length findings obtained (in syllables) appeared to be consistent with values for their chronologic age peers reported in previous studies (as summarized in Flipsen, 2002b). Values in phones, however, appeared to be somewhat low compared to chronological age expectations. They did appear to be consistent with age expectations if compared based on amount of implant use. Taken together, these findings support the notion of improved outcomes for children with severe or profound hearing impairments who are fitted with CIs compared to what might have been obtained with hearing aids. Clearly, some speech production issues remain suggesting the need for continued work in this area.

Correlational Analysis

As indicated in Table 10–7, more than 60% (32/52) of the variables examined were significantly correlated with II. As in previous studies of the speech of the individuals with hearing impairments, both segmental and suprasegmental variables were implicated as potentially affecting intelligibility.

The strongest correlations with II were those related to segmental variables, particularly those related to consonant accuracy. Interestingly the correlation coefficient obtained for PCC (.696) is strikingly similar to

that obtained by both Hudgins and Numbers (1942) and Smith (1975) who both reported correlations between intelligibility and consonant accuracy of .70. Findings for the correlations between vowel accuracy and intelligibility were not so similar however, as Hudgins and Numbers reported .585 and Smith reported .75 compared to the PVC value of .428 obtained in the current study. The lower value in the current study likely reflected the fact that vowels were much less of an issue for the children in the current study than we have historically seen in this population. The limited variability in vowel accuracy observed in the current study also suggests that some ceiling effects may have been operating.

Consonant accuracy was more strongly correlated with II than vowel accuracy. This contrasts with the findings of Maassen and Povel (1985) who suggested that vowel errors had a greater impact on intelligibility than consonant errors. This is consistent with the lower accuracy (and particularly the greater variability) of consonant production compared to vowels.

All three of the developmental sound classes of consonants were significantly correlated with II. The weakest correlations were with the Early 8 which, like the situation with vowels, may have reflected their high level of accuracy and therefore possible ceiling effects. The strongest correlations appeared to be related to the Middle 8 consonants.

The large number of significant segmental variables at the top of Table 10–7 may have been partly an artifact of the nature of the variables used. PCC, PCCR, and PCCA (and their variants) differ only to the degree that they deal with distortion errors and thus are not fully orthogonal with each other (they are effectively a "nested series"; Gruber, 1997, personal communication). As well, the differences among the three scores were relatively small. Not surprisingly, these variables were highly correlated with each other, and so it should not be surprising that their correlations with II were so close to each other in magnitude.

Of the nine phonological error patterns that were significantly correlated with II, six represented non-developmental patterns. This is particularly interesting in light of the relatively low level of occurrence of the nondevelopmental patterns (see Table 10–4). One interpretation of this finding is that atypical error patterns, when they occur, may focus the attention of the listener away from the intended message (i.e., act as a distraction). This possibility is supported by the fact that all three of the error patterns related to vowels were significantly correlated with II (again despite the low frequency of vowel errors). Indeed, the two error patterns most strongly correlated with II were Vowel Substitution and Diphthong Simplification. Note that all three of the vowel-related error patterns reflected omission and/or substitution errors. Vowel distortions did not appear to influence II as much, however, as PVCR (which assumes distortions to be correct) was more strongly correlated with II than PVC.

Four of the seven prosody and voice variables were significantly correlated with II. Three of these variables (Stress; Laryngeal Quality; Resonance Quality) were the variables that were the most problematic for the participants. The one other (Pitch) was somewhat surprising given an average of 97.6% appropriate utterances across the samples (see Table 10–5). Although none of the samples had fewer than 80% appropriate utterances, an examination of individual sample data suggested that lower values for Pitch were obtained from Participants 4 and 6 who also happened to produce speech that was the least intelligible. This suggested that small differences in pitch may

have had a significant impact on II, at least for some participants. Neither of the rate measures (whether from the PVSP or the instrumental measures) was significantly correlated with II. Thus, relative to rate, the instrumental analysis appeared to confirm the perceptual analysis of the PVSP. Slow speaking rate has been previously identified as a problem with the speech of the hearing impaired, but the measures used in the current study may not have been well suited to comparisons with previous research; Stathopoulos, Duchan, Sonnenmeier, and Bruce (1986) noted reduced speaking rate in their study and attributed the reductions to both slower articulation and longer pauses. Both of the measures used in the current study ignored most pauses. The PVSP evaluates rate on an utterance by utterance basis, and thus would only consider within-utterance pauses. The instrumental analysis used herein specifically looked at articulation rate with the phonetic phrase being used as the unit of analysis; the phonetic phrase completely ignores pauses. This would suggest that while the speed with which children with CIs articulate speech sounds appears to have little or no impact on their intelligibility, pausing (particularly between utterance pauses) still needs to be considered.

Phonetic phrase length in phones was significantly correlated with II. The direction of the correlation was positive indicating that as the number of phones in the phonetic phrase increased, intelligibility increased. However, phonetic phrase length in syllables was not significantly correlated with II. This suggests that as intelligibility was increasing, the participants were expanding existing syllable forms. This possibility is supported by the significant (and negative) correlations between II and several error patterns that reflect deletion errors (Initial Consonant Deletion, Cluster Reduction, and Final Consonant Deletion).

Regression Analysis

The regression analysis reduced the set of 32 potentially interacting variables to a combination of six variables that in combination accounted for 60% of the adjusted variance in II. The combination included overall consonant accuracy (PCC), accuracy specific to early developing consonants (PCC-E), two voice variables (Pitch and Laryngeal Quality), and two nondevelopmental error pattern variables (Backing–Initial and Glottal Stop Substitution–Medial). The number and variety of variables included in the model highlights the caution by Smith (1975) that reductions in the intelligibility of speech producing by individuals with hearing impairment likely involves a complex interaction of multiple factors.

Within the context of the regression model, PCC accounted for, by far, the largest portion (48.4%) of the adjusted variance in II. This seems intuitively reasonable as vowel accuracy was consistently high in the current sample and accuracy of the remaining segments (i.e., consonants) would seem crucial to conveying meaning to the listener.

Five other variables accounted for significant amounts of the variance in II, but none of them accounted for more than 3.1%. This would suggest that none of these variables would qualify as needing a significant amount of clinical attention. Interestingly, in each case these other variables could be seen as unusual or atypical. The most obvious of these are the nondevelopmental pattern variables which were discussed previously as potential distractions for the listener. The two voice variables could be seen in the same light as they reflected the percentage of utterances rated as "appropriate." The one remaining variable (PCC-E) might also reflect a similar possibility as difficulties with the earliest sounds might also call attention to themselves. Alternatively, or perhaps in addition, such segmental errors may simply not trigger word recognition.

One omission from the model that might be seen as surprising was Resonance Quality because, as with the nondevelopmental patterns, abnormal resonance might have been a particular distraction for the listener. As indicated in Table 10–5, this was the PVSP variable that was the most problematic for the children in the current study group. Anecdotal impressions however, were that the resonance quality observed in the current samples was not typical of that usually expected from the speech of individuals with severe or profound hearing impairments. Utterances in the current study which were rated as "not appropriate" on this variable would not have met the classic expectations for "cul-de-sac" resonance usually observed in the speech of individuals with severe or profound hearing impairments. This points out a notable limitation of the PVSP approach of simply rating utterances as "appropriate" or "not appropriate" on each of the variables. Admittedly however, a limited search failed to uncover a documented approach to quantifying cul-de-sac resonance. Thus, no other option appears to be currently available.

Conclusions

It would appear that consonant accuracy is the largest single variable contributing to the remaining intelligibility deficits in children fitted with CIs. Five other variables each contributed a significant but very small amount of variance (3.1% or less). This would suggest that, if these findings can be replicated with other members of this population, therapy aimed at improving intelligibility for these children should focus largely on improving consonant production.

Shortcomings and Future Directions

Clearly, the current study is limited by its small sample size of six children. As well, the sample included a disproportionate number of females (5). Thus, on both dimensions it is not clear that it is fully representative of the population. Findings, therefore, should be generalized with great care. In addition, as noted previously, this sample did not represent those who would be referred to as implanted early as the age of implantation limits have been lowered since these participants were recruited. The current study also did not consider language skill or fluency which may well have affected the intelligibility of the message. Another problem is that the longitudinal samples in the current study were each treated as separate data sets, even though they represented performance by six participants over time; thus time was not considered as a factor. It would certainly be valuable in future studies to learn whether the factors that affect intelligibility change over time. Finally, the current study suffers from the usual correlation-causation problem as all correlational approaches. More direct studies such as the simulations conducted by Maassen and Povel (1985) might be of great value in this regard.

This preliminary study clearly requires replication with a larger group of participants. Given that under ideal conditions, children would be identified at birth (or sooner if that becomes feasible) and receive their implants as soon as practicable, future studies should look at such children. On the other hand, lacking such ideal conditions, studies should also be conducted of children implanted over a wider range of ages. Future studies might also focus on children whose hearing losses are tied to specific etiologies (e.g., cytomegalovirus, meningitis) as outcomes may differ. Recent trends in implantation include providing bilateral implants as well as providing implants for children who do not fit typical eligibility requirements (e.g., those with other handicapping conditions). Studies such as the current one (as well as general outcome studies) are certainly also needed for those children. Finally, the current study only looked at conversational speech, and future studies might also investigate whether factors affecting intelligibility differ at other linguistic levels.

The Bigger Picture

The measurement and application of the construct of intelligibility clearly is not limited to the study of the speech of individuals with hearing impairment. It appears to lie at the heart of much of what those of us who study speech sound disorders in children are about. Indeed, questions about intelligibility can easily be associated with the focus of many of the other chapters in this volume. For example, children with significantly reduced speech intelligibility make up a sizable portion of the preschool children encountered in speech-language pathology practice. Where do such deficits originate? Although some data suggest that the source of the problem for up to 60% of such children may be genetic, will this knowledge ultimately lead us to preventive measures? Will in utero gene therapy, for example, be the answer? What about the large group of children whose speech delay appears to be related to a history of frequent otitis media with effusion (Shriberg's SD-OME category)? Why does the speech of many children with these histories stand out because of a somewhat unique intelligibility-speech gap (Shriberg, Flipsen, Kwiatkowski, & McSweeny, 2003) or a high frequency of backing errors (Shriberg, Kent, Karlsson, McSweeny, Nadler, & Brown, 2003)? Does significantly reduced speech intelligibility place children at increased risk for comorbid disorders in other communication domains? Or might disorders in other domains lead to intelligibility problems? Are acoustic analysis approaches (whether carried out manually or through computer automated methods; see also Chapters 5 and 6) better suited to quantifying intelligibility or identifying the sources of intelligibility deficits compared to the largely perceptual methods used herein and in most other studies of this kind? Clearly, much work remains to be done in understanding the role of intelligibility in speech sound disorders.

References

Allen, G. D., & Arndorfer, P. M. (2000). Production of sentence-final intonation contours by hearing-impaired children. *Journal of Speech, Language, and Hearing Research*, 43, 441–455.

Allen, M. C., Nikolopoulos, T. P., & O'Donoghue, G. M. (1998). Speech intelligibility in children after cochlear implantation. *American Journal of Otology*, 19, 742–746.

Angelocci, A. A., Kopp, G. A., & Holbrook, A. (1964). The vowel formants of deaf and normal-hearing eleven- to fourteen-year-old boys. *Journal of Speech and Hearing Disorders*, 29, 156–170.

Bakhshaee, M., Ghasemi, M. M., Shakeri, M. T., Razmara, N., Tayarani, H., & Tale, M. R. (2007). Speech development in children after cochlear implantation. *European Archives of Otolaryngology*, 264(11), 1263–1266.

Beadle, E. A. R., McKinley, D. J., Nikolopoulos, T. P., Brough, J., O'Donoghue, G. M., & Archbold, S. M. (2005). Long-term functional outcomes and academic-occupational status in implanted children after 10 to 14 years of cochlear implant use. *Otology and Neurotology*, 26, 1152–1160.

Boone, D. R. (1966). Modification of the voices of deaf children. *Volta Review*, 68, 686–692.

Bracken, B. (1998). *Bracken Concept Development Program-Revised*. San Antonio, TX: Psychological Corporation.

Calmels, M-N., Saliba, I., Wanna, G., Cochard, N., Fillaux, J., Deguine, O., et al. (2004). Speech perception and speech intelligibility in children after cochlear implantation. *International Journal of Pediatric Otorhinolaryngology*, 68, 347–351.

Chin, S. B., Finnegan, K. R., & Chung, B. A. (2001). Relationships among types of speech intelligibility in pediatric users of cochlear implants. *Journal of Communication Disorders*, 34, 187–205.

Chin, S. B., Tasi, P. L., & Gao, S. (2003). Connected speech intelligibility of children with cochlear implants and children with normal hearing. *American Journal of Speech-Language Pathology*, 12, 440–451.

Connor, C. M., Craig, H. K., Raudenbush, S. W., Heavner, K., & Zwolen, T. E. (2006). The age at which young deaf children receive cochlear implants and their vocabulary and speech production growth: Is there an added value for early implantation? *Ear and Hearing*, 27, 628–644.

Coplan, J., & Gleason, J. R. (1988). Unclear speech: Recognition and significance of unintelligible speech in preschool children. *Pediatrics*, 82, 447–452.

Dawson, P. W., Blamey, P. J., Dettman, S. J., Rowland, L. C., Barker, E. J., Tobey, E. A., et al. (1995). A clinical report on speech production of cochlear implant users. *Ear and Hearing*, 16, 551–561.

Dollaghan, C. A., Biber, M. E., & Campbell, T. F. (1993). Constituent syllable effects in a nonsense-word repetition task. *Journal of Speech and Hearing Research*, 36, 1051–1054.

Dunn, L. M., & Dunn, L. M. (1997). *Peabody Picture Vocabulary Test-Third Edition*. Circle Pines, MN: American Guidance Service.

Dykstra, A. D., Hakel, M. E., & Adams, S. G. (2007). Application of the ICF in reduced speech intelligibility in dysathria. *Seminars in Speech and Language*, 28, 301–311.

Flipsen, P., Jr. (1999). *Articulcation rate and speech-sound normalization following speech delay*. Unpublished doctoral dissertation, University of Tennessee, Knoxville.

Flipsen, P., Jr. (2002a). *Causes and speech sound disorders. Why worry?* Presentation at the Speech Pathology Australia National Conference: Alice Springs, Northern Territory, Australia.

Flipsen, P., Jr. (2002b). Longitudinal changes in articulation rate and phonetic phrase length in children with speech delay. *Journal of Speech, Language, and Hearing Research, 45*(1), 100–110.

Flipsen, P., Jr. (2006). *Articulation rate in young children with cochlear implants.* Poster presentation at the Annual Convention of the American Speech-Language-Hearing Association (ASHA), Miami, FL.

Flipsen, P., Jr., (2008). Intelligibility of spontaneous conversational speech produced by children with cochlear implants: A review. *International Journal of Pediatric Otorhinolaryngology, 72*(5), 559–564.

Flipsen, P., Jr., & Colvard, L. G. (2006). Intelligibility of conversational speech produced by children with cochlear implants. *Journal of Communication Disorders, 39,* 93–108.

Flipsen, P., Jr., Khwaileh, F., & Erickson, M. (2007). *Transcription vs. multiple choice scoring on the CSIM.* Poster presentation at the Annual Convention of the American Speech-Language-Hearing Association (ASHA), Boston, MA.

Flipsen, P., Jr., & Parker, R. G. (2008). Phonological patterns in the speech of children with cochlear implants. *Journal of Communication Disorders, 41*(4), 337–357.

Geers, A. E. (2004). Speech, language, and reading skills after early cochlear implantation. *Archives of Otolaryngology, Head and Neck Surgery, 130,* 634–638.

Gold, T. (1980). Speech production in hearing-impaired children. *Journal of Communication Disorders, 13,* 397–418.

Horga, D., & Liker, M. (2006). Voice and pronunciation of cochlear implant speakers. *Clinical Linguistics and Phonetics, 20,* 211–217.

Hudgins, C. V., & Numbers, F. C. (1942). An investigation of the intelligibility of the speech of the deaf. *Genetic Psychology Monographs, 25,* 289–392.

Hustad, K. C. (2007). Effects of speech stimuli and dysarthria severity on intelligibility scores and listener confidence ratings for speakers with cerebral palsy. *Folia Phoniatrica et Logopedica, 59,* 306–317.

Inscoe, J. (1999). Communication outcomes after paediatric cochlear implantation. *International Journal of Pediatric Otorhinolaryngology, 47,* 195–200.

Iosub, S., Fuchs, M., Bingol, N., & Gromisch, D. S. (1981). Fetal alcohol syndrome revisited. *Pediatrics, 68*(4), 475–479.

Jensema, C. J., Karchmer, M. A., & Trybus, R. J. (1978). *The rated speech intelligibility of hearing impaired children: Basic relationships and a detailed analysis.* Washington, DC: Office of Demographic Studies, Gallaudet College.

Kent, R. D. (1992). *Intelligibility in speech disorders.* Amsterdam: John Benjamins.

Kent, R. D. (1993). Speech intelligibility and communicative competence in children. In A. P. Kaiser, & D. B. Gray, (Eds.), *Enhancing children's communication. Research foundations for intervention* (pp. 223–239). Baltimore: Paul H. Brookes.

Kent, R. D., Miolo, G., & Bloedel, S. (1994). The intelligibility of children's speech: A review of evaluation procedures. *American Journal of Speech-Language Pathology, 3*(2), 81–95.

Kumin, L. (1994). Intelligibility of speech in children with Down syndrome in natural settings: Parents' perspective. *Perceptual and Motor Skills, 78,* 307–313.

Lenden, J. M. (2005). *Prosody and voice characteristics of children with cochlear implants.* Unpublished undergraduate honors thesis. Knoxville, TN: University of Tennessee.

Lenden, J. M., & Flipsen, P., Jr. (2007). Prosody and voice characteristics of children with cochlear implants. *Journal of Communication Disorders, 40*(1), 66–81.

Levitt, H., & Stromberg, H. (1983). Segmental characteristics of the speech of hearing-impaired children: Factors affecting intelligibility. In I. Hochberg, H. Levitt, & M. J. Osberger, (Eds.), *Speech of the hearing impaired. Research, training, and personnel preparation* (pp. 53–73). Baltimore: University Park Press.

Löhle, E., Fischmuth, S., Holm, M., Becker, L., Flamm, K., Laszig, R., et al. (1999). Speech recognition, speech production and speech intelligibility in children with hearing aids versus implanted children. *International Journal of Pediatric Otorhinolaryngology*, *47*, 165–169.

Loundon, N., Busquet, D., Roger, G., Moatti, L., & Garabedian, E. N. (2000). Audiophonological results after cochlear implantation in 40 congenitally deaf patients: Preliminary results. *International Journal of Pediatric Otorhinolaryngology*, *56*, 9–21.

Maassen, B., & Povel, D-J. (1985). The effect of segmental and suprasegmental corrections on the intelligibility of deaf speech. *Journal of the Acoustical Society of America*, *78*, 877–886.

Manrique, M., Cervera-Paz, F. J., Huarte, A., & Molina, M. (2004). Advantages of cochlear implantation in prelingual deaf children before 2 years of age when compared to later implantation. *Laryngoscope*, *114*, 1462–1469.

Markides, A. (1970). The speech of deaf and partially-hearing children with special reference to factors affecting intelligibility. *British Journal of Disorders of Communication*, *5*, 126–140.

Miyamoto, R. T., Iler Kirk, K., Robbins, A. M., Todd, S., & Riley, A. (1996). Speech perception and speech production skills in children with multichannel cochlear implants. *Acta Otolaryngologica (Stockholm)*, *116*, 240–243.

Miyamoto, R. T., Iler Kirk, K., Svirsky, M. A., & Sehgal, S. T. (1999). Communication skills in pediatric cochlear implant recipients. *Acta Otolaryngologica (Stockholm)*, *119*, 219–224.

Mondain, M., Sillon, M., Vieu, A., Lanvin, M., Reuillard-Artieres, F., Tobey, E., et al. (1997). Speech perception skills and speech production intelligibility in French children with prelingual deafness and cochlear implants. *Archives of Otolaryngology, Head and Neck Surgery*, *123*, 181–184.

Nicholas, J. G., & Geers, A. E. (2007). Will they catch up? The role of age at cochlear implantation in the spoken language development of children with severe to profound hearing loss. *Journal of Speech, Language, and Hearing Research*, *50*, 1048–1062.

Osberger, M. J. (1992). Speech intelligibility in the hearing impaired: Research and clinical implications. In R. D. Kent (Ed.), *Intelligibility in*

speech disorders (pp. 233–264). Amsterdam: John Benjamins.

Osberger, M. J., Robbins, A. M., Todd, S. L., Riley, A. I., & Miyamoto, R. T. (1994). Speech production skills of children with multichannel cochlear implants. In I. J. Hochmair-Desoyer, & E. S. Hochmair, (Eds.), *Advances in cochlear implants* (pp. 503–508). Manz: Wien.

Parker, R. G. (2005). *Phonological process use in the speech of children fitted with cochlear implants*. Unpublished master's thesis. Knoxville, TN: University of Tennessee.

Parkhurst, B. G., & Levitt, H. (1978). The effect of selected prosodic errors on the intelligibility of deaf speech. *Journal of Communication Disorders*, *11*, 249–256.

Peng, S-C., Spencer, L. J., & Tomblin, J. B. (2004). Speech intelligibility of pediatric cochlear implant recipients with 7 years of device experience. *Journal of Speech, Language, and Hearing Research*, *47*, 1227–1236.

Ramirez Inscoe, J., & Nikolopoulos, T. P. (2004). Cochlear implantation in children deafened by cytomegalovirus: Speech perception and speech intelligibility outcomes. *Otology and Neurotology*, *25*, 479–482.

Schiavetti, N. (1992). Scaling procedures for the measurement of speech intelligibility. In R. D. Kent (Ed.), *Intelligibility in speech disorders* (pp. 11–34). Amsterdam: John Benjamins.

Shriberg, L. D. (1986). *PEPPER: Programs to examine phonetic and phonologic evaluation records* [Computer program]. Madison: University of Wisconsin-Madison.

Shriberg, L. D., Allen, C. T., McSweeny, J. L., & Wilson, D. L. (2001). *PEPPER: Programs to examine phonetic and phonologic evaluation records* [Computer program]. Madison: University of Wisconsin.

Shriberg, L. D., Austin, D., Lewis, B. A., McSweeny, J. L., & Wilson, D. L. (1997). The percentage of consonants correct (PCC) metric: Extensions and reliability data. *Journal of Speech, Language, and Hearing Research*, *40*, 708–722.

Shriberg, L. D., Flipsen, P., Jr., Kwiatkowski, J., & McSweeny, J. L. (2003). A diagnostic marker for speech delay associated with otitis media with effusion: The intelligibility-speech gap. *Clinical Linguistics and Phonetics*, *17*(7), 507–528.

Shriberg, L. D., & Kent, R. D. (1995). *Clinical phonetics* (2nd ed.). New York: MacMillan.

Shriberg, L. D., Kent, R. D., Karlsson, H. B., McSweeny, J. L., Nadler, C. J., & Brown, R. L. (2003). A diagnostic marker for speech delay associated with otitis media with effusion: Backing of obstruents. *Clinical Linguistics and Phonetics, 17*, 529–547.

Shriberg, L. D., & Kwiatkowski, J. (1980). *Natural process analysis (NPA): A procedure for phonological analysis of continuous speech samples.* New York: Macmillan.

Shriberg, L. D., & Kwiatkowski, J. (1982). Phonological disorders III: A procedure for assessing severity of involvement. *Journal of Speech and Hearing Disorders, 47*, 256–270.

Shriberg, L. D., Kwiatkowski, J., & Rasmussen, C. (1990). *Prosody-voice screening profile [pvsp].* Tuscon, AZ: Communication Skill Builders.

Smith, C. R. (1975). Residual hearing and speech production in deaf children. *Journal of Speech and Hearing Research, 18*, 795–811.

Stathopoulos, E. T., Duchan, J. F., Sonnenmeier, R. M., & Bruce, N. V. (1986). Intonation and pausing in deaf speech. *Folia Phoniatrica, 38*, 1–12.

Tye-Murray, N., Spencer, L., & Woodworth, G. G. (1995). Acquisition of speech by children who have prolonged cochlear implant experience. *Journal of Speech and Hearing Research, 38*, 327–337.

Uziel, A. S., Sillon, M., Vieu, A., Artieres, F., Piron, J-P., Daures, J-P., et al. (2007). *Otology and Neurotology, 28*, 615–628.

Vieu, A., Mondain, M., Blanchard, K., Sillon, M., Reuillard-Artieres, F., Tobey, E., et al. (1998). Influence of communication mode on speech intelligibility and syntactic structure of sentences in profoundly hearing impaired French children implanted between 5 and 9 years of age. *International Journal of Pediatric Otorhinolaryngology, 44*, 15–22.

Vollrath, M. A., Kwan, K. Y., & Corey, D. P. (2007). The micromachinery of microtransduction in hair cells. *Annual Reviews of Neuroscience, 30*, 339–365.

Von Berg, S., McColl, D., & Brancamp, T. (2007). Moebius syndrome: Measures of observer intelligibility with versus without visual cues in bilateral facial paralysis. *Cleft Palate-Craniofacial Journal, 44*, 518–522.

Wagner, C. R., Nettelbladt, U., Sahlen, B., & Nilholm, C. (2000). Conversation versus narration in pre-school children with language impairment. *International Journal of Language and Communication Disorders, 35*, 83–93.

Whitehill, T. L. (2002). Assessing intelligibility in speakers with cleft palate: A critical review of the literature. *Cleft Palate-Craniofacial Journal, 39*, 50–58.

Wilson, B. S. (2000). Cochlear implant technology. In J. K. Niparko, K. I. Kirk, N. K. Mellon, A. M. Robbins, D. L. Tucci, et al. (Eds.), *Cochlear implants. Principles and practices* (pp. 109–119). Philadelphia: Lippincott Williams & Wilkins.

Yorkston, K. M., & Beukelman, D. R. (1978). A comparison of techniques for measuring intelligibility of dysarthric speech. *Journal of Communication Disorders, 11*, 499–512.

Index

A

Acoustic SSD analysis
  boundary cues, 97
  coarticulation, 106
  digital signal processing (DSP), 94, 110
  eccentric acoustic-phonetic children's
      patterns, 96
  frequency range of child speech, 95
  future of, 93–95
  harmonics of child speech, 96
  idiosyncratic acoustic-phonetic children's
      patterns, 96
  maturation, variability as index of, 107–109
  meter, 97–98
  normative children's speech behavior
      adequacy, 96
  overview, 93
  pattern variability of child speech, 96
  pediatric speech science factors, 95–96
  phonetic biases as confounding, 95
  precision, variability as index of, 107–109
  proficiency in, 95
  prosodic patterns, 96–97
  rhythm, 97–98
  segmental analysis, 98–106
  sensitivity of, 109
  speaker intelligibility acoustic correlates,
      106–107
  spectral patterns, segmental analysis,
      101–104
  spectrotemporal liquid/glide patterns,
      segmental analysis, 104–106
  temporal patterns, segmental analysis,
      98–101

variability and precision/maturation,
    107–109
velopharyngeal function in children, 96
and vocal tract developmental aspects, 96
ADHD (attention-deficit hyperactivity
    disorder), 51, 61
AOS (apraxia [acquired adult] of speech).
    See also CAS (childhood apraxia of
    speech)
  classification, 23–24, 144
ARC protein, 46
Articulation disorders *versus* phonological
    disorders dichotomy, 2
ASD (autism spectrum disorders), 25, 61, 137
  HFA (high functioning autism), 143. *See
    also* ASD (autism spectrum disorders)
    main entries
  motor deficits, 141–144. *See also* MSD
    (motor speech disorder) *main entry*
  overview, 141, 181
  studies
    acoustics: ASD, 156–171
    acoustics: CAS, 152–156
    conclusion, 175
    discussion, 171–175
    parent survey (ASD), 150–152
ASD toddler vocal production
  acoustic analysis of nonlinguistic
      vocalization study
    acoustic analysis, 185–187
    discussion, 200–202
    pitch information results, 187–189
    results, 187–189
    study protocols, 182–185
    vocalization duration results, 187

ASD toddler vocal production *(continued)*
  articulation development, 182
  developmental vocal deviancies,
      181–182
  perceptual analysis of speech/nonspeech
      vocalizations study
    communicativeness results, 197–198
    discussion, 200–202
    nonspeech vocalization results, 196–197
    nonspeech vocalization statistical
        comparisons, 198–200
    results, 194–200
    speechlike vocalization statistical
        comparisons, 198
    speech sound inventory results, 194–195
    speech stage results, 195
    study protocols, 189–194
    syllable structure complexity results,
        195
    word production results, 196, 197
  phonological development, 182
  prelinguistic vocalization, 181–182. *See
      also* acoustic analysis of nonlinguistic
      vocalization study *in this section*
ASHA (American Speech-Language-Hearing
      Association)
  on CAS (childhood apraxia of speech),
      147
  SSD (speech sound disorders) term
      adoption, 2–3
Asperger disorder, 141, 143. *See also* ASD
      (autism spectrum disorders) *main
      entries*
Autism spectrum disorders. *See* ASD (autism
      spectrum disorders) *entries*

B

BDNF (brain-derived neurotrophic factor)
      learning example, 45–46, 47
  example, 45–46
  and LTP (long-term potentiation), 46

C

CAS (childhood apraxia of speech), 73, 136.
      See also AOS (apraxia [acquired
      adult] of speech)
  acoustic investigations, 148–150

and ASD dysarthria symptoms, 144, 147
  ASHA (American Speech-Language-
      Hearing Association) on, 147
  computer processing, speech disorder
      analysis, 136
  encoding, 144–145
Case example
  speech with language impairment, 81–84
Causality research timeline, 3
Childhood SSD (speech sound disorders)
      overview
  classification system, 71–72
    etiologically based, 72
    need for, 3–4
    speech symptomatology/
        psycholinguistic theory, 72–73
  comorbidity of language disorder, 11
  epidemiology, 7–11
  etiologic classification system, 3–7
  normalization/persistence, 11
  onset of speech, 11
  overview, 2–4
  persistence/normalization, 11
  prevalence/persistence
    clinical prevalence, 10
    sex ratios, 10–11
  prevalence/persistence, 7–8
  SSD (speech sound disorders) as term, 2
Chromosome translocations, 25
Clinical Phonetics (Shriberg & Kent), 109
Cochlear implants (CI)/conversational
      intelligibility
  Deaf speech/intelligibility, 228–229
  future research directions, 242
  intelligibility beyond CI and hearing
      impairment, 242–243
  intelligibility factors, in general, 226–227
  overview, 225–226, 229–231
  PEPPER (Programs to Examine Phonetic
      and Phonologic Evaluation Records),
      234, 236
  study
    conclusions, 241
    correctional analysis, 239–240
    discussion, 238–241
    findings, 234–239
    individual variables, 234–237
    performance, overall, 238–239
    protocol, 231–234

rationale, 231
  regression analysis, 241
  regression model, 238
  shortcomings, 242
  zero-order correlations, 237–238
Coffin-Siris syndrome, 25
Comorbidity, 11
  domain relationships, speech deficits, 76
  and genetic influences, 51, 53, 54, 55–58,
      63. *See also* Genetic influences on
      SSD *main entry*
  of language deficits, 74–75
  reading deficits, 54, 55–58, 63, 76–77
  of speech deficits, 75–76
Computer processing, speech disorder
      analysis
  accuracy measurement, 134–135
  application of, 135–137
  ASR (automatic speech recognition), 130,
      134, 135, 136
  and assertive devices, 137
  autocorrelation technique, 127
  CAS (childhood apraxia of speech)/CVR,
      136
  cepstral technique, 127–128
  cepstrum measurement, 123–125
  computer models, speech
      recognition/classification, 129–135
  computers as tools, 115
  CVR (coefficient of variation ratio)/ CAS,
      136
  data analysis, 120
  data collection, 118–120
  dysarthric speech intelligibility
      improvement, 137
  energy measurement, 121–122
  F_0 (fundamental frequency), 127–129
  formants, 126
  glottal source, 126–127
  harmonic sieve theory of pitch
      perception, 129
  HMM (hidden Markov models), 131–134
    detecting /r/ pronunciation errors,
      136–137
  intelligibility improvement, dysarthric
      speech, 137
  inverse-filtering technique, 128–129
  LPC (linear predictive coefficients), 125
  measurement reliability, 115–116

motivation for, 115–118
  MultiSpeech software, 120
  overview, 137
  PEPPER (Programs to Examine Phonetic
      and Phonologic Evaluation Records),
      120, 233, 234, 236
  PLP (perceptual linear prediction, 125
  rationale/motivation for, 135–136
  reliability of measurement, 115–116
  and SMI (speech motor involvement),
      136
  software for data collection, 119–120
  SPA (Speech Paul Algorithm) software,
      136
  spectrum measurement, 122–123
  speech recognition challenge, 129–130
  speech signal, 121–125
  speech signal feature automatic
      measurement, 121–129
  speech-specific considerations, 117–118
  strengths of, 116–117
  weaknesses of, 117
Conversational intelligibility. *See* Cochlear
      implants (CI)/conversational
      intelligibility; Intelligibility

D

sDAS (suspected developmental apraxia of
      speech), 97
Descriptivism, 37
Developmental communication disorders
  challenge of explanation, 36–37
  ERPs (event-related potentials), 42
  explanatory account alternative approach,
      37–38
  fMRI (functional magnetic resonance
      imaging), 42
  mechanistic explanations, individual
      differences, 44–45
  multifaceted explanatory accounts, 47
  multiple systems and individual
      differences explanations, 42–43
  NIRS (near-infrared spectroscopy), 42
  reductionist explanations, individual
      differences, 43–44
  Shriberg, Lawrence work on, 35–36, 47
  social values as explanatory route, 38–40
Down syndrome (trisomy 21), 25, 146

Dysarthria
  childhood form underdiagnosis,
    145–146
  MSD (motor speech disorder)
    childhood form underdiagnosis,
      145–146
  Parkinson disease, 146
  symptoms and CAS, 144, 147
Dyslexia
  genetics, 51, 59–60, 61

E

Epilepsy, rolandic, 25
ERPs (event-related potentials)
  brain function measurement, 42

F

fMRI (functional magnetic resonance
    imaging)
  brain function measurement, 42
  genetic influences on SSD, 60–62
Fragile X syndrome, 25, 145

G

Genetic influences on SSD, 42–43
  and academic difficulties, 63–64
  and behavioral difficulties, 62–63
  candidate genes/cognitive-linguistic traits,
    58–62
  challenges to study of, 53
  and chromosome 3 locus, 54
  and chromosome 6 (6p22), 55, 59
  and chromosome 15 (15p21), 55
  and chromosome 15 (DYXI), 55
  cognitive-linguistic traits/candidate genes,
    58–62
  and comorbidities, SSD, 51, 53, 63
    LI (language impairment), 54, 55, 63
    RD (reading disorders), 54, 55–58, 63
  core domains genetic evidence, 57
  DCDC2, 59–60
  DCX, 60
  developmental trajectory of, 57
  doublecortin 2, 59–60
  DYX1C1, 60
  endophenotype genetic evidence, 57
  endophenotypes
    phonological memory, 57

endophenotypes for SSD, RD, LI, 55–58
  motor skills, 56
  phoneme awareness, 56
  phonological memory, 56
  processing speed, 56, 58
and etiologic subgroups, 71
and fMRI (functional magnetic resonance
    imaging) studies, 60–62
FOXP2 gene, 3, 53, 59, 62
future directions, 64
KIAA0319, 59–60
and language, 57
MIM (Mendelian Inheritance in Man)
    entry, 12, 13
and motor skills, 56
and MRI studies, 60–62
and neuronal migration, 60
and occupational difficulties, 62–63
and oral motor skills, 57
and outcomes, 62–64
overview, 51, 64
Pennington's multiple deficit
    developmental disorders model, 55
phenotypes for SSD, 54–55
and phoneme awareness, 56
and phonological awareness, 57
and phonological encoding, 56
and phonological memory, 56, 57
and processing speed, 56
and proposed subtypes, 73
reading, 57
ROBO1 (roundabout 1), 59
and speech sound production, 57
study rationale, 52–53
  challenges to, 53
written/spoken language shared
    processing, 54–55
Glactosemia, 25
Goldman-Fristoe Test of Articulation (GFTA),
    55

H

Hippocampus as learning locus, 46
Human Genome Project, 3

I

Intelligibility. *See* Cochlear implants
    (CI)/conversational intelligibility

beyond hearing impairment, 242–243
and cochlear implants (CI) in young
    children, 229–243. *See also* Cochlear
    implants (CI)/conversational
    intelligibility
and deaf speech, 228–229
factors affecting, 226–227
speaker intelligibility acoustic correlates,
    106–107

J

Joubert syndrome, 25

L

Learning (declarative/Hebbian), 46
LI (language impairment), 53
    and neuronal migration, 60
LTP (long-term potentiation), BDNF
    (brain-derived neurotrophic factor)
    learning example, 46

M

Mechanistic explanations of developmental
    communication disorders, 46–47
MIM (Mendelian Inheritance in Man)
    SSD (speech sound disorder) entry, 12, 13
Motor speech disorder. *See* MSD (motor
    speech disorder)
Learning (declarative/Hebbian), 46
MRI studies, genetc influences on SSD, 60–62
MSD (motor speech disorder), 25
    AOS (apraxia [acquired adult] of speech),
        144–145
    Asperger disorder, 141
        phonetic deficits, 143
    in autism, 141–175. *See also* ASD (autism
        spectrum disorders) motor speech
        disorders (MSD) *main heading for
        details*
    CAS (childhood apraxia of speech)
        encoding, 144–145
        acoustic investigations, 148–150
    defined, 6
    dysarthria
        neuromotor effects of, 146
        symptoms and CAS, 144, 147

HFA (high functioning autism)
    articulation deficits, 143
    phonetic deficits, 143
    phonological deficits, 143
    overview, 144–150
MultiSpeech software, 120
Multisyllabic Word Repetition, 55

N

Neutralism, 37
NIRS (near-infrared spectroscopy) brain
    function measurement, 42
Nonsense Word Repetition, 55

P

Parkinson's disease dysarthria, 146
PDD (pervasive developmental disorder),
    141. *See also* ASD (autism spectrum
    disorders) *main entries*
Pediatric speech science factors, 95–96
PEPPER (Programs to Examine Phonetic and
    Phonologic Evaluation Records)
    software, 120, 233, 234
Percent Consonants Correct (PCC), 55. *See
    also under* Speech change after
    severe TBI (traumatic brain injury)
Prader-Willi syndrome, 145–146
Production, vocal. *See* ASD toddler vocal
    production

R

Rapid Naming of Colors, 55
RD (reading disorder)
    genetics, 53, 54, 55–58, 59–60
    and neuronal migration, 60
Rett syndrome, 25
Rolandic epilepsy, 25
Russell-Silver syndrome, 25

S

SALT (Systematic Analysis of Language
    Transcripts) software, 120. *See also*
    PEPPER (Programs to Examine
    Phonetic and Phonologic Evaluation
    Records) software

SBH (spina bifida with hydrocephalus), 145
SDCS (speech disorders classification system)
  emerging research from framework speech delay–genetic (SD-GEN), 12–18
  epidemiology, 7–11
  etiology (SDCS-E), 4
    subtypes, 5, 6–7
  framework
    chart, 5
    emerging research from, 11–24. *See also* emerging research from framework *in this section*
    and risk factors/markers, 27
  framework chart, 5
  markers/risk factors (framework), 27–28
  speech delay–developmental psychosocial involvement (SD-DPI) research
    diagnostic markers, 22
    literature review, 21–22
  speech delay–genetic (SD-GEN) emerging research
    children's diagnostic marker, 15–16
    diagnostic markers, 15–18, 73
    endophenotypes, verbal trait disorders, 14–15
    literature review, 12–13
    MIM (Mendelian Inheritance in Man) entry, 12, 13
    phenotypes, 13–14
    residual speech error phenotype recovery acoustic markers, 16–18
  speech delay–otitis media with effusion (SD-OME)
    literature review, emerging research, 18–21, 225
    research directions, 21
  typology (SDCS-T), 4, 5
  USSD (undifferentiated speech sound disorders), 7
7q32-34 deletion, 25
Sickle cell anemia, 45
SLI (specific language impairment), 59, 61
Speech change after severe TBI (traumatic brain injury)
  challenges of studying, 206
  overview, 205–206
  PCC performance curve

applications of, potential, 216–217
  calculation steps, 211–213
  overview, 217
  PCC *versus* PCC-R, 213, 214
  validity, 213, 215–216
  studies
    changes in PCC after pediatric TBI, 207–209
    performance curve approach to change after severe TBI, 209–211
Spina bifida with hydrocephalus (SBH), 145
SSD (speech sound disorder)
  improving service delivery to children, 26
  MIM (Mendelian Inheritance in Man) entry, 12, 13
  programmatic study needs, 25–26
  translational needs, 24–28
  why etiologic classification?, 24–25
Stuttering, 61

T

TBI (traumatic brain injury). *See* Speech change after severe TBI (traumatic brain injury)
Toddlers. *See* ASD toddler vocal production
Traumatic brain injury. *See* Speech change after severe TBI (traumatic brain injury)
Treatment
  and capability-focus of patient (goodness-of-fit), 85–86
  case example
    speech with language impairment, 81–84
  decision making, ongoing, 83–86
  decision making/long-term outcomes, 86–87
  empirical bases, 78–81
  generalization across domains *versus* specificity, 77–78
  indirect gains, 80–81
  long-term outcome expectations, 77–78
  monitoring change, multiple domains, 84
  multiple-deficit scheduling, 79–80
  outcomes, long-term, 83–86

scheduling multiple-deficit areas, 79–80
theoretical basis, 78
22q11.2 deletion, 25

V

Velocardiofacial syndrome, 25

Vocal production. *See* ASD toddler vocal
production

W

Williams-Beuren locus duplication
(7q11.28), 25